Review of
Intensive Care Medicine

2nd Edition

Review of Intensive Care Medicine

2nd Edition

Nicholas A. Smyrnios, M.D.
Associate Professor of Medicine
University of Massachusetts Medical Center
Director, Medical Intensive Care Unit
Division of Pulmonary, Allergy, and Critical Care Medicine
UMass Memorial Healthcare
Worcester, Massachusetts

Richard S. Irwin, M.D.
Professor of Medicine
University of Massachusetts Medical School
Director, Division of Pulmonary, Allergy, and Critical Care Medicine
UMass Memorial Healthcare
Worcester, Massachusetts

Frank B. Cerra, M.D.
Senior Vice President for Health Sciences and Professor of Surgery
University of Minnesota
Minneapolis, Minnesota

James M. Rippe, M.D.
Associate Professor of Medicine (Cardiology)
Tufts University School of Medicine
Boston, Massachusetts
Director, The Center of Clinical and Lifestyle Research
Shrewsbury, Massachusetts

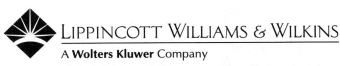
LIPPINCOTT WILLIAMS & WILKINS
A **Wolters Kluwer** Company
Philadelphia • Baltimore • New York • London
Buenos Aires • Hong Kong • Sydney • Tokyo

Acquisitions Editor: R. Craig Percy
Developmental Editor: Selina M. Bush
Production Editor: Steven P. Martin
Manufacturing Manager: Colin J. Warnock
Cover Designer: Christine Jenny
Compositor: Circle Graphics
Printer: Vicks Litho

Printed in the USA

Library of Congress Cataloging-in-Publication Data

Review of intensive care medicine / Nicholas A. Smyrnios . . . [et al.].—2nd ed.
    p.; cm.
  Rev. ed. of: Review for intensive care medicine.
  Companion v. to: Irwin and Rippe's intensive care medicine.
  ISBN 0-7817-2021-4 (pbk.)
  1. Critical care medicine—Examinations, questions, etc. I. Smyrnios, Nicholas A. II. Sebastian, Mark W. Review for intensive care medicine. III. Title.
  [DNLM: 1. Critical Care—Examination Questions. 2. Critical Illness—Examination Questions. WX 18.2 R454 2000]
  RC86.9.S43 2000
  616′028′076—dc21

                                                                            99-05386

Care has been taken to confirm the accuracy of the information presented and to describe generally accepted practices. However, the authors, editors, and publisher are not responsible for errors or omissions or for any consequences from application of the information in this book and make no warranty, expressed or implied, with respect to the currency, completeness, or accuracy of the contents of the publication. Application of this information in a particular situation remains the professional responsibility of the practitioner.

The authors, editors, and publisher have exerted every effort to ensure that drug selection and dosage set forth in this text are in accordance with current recommendations and practice at the time of publication. However, in view of ongoing research, changes in government regulations, and the constant flow of information relating to drug therapy and drug reactions, the reader is urged to check the package insert for each drug for any change in indications and dosage and for added warnings and precautions. This is particularly important when the recommended agent is a new or infrequently employed drug.

Some drugs and medical devices presented in this publication have Food and Drug Administration (FDA) clearance for limited use in restricted research settings. It is the responsibility of the health care provider to ascertain the FDA status of each drug or device planned for use in their clinical practice.

10 9 8 7 6 5 4 3 2 1

Contents

Preface

We are delighted to present the second edition of *Review of Intensive Care Medicine*. We hope and believe that this edition will continue the excellent tradition established by the first edition of this book, which was edited by Drs. Sebastian, Fulkerson, and Reed, and provide useful information in an interactive mode for practitioners of intensive care medicine.

We are pleased to be joined in the second edition of the *Review* book by Dr. Nicholas Smyrnios. It is Dr. Smyrnios who has led the effort to generate this current edition.

A number of changes and additions have been made to the second edition of the *Review* book to make it a more useful learning tool for practitioners of intensive care at all levels. First and foremost, all information in the second edition of *Review of Intensive Care Medicine* has been updated to reflect advances in critical care medicine and to make the book consistent with its parent book, the 4th edition of *Irwin and Rippe's Intensive Care Medicine* (Lippincott Williams & Wilkins, Philadelphia, 1999). Thus, the *Review* book becomes a particularly timely and accurate source of information in all areas of intensive care medicine.

A number of editorial features have been added to clearly link the *Review* book to its parent textbook. Specifically, in the *Review* book, the page in the parent textbook where the answer can be found is clearly stated in the answer to each question. Also, all questions and answers have been updated where knowledge has changed either in nuance or substance, since the previous edition.

In addition, new questions were developed for approximately 40 chapters, which were either new in the 4th edition of *Irwin and Rippe's Intensive Care Medicine* or in instances where chapters did not have questions written in the first edition of *Review of Intensive Care Medicine*. As a result, in the new edition of this book there is at least one question for every chapter from the parent textbook. Many of the questions have been rewritten to make them more clear and concise.

By linking the *Review* book even more closely to *Irwin and Rippe's Intensive Care Medicine (4th edition)*, we hope that the net result of this substantial editorial work is to make the second edition of the *Review of Intensive Care Medicine* an even more valuable teaching tool than the first edition.

In the 12 years since the first edition of *Intensive Care Medicine* was published, the field of intensive care medicine and the literature and knowledge used by practitioners of intensive care have undergone great change. The challenge in editing books in this area has always been to provide readers with state-of-the-art, user-friendly, and clinically relevant information. Now with the publication of the second edition of *Review of Intensive Care Medicine*, the basic body of information contained in the 4th edition of *Irwin and Rippe's Intensive Care Medicine*, can be viewed in seven different perspectives, through answering board review type questions. The accuracy and timeliness of this book are assured by the experience and knowledge of not only Dr. Smyrnios, but the participation of contributors to the parent book.

We hope that Review of *Intensive Care Medicine (2nd Edition)*, will thus join *Irwin and Rippe's Intensive Care Medicine* as a useful, authoritative resource to guide the practice of modern, intensive, and critical care. We hope that our readers will continue to find this body of information useful as they devote their efforts to treating the desperately ill individuals typically found in intensive and critical care units.

J.M.R.
N.A.S.
R.S.I.
F.B.C.

Review of
Intensive Care Medicine

2nd Edition

I. Procedures and Techniques

1. Airway Management and Endotracheal Intubation

True or False

1. The hard palate defines the beginning of the oropharynx, which extends inferiorly to the epiglottis.
2. The thyroid, cricoid, epiglottic, cuneiform, and corniculate cartilages compose the laryngeal skeleton.
3. The cricoid cartilage defines the narrowest portion of the airway in an adult.
4. The indications for endotracheal intubation can be divided into four basic categories: acute airway obstruction, excessive pulmonary secretions or inadequate ability to clear secretions, loss of protective reflexes, and respiratory failure.

Select the best answer

5. Regarding intubation in a patient with suspected cervical spine injury:

   A. Cervical spine injury must be confirmed radiologically before manipulation, and airway management should be performed.
   B. Nasal intubation is uniformly preferred for a patient with suspected cervical spine injury.
   C. If oral intubation is needed in the treatment of a patient with suspected cervical spine injury, an assistant is required to maintain the neck in the neutral position.
   D. Cervical collars should be removed before oral or nasotracheal intubation in the treatment of a patient with suspected cervical spine injury.

6. Regarding complications of endotracheal intubation:

   A. The most serious complication of extubation is laryngeal spasm.
   B. The decision to extubate is based on multiple laboratory values.
   C. Female patients are more likely than male patients to experience vocal cord paralysis after intubation.
   D. Laryngeal edema rarely accompanies smooth endotracheal intubation.

7. Regarding techniques of endotracheal intubation, which statement is *false*?

   A. When the laryngeal scope blade is in place, the operator should lift at the handle, keeping the left wrist stiff.
   B. The endotracheal tube is held in the right hand and is inserted at the right corner of the mouth in a plane that intersects with the laryngeal scope blade at the level of the glottis.

1

C. If the vocal cords cannot be visualized, no attempt at intubation can be made.

D. A stylet can be used with a light to aid in intubation.

8. Regarding alternative airway management:

A. Nasotracheal intubation is the preferred approach to intubation of a patient with extensive facial trauma.

B. Cerebrospinal rhinorrhea is an indication for nasopharyngeal airway.

C. The laryngeal mask airway can be positioned without direct visualization of the vocal cords.

D. Nasotracheal intubation should be performed on an obtunded and apneic patient.

2. Central Venous Catheters

True or False

1. The ideal location for the catheter tip for central venous catheterization is in the distal innominate or proximal superior vena cava, 3 to 5 cm proximal to the caval atrial junction.

2. Once a catheter is properly placed, migration of the catheter tip is uncommon.

3. After electrocardiogram (ECG) leads are used to ensure accurate catheter tip location, a chest radiograph is not necessary.

4. An important complication resulting from antecubital central venous catheterization is pericardial tamponade.

5. Regarding the basic principles of central venous catheterization, which of the following statements is *false*?

A. Volume resuscitation alone is not an indication for central venous catheterization.

B. Peripheral vein cannulation may be impossible in the treatment of hypovolemic patients.

C. The femoral vein may be a reasonable alternative for resuscitation of a hypovolemic patient.

D. Central venous access may be needed for infusion of irritant medications such as potassium chloride or for infusion of vasoactive agents.

E. Internal jugular vein cannulation can be achieved most easily during cardiopulmonary resuscitation, although subclavian vein cannulation requires less interruption of chest compressions.

Select the best answer

6. Regarding emergency transvenous pacemaker insertion:

A. Emergency transvenous pacemakers are best inserted through the right subclavian vein.

B. In treatment of patients with coagulopathy, the external jugular vein, although accessible, should not be used.

C. Catheters inserted from the right subclavian vein follow a more natural curve than those inserted from the left subclavian vein, traversing the right ventricle into the right pulmonary artery.

D. Emergency transvenous pacemakers are best inserted through the right internal jugular vein because of the direct path to the right ventricle.

Select the *false* statement

7. Regarding the structures neighboring the internal jugular vein:

   A. The internal carotid artery runs medial to the internal jugular vein, in general.
   B. The stellate ganglion and the cervical sympathetic trunk lie within the carotid sheath posterior to the internal carotid artery.
   C. The dome of the pleura, which is higher on the left, is caudal to the junction of the internal jugular vein and subclavian vein.
   D. The cholinergic and vagus nerves course posteriorly at the route of the neck.
   E. The thoracic duct lies behind the left internal jugular vein and enters the superior margin of the subclavian vein near the jugulosubclavian junction.

3. Arterial Line Placement and Care

True or False

1. The result of an Allen test is a reliable predictor that the blood supply to the hand will not be compromised by percutaneous radial placement of an arterial line.
2. Brachial artery catheterization is commonly performed in large medical centers.

Select the best answer

3. Regarding complications of use of intraarterial lines:

   A. The femoral artery site has the highest rate of thrombotic complications.
   B. Infection is the most common complication of use of intraarterial lines.
   C. Forward arterial blood flow prevents embolization of air or fluid infused through an intraarterial catheter from reaching the cerebral circulation.
   D. *Staphylococcus* species are the most common cause of intraarterial catheter infections.
   E. The heparin dose used for continuous flushing of intraarterial catheters is not sufficient to induce thrombocytopenia.

4. Pulmonary Artery Catheters

True or False

1. The inflation of the distal balloon in the pulmonary artery catheter can be with air or liquid.
2. Anticoagulation or deranged coagulation values are a contraindication to hemodynamic monitoring.
3. Because it is difficult to estimate true transmitted vascular pressure when a patient is undergoing positive end-expiratory pressure (PEEP), disconnecting PEEP to measure wedge pressure is recommended.
4. Within the setting of acute mitral regurgitation, a V wave is generated that affects the pulmonary arterial waveform and produces a bifid pulmonary artery waveform that persists with catheter wedging.
5. A mean pulmonary arterial pressure greater than 40 mm Hg defines pulmonary hypertension.

Select the best answer

6. Regarding catheter placement for pulmonary arterial catheters:

    A. During insertion, catheter advancement proceeds with the balloon inflated until tracing is seen on the monitor and then the balloon is deflated.

    B. The initial access of the pulmonary arterial catheter to the central venous circulation proximal to the right atrium is the most risky time for generation of arrhythmias.

    C. If arrhythmias are encountered in passage of the right ventricle, transient deflation of the balloon minimizes right ventricular irritation.

    D. With the catheter in the right pulmonary artery, a chest radiograph should be obtained to confirm catheter position, and whatever the placement, catheter position should be documented and confirmed with daily chest radiographs.

7. Regarding right atrial pressures:

    A. Normal resting right atrial pressure is 10 to 14 mm Hg.

    B. Two major positive atrial pressure waves, the A wave and the B wave, can usually be recorded.

    C. Once a multilumen pulmonary arterial catheter is in position, it is possible to sample right atrial blood and monitor right atrial pressure using the proximal lumen.

    D. The V wave represents the pressure generated by venous filling of the right atrium with the tricuspid valve open.

8. Regarding the right ventricle and right ventricular pressure:

    A. The normal resting right ventricular pressure is 30 to 35 mm Hg over 6 to 10 mm Hg recorded when the pulmonary arterial catheter crosses the tricuspid valve.

    B. Right ventricular systolic pressure always equals pulmonary arterial systolic pressure.

    C. Right ventricular monitoring is being increasingly used in the surgical critical care setting.

    D. Right ventricular pressure exceeds mean right atrial pressure during diastole when the tricuspid valve is open.

9. Regarding the pulmonary artery during use of a pulmonary arterial catheter:

    A. Normal resting pulmonary arterial pressure is 15 to 30 mm Hg over 5 to 13 mm Hg with a normal mean pressure of 10 to 18 mm Hg.

    B. The pulmonary arterial waveform is characterized by systolic peak and diastolic trough with a smooth decline from peak to trough.

    C. The peak pulmonary arterial systolic pressure occurs within the QRS complex of a simultaneously recorded electrocardiogram.

    D. Pulmonary arterial diastolic pressure is closely related to mean pulmonary arterial wedge pressure and can be reliably used as an index of left ventricular filling pressure.

10. Regarding pulmonary arterial wedge pressure:

    A. Pulmonary arterial wedge pressure correlates poorly with left ventricular filling pressure.

    B. A valid pulmonary arterial wedge pressure is obtained if the catheter tip lies in zone 1 of the lung.

C. Pulmonary arterial wedge pressure is an acceptable measurement for estimating capillary hydrostatic filtration pressure and is an absolute indication for the formation of pulmonary edema.

D. Pulmonary arterial wedge pressure should be measured at end expiration for a reliable reference point for interpretation.

5. *Temporary Cardiac Pacing*

Select the best answer

1. Regarding use of temporary cardiac pacing in acute myocardial infarction:

   A. Bradyarrhythmias unresponsive to medical treatment resulting in hemodynamic compromise are an indication for temporary pacing.

   B. Patients with anterior infarction and bifascicular block or second degree atrioventricular block do not need temporary pacemaker.

   C. Ventricular pacing may be essential for preservation and maintenance of effective stroke volume in the treatment of certain patients and should be the mode of choice.

   D. Prophylactic transvenous cardiac pacing is indicated in the treatment of patients who are to undergo thrombolytic therapy.

2. Which of the following is not a complication of transvenous pacemaker placement?

   A. Left ventricular perforation
   B. Arrhythmia
   C. Infection
   D. Pneumothorax
   E. Pericardial tamponade

6. *Cardioversion and Defibrillation*

True or False

1. The term *cardioversion* is used to describe electrical countershock to terminate ventricular fibrillation.
2. Defibrillation is the process of electrically depolarizing the myocardium in an effort to terminate ventricular fibrillation.
3. Cardioversion of paroxysmal supraventricular tachycardia or atrial fibrillation is contraindicated in pregnancy.
4. Which of the following is the appropriate energy setting for initial defibrillation of a 100 kg patient?

   A. 200 J
   B. 300 J
   C. 360 J
   D. 400 J

7. *Echocardiography in the Intensive Care Unit*

True or False

1. The use of transthoracic echocardiography (TTE) in the intensive care unit (ICU) is not indicated because of considerations of mechanical ventilation, chronic obstructive pulmonary disease, and the presence of bandages on the thorax.
2. Ejection fraction estimated by means of visual inspection of the two-dimensional echocardiographic images has been found to be inferior to computation of left ventricular end-diastolic and end-systolic volumes.

Select the best answer

3. Regarding echocardiography of the left ventricle:

   A. Left ventricular chamber dimensions and volumes may be estimated visually or by means of quantitative analysis.
   B. Echocardiography cannot be used to diagnose hypovolemia.
   C. A reduction of coronary flow of 50% is necessary to see regional wall motion abnormalities.
   D. Echocardiographic findings rarely lead to dramatic changes in treatment of the hypotensive patient.

Select the *false* statement

4. Regarding echocardiography in patients with congestive heart failure.

   A. Studies on patients with congestive heart failure referred for echocardiography show findings that are worse than clinically suspected in some patient populations.
   B. Echocardiography leads to changes in clinical management among approximately one third of patients.
   C. In clinical heart failure among patients with acute myocardial infarction, there is a restricted mitral inflow pattern indicative of abnormally elevated left ventricular diastolic pressure.
   D. In clinical congestive heart failure, diastolic filling variables become unrelated to systolic function.

5. Regarding special techniques of echocardiography:

   A. Continuous wave Doppler may be used to measure peak velocity and estimate pressure gradients across cardiac valves.
   B. Doppler-derived pressure gradients correlate closely with invasive determinants.
   C. Transesophageal echocardiography (TEE) is more sensitive than TTE for sensitivity and specificity in bacterial endocarditis.
   D. TEE has replaced TTE as a diagnostic technique in endocarditis.

8. *Pericardiocentesis*

True or False

1. Patient position during pericardiocentesis has relatively little influence on successful aspiration of pericardial fluid.

Select the best answer

2. Regarding the anatomy of the pericardium:

   A. The multiple attachments of the parietal pericardium are attached directly to the epicardium at the borders of the entrance at the inferior and superior venae cavae and pulmonary veins.
   B. The anchoring of the parietal pericardium results in a distensible large space between the visceral and parietal areas.
   C. The pericardial space, or sac, usually contains no fluid.
   D. The effusions that collect slowly over days to weeks may cause hemodynamic compromise with volumes less than 200 mL.

3. After successful pericardiocentesis:

   A. Recurrent tamponade is an infrequent event after successful pericardiocentesis.
   B. A small effusion is associated with a decreased incidence of complications after pericardiocentesis.
   C. Localized pericardial effusion is associated with increased risk for complications.
   D. A chest radiograph obtained immediately after the procedure is the only monitoring necessary after pericardiocentesis.

4. The following is not an indication for surgical treatment after pericardiocentesis:

   A. Pericardial disease with constrictive physiologic characteristics
   B. Known loculated or posteriorly located effusions not amenable to pericardiocentesis
   C. Suspected purulent pericarditis
   D. Effusions not successfully drained by means of pericardiocentesis
   E. Metastatic disease of the pericardium

9. The Intraaortic Balloon and Counterpulsation

True or False

1. The intraaortic balloon pump requires no minimum cardiac output to function effectively.
2. Intraaortic balloon counterpulsation is effective in stabilizing the condition of patients with mechanical intracardiac defects complicating myocardial infarction.
3. Other indications for intraaortic balloon counterpulsation are management of unstable angina, gradual discontinuation of cardiopulmonary bypass, preoperative use as a bridge to transplantation, and use during percutaneous coronary angioplasty.

Select the *false* statement

4. Regarding contraindications to balloon pump use:

   A. The use of intraaortic balloon counterpulsation to control ventricular arrhythmia is decreasing in frequency.
   B. Aortic valvular insufficiency is not a contraindication to intraaortic balloon pump counterpulsation.
   C. Aortic dissection is an absolute contraindication to counterpulsation.
   D. Severe aortoiliac disease is a contraindication to counterpulsation.

Select the best answer

5. Regarding weaning from counterpulsation:

   A. Weaning from counterpulsation requires three steps: weaning, inotropic support, and removal of the device.
   B. The only method of weaning involves counterpulsation ratios of 1:1, 1:2, and 1:3 based on the cardiac cycle.
   C. Heparin infusion should be continued through removal of the intraaortic balloon pump to avoid reocclusion of the coronary arteries.
   D. Once a patient has been weaned to a ratio of 1:3 and his or her condition has been stable for a few hours, the intraaortic balloon pump may be removed.

10. Temporary Mechanical Assistance of the Failing Left Ventricle

True or False

1. Indications for use of a left ventricular assist device include criteria such as cardiac index of less than 1.8 L/m^2/min, mean arterial pressure less than 60 mm Hg, left atrial pressure or right atrial pressure greater than 20 mm Hg, urine output less than 20 mL/h, and systemic vascular resistance greater than 2,100 dyne/s/cm^5.

Select the best answer

2. Contraindications to a ventricular assist device do not include the following:

   A. The presence of massive myocardial infarction
   B. Sepsis
   C. End stage renal disease
   D. Age younger than 12 years

3. Which of the following is not a sign of potential success in gradual discontinuation of use of a left ventricular assist device?

   A. Less than 75 hours of left ventricular assist device pump support
   B. No evidence of postoperative myocardial infarction
   C. Some evidence of left ventricular recovery
   D. Control of bleeding
   E. Right ventricular failure

11. Chest Tube Insertion and Care

True or False

1. The lung fills all but approximately 10 mL of the hemithorax in the normal physiologic state.
2. Up to 100 mL of fluid is present in the pleural space under normal conditions.

Select the best answer

3. Regarding timing of operation for traumatic hemothorax:

   A. Pulmonary parenchymal hemorrhage often is life threatening because of the high volume of blood flow through the pulmonary vasculature.

B. Systemic arterial sources of bleeding, such as the intercostal, internal mammary, or subclavian arteries or the heart, rarely cause hemothorax.

C. Tube thoracostomy is not indicated in the initial management of hemothorax due to trauma.

D. Indications for open thoracotomy after thoracostomy include blood loss of more than 1500 mL, more than 500 mL blood loss over the first hour, more than 200 mL blood loss per hour after 2 to 4 hours, or more than 100 mL per hour after 6 to 8 hours, or treatment of a patient in unstable condition not responding to volume resuscitation.

4. The following statement regarding chylothorax is *not true*:

A. The primary causes of chylothorax are trauma, malignant disease, congenital abnormalities, and miscellaneous conditions, such as infection.

B. The surgical procedures most often implicated in iatrogenic injuries include those involving mobilization of the aortic arch and esophageal resection.

C. The appearance of chyle in the pleural space is immediate after injury.

D. Treatment consists of tube drainage and aggressive maintenance of nutritional status.

12. Bronchoscopy

True or False

1. Patients with documented postrheumatic valvular heart disease should receive antibiotic prophylaxis against infective endocarditis before flexible bronchoscopy.

2. Flexible bronchoscopy is contraindicated for 6 weeks after acute myocardial infarction.

Select the best answer

3. Regarding flexible bronchoscopy:

A. The site and cause of hemoptysis are determined for approximately 50% of patients when bronchoscopy is performed before bleeding ceases.

B. Bronchoalveolar lavage and transbronchial lung biopsies have a sensitivity of greater then 90% for the detection of *Pneumocystis carinii* pneumonia.

C. Bronchoscopy performed through an endotracheal tube requires a tube at least 7 mm in internal diameter.

D. The most common complication following bronchoscopy is pneumothorax.

13. Methods of Obtaining Lower Respiratory Tract Secretions in Pneumonia

True or False

1. To define an optimal expectorated sputum sample, both number of white cells and presence of epithelial cells are required.

2. Transtracheal aspiration is commonly performed in the intensive care unit for the isolation of anaerobic and aerobic pulmonary pathogens.

3. Bronchoalveolar lavage samples a smaller, but more representative amount of the lower respiratory tract than protected brush specimen collection does.

Select the best answer

4. Regarding expectorated sputum samples for diagnosis of pneumonia:

    A. Findings from routinely processed expectorated sputum samples are both sensitive and specific for diagnosis of bacterial pneumonia.
    B. Direct immunofluorescence for *Legionella* species has a low specificity (50%) but a high sensitivity (94%).
    C. Potassium chloride wet mount may be useful in the diagnosis of certain gram-negative bacterial infections.
    D. Although approximately 80% of patients can produce a sputum sample when requested, only 50% of the samples are adequate for analysis.

14. Thoracentesis

Select the best answer

1. Regarding a cell count and differential for thoracentesis in a grossly bloody effusion:

    A. A red blood cell count of 50,000 cells per cubic millimeter must be present for fluid to appear pink.
    B. The presence of effusions containing more than 100,000 red blood cells per cubic millimeter are consistent with trauma alone.
    C. To differentiate traumatic thoracentesis from preexisting hemothorax, one can allow the blood sample to stand. If a clot forms, the patient has a preexisting hemothorax.
    D. Traumatic thoracentesis is suggested when pleural fluid and blood hematocrit values are identical.

2. Regarding malignant pleural effusions, the following statement is incorrect:

    A. Malignant tumors can produce pleural effusions by means of two basic mechanisms: implantation of malignant cells on the pleural surface or impairment of lymphatic drainage because of tumor obstruction.
    B. The most common tumors that cause pleural effusions are lung cancer, breast cancer, and lymphoma.
    C. Cytologic examination of pleural fluid should be performed for a transudative effusion of unknown cause.
    D. Heparin should be added to a container when a suspected malignant effusion is present to prevent clotting of the fluid.

15. Arterial Puncture for Blood Gas Analysis

True or False

1. Arterial blood gas analysis is indicated whenever there is a reason to rule in or out the presence of a respiratory or metabolic disturbance and to assess the nature, progression, or severity of a respiratory or metabolic disorder.
2. After puncture of the radial artery, pressure should be applied to the puncture site for a full 2 minutes.
3. P_{O_2} greater than 50 mm Hg indicates an arterial sample.

Select the best answer

4. Which of the following is true regarding arterial puncture for blood gas analysis?

   A. Complications occur in approximately 2% to 4% of cases.
   B. Thirty-five seconds of breath holding has been associated with a fall in PaO_2 of 50 mm Hg and pH of 0.07, and a rise in $PaCO_2$ of 10 mm Hg.
   C. Normal value for the PaO_2 of a nonsmoking adult is 90 to 100 mm Hg.
   D. In cases of total occlusion of the radial artery, the ulnar artery provides adequate blood flow to the hand 50% of the time.

16. Tracheotomy

True or False

1. Tracheotomy performed in the intensive care unit is an uncommon procedure.
2. The cricothyroid space is larger in its vertical dimension than the diameter of most tracheotomy tubes.

Select the best answer

3. Regarding delayed hemorrhage after tracheotomy:

   A. Late hemorrhage after tracheotomy is usually caused by erosion into adjacent venous collateral vessels.
   B. In some early series, it was reported that tracheotomy bleeding more than 48 hours after the procedure was due to rupture of the innominate artery.
   C. Exsanguination from trachea–innominate artery fistula has been eliminated with the advent of low-pressure, high-volume cuffs.
   D. Trachea–innominate artery fistulas are still described in the literature and carry a mortality of 30%.

4. Regarding percutaneous dilational elective tracheotomy in the intensive care unit:

   A. The risk for posterior perforation of the trachea into the esophagus is increased in comparison with the risk of surgical tracheotomy.
   B. It is somewhat slower to perform than conventional tracheotomy.
   C. The kit is less expensive than operating room expense and personnel.
   D. There is increased dissection compared with that during operative tracheotomy.
   E. Upper airway endoscopy is contraindicated during the procedure.

17. Extracorporeal Life Support for Cardiac and Respiratory Failure

Select the best answer

1. Regarding extracorporeal life support (ECLS):

   A. ECLS has made little progress in recent years.
   B. ECLS is more successful when used as an early intervention before the appearance of irreversible organ damage.

C. Early clinical trials with extracorporeal membrane oxygenation (ECMO) compared conventional mechanical ventilation with ECMO as therapy for adult respiratory distress syndrome, and showed a survival advantage with ECMO.

D. To date, approximately 900 patients have been treated with ECLS in the United States at 90 centers.

2. Which of the following is not considered a contraindication to the use of ECLS?

A. Potential for severe bleeding
B. Necrotizing pneumonia
C. Age older than 60 years
D. Time on mechanical ventilation less than 5 days
E. Expected poor quality of life

18. Gastrointestinal Endoscopy

Select the best answer

1. Regarding lower gastrointestinal endoscopy:

A. Lower gastrointestinal endoscopy can help identify a colonic source of acute bleeding with 90% accuracy.
B. Colonic decompression is indicated as primary therapy for pseudoobstruction among patients in intensive care units.
C. Endoscopic colonic decompression has been advised for right colonic diameter dilatations exceeding 12 cm.
D. Relapse is uncommon after colonic decompression.

19. Paracentesis and Diagnostic Peritoneal Lavage

True or False

1. Diagnostic peritoneal lavage has 95% to 100% sensitivity in the detection of hemoperitoneum among patients who have had abdominal trauma.
2. The most common complication of abdominal paracentesis is introduction of infection into the peritoneal cavity.

Select the best answer

3. Which of the following is not consistent with a positive finding in diagnostic peritoneal lavage after blunt abdominal trauma?

A. Red blood cell count 1,000/mL
B. White blood cell count 1,000/mL
C. Amylase 500 units/100 mL

D. Return of lavage fluid through urinary catheter

E. Return of food particles

---

20. *Management of Acute Esophageal Variceal Hemorrhage with Gastroesophageal Balloon Tamponade*

Select the best answer

1. Regarding complications of gastric balloon tamponade of variceal bleeding:

   A. The most common complication is acute laryngeal obstruction.

   B. The most severe complication is aspiration pneumonia.

   C. Migration of the tube may lead to esophageal perforation.

   D. Mucosal ulceration of the gastroesophageal junction is rare but is related to prolonged traction time.

2. Regarding the insertion and maintenance of gastroesophageal balloon tamponade tubes:

   A. Endotracheal intubation should be performed before tube insertion.

   B. The esophageal balloon must be deflated for 30 minutes each day.

   C. After confirmation of tube position by means of auscultation in the epigastrium while a flush of air is injected through the gastric lumen, the gastric balloon is inflated with no more than 80 mL.

   D. The esophageal balloon should be inflated with a bedside manometer to approximately 90 mm Hg.

---

21. *Endoscopic Placement of Feeding Tubes*

True or False

1. Maneuvers used for clearance of clogged feeding tubes include irrigation with warm saline solution, with carbonated liquid, with cranberry juice, or with an enzyme solution.

Select the best answer

2. Regarding the placement of nasoenteric feeding tubes:

   A. A tube 30 to 36 inches (76 to 91 cm) long is needed for placement of the tip in the duodenum.

   B. Metoclopramide has not been shown to assist with the passage of the tube tip into the duodenum.

   C. Erythromycin administered 30 minutes before tube insertion has been shown to improve the success of postpyloric tube placement.

   D. Tube feeding may begin after the tube position has been confirmed by means of auscultation in the epigastrium while a flush of air is injected through the gastric lumen.

   E. Placement of a tube into a jejunal location eliminates risk for aspiration.

22. *Therapeutic Hemapheresis*

True or False

1. Hemapheresis involves removal of a specific blood component and reinfusion of the remaining blood.

Select the best answer

2. The disease entity that is not indicated for treatment with therapeutic plasma exchange is:

   A. Guillain-Barré syndrome
   B. Idiopathic thrombocytopenic purpura
   C. Myasthenia gravis
   D. Thrombotic thrombocytopenic purpura

23. *Cerebrospinal Fluid Aspiration*

True or False

1. Postdural puncture headache typically develops within 72 hours and lasts 3 to 5 days.
2. Appropriate needle placement in children is at L4-5 or L5-S1.

Select the best answer

3. Which of the following is most indicative of a subarachnoid hemorrhage?

   A. A decreasing red blood cell count in tubes collected serially during lumbar puncture
   B. Presence of a fibrinous clot in the collected specimen
   C. Breakdown products of red blood cells in cerebrospinal fluid
   D. A leukocyte to erythrocyte ratio of 1:700

24. *Neurologic and Intracranial Pressure Monitoring*

Provide the answer

1. What is the Glasgow Coma Scale Score for a patient with the following examination findings: opens eyes to painful stimulus, plantar reflex with toes downgoing, speaks isolated, inappropriate words, pupils equal and reactive, extremity movements attempt to push away painful stimulus?

   A. 6
   B. 8
   C. 10
   D. 12
   E. 14

True or False

2. Retrograde cannulation of the jugular bulb is a high-risk, technically demanding procedure that yields consistently sensitive analysis of cerebral oxygen demand through measurement of mixed cerebral venous blood oxygen levels.

25. *Percutaneous Cystostomy*

True or False

1. Complications of percutaneous cystostomy are limited to the following: bladder spasms, hematuria, postobstructive diuresis.

Select the best answer

2. Which of the following is not a contraindication to percutaneous cystostomy?

   A. Bladder cancer
   B. Prostate cancer
   C. Nonpalpable bladder
   D. Coagulopathy
   E. Clot retention

26. *Aspiration of Joints*

True or False

1. The viscosity of synovial fluid is a measure of the protein present in the fluid.

Select the best answer

2. Regarding management of arthritis in the intensive care unit:

   A. Periarticular inflammation with arthralgia is an indication for arthrocentesis.
   B. Bursitis and tendonitis may mimic true joint arthritis.
   C. A patellar tap may be useful with small effusions as a diagnostic technique.
   D. Arthrocentesis is a diagnostic technique only.

27. *Anesthesia for Bedside Procedures*

True or False

1. Return of consciousness can be seen within minutes after termination of an 8-hour propofol infusion, although the elimination half-life of propofol is 5 hours.
2. Recent data suggest that reversal of an opioid with an opioid agonist-antagonist such as nalbuphine may be safer than administration of naloxone.

3. Etomidate has beneficial effects on cerebral oxygen kinetics, similar to those seen with barbiturates; however, it carries significantly increased risk for cardiovascular side effects.

4. The most important aspect of pain and anxiety control in the intensive care unit (ICU) is sedative administration.

Select the best answer

5. Which of the following statements best describes the use of naloxone in the intensive care unit?

   A. Administering small doses of naloxone (0.04 mg) to patients to reverse respiratory depression of narcotic overdose in the ICU has been shown to be safe and effective.

   B. Opiate side effects such as vomiting, delirium, arrhythmia, pulmonary edema, cardiac arrest, and sudden death may be avoided by means of reversal with naloxone.

   C. The administration of small doses of naloxone is relatively contraindicated in the ICU because of the large number and severity of side effects.

   D. Naloxone levels decline more slowly than do morphine levels, leading to complications of analgesia and respiratory status in the ICU.

6. Which of the following statements best describes the use of midazolam in the intensive care unit?

   A. Midazolam provides excellent anterograde amnesia.
   B. Midazolam produces considerable pain on injection.
   C. Midazolam is approximately one-half protein-bound.
   D. The elimination half-life of midazolam is approximately 12 hours.

28. Routine Monitoring of Critically Ill Patients

True or False

1. New methods of automated noninvasive blood pressure monitoring approximate the accuracy of invasive measurements and may be used interchangeably with invasive monitoring.

Select the best answer

2. Regarding gastric intramucosal pH monitoring:

   A. Intramucosal pH monitoring is used to monitor trends in tissue pH in response to local oxygen delivery and metabolism.

   B. These trends have not yet been used in predicting intensive care unit outcome.

   C. The technique is used to measure P_{CO_2} and pH in a gas state in a balloon placed in the lumen of a viscus, usually the stomach, the sigmoid colon, and the bladder.

   D. The use of gastric intramucosal pH monitoring has been shown to confer a postoperative survival advantage among patients who have undergone cardiac operations.

3. Regarding temperature monitoring:

  A. Bladder, sublingual, tympanic, and great-vessel measurements provide accurate core temperature readings.
  B. Perforation of the tympanic membrane has been reported after tympanic temperature measurement.
  C. Measurement of mixed venous temperature necessitates placement of a separate probe.
  D. All critically ill patients should have temperature measured hourly.

29. Indirect Calorimetry

Select the best answer

1. Which of the following values is routinely measured directly by means of indirect calorimetry?

  A. Oxygen consumption
  B. Carbon dioxide production
  C. Exhaled minute ventilation
  D. Inhaled minute ventilation
  E. Energy expenditure

30. Interventional Radiology Drainage Techniques

True or False

1. Infection accompanied by fluid accumulation is effectively managed with antibiotics.
2. After catheter insertion into a fluid collection requiring drainage, the aftercare of the catheter consists of continuous wall suction.
3. Cholestasis is uncommon in the intensive care unit.

Answers
Chapter 1

1. False. The soft palate defines the beginning of the oropharynx, which extends inferiorly to the epiglottis. The oropharynx connects the posterior portion of the oral cavity to the hypopharynx. (*See textbook page* 3.)
2. False. The thyroid, cricoid, epiglottic, cuneiform, corniculate, and arytenoid cartilages compose the laryngeal skeleton. The thyroid and cricoid cartilages are readily palpated in the anterior neck. The cricoid cartilage articulates with the thyroid cartilage and is joined to it by the cricothyroid ligament. With extension of the head, the cricothyroid ligament may be pierced with a scalpel or a large-bore needle, providing an emergency airway. (*See textbook page* 3.)

3. **False.**   The glottis is the narrowest space in the adult upper airway, and in children the cricoid cartilage is the narrowest portion of the airway. (*See textbook page* 3.)

4. **True.**   Indications for endotracheal intubation can be divided into four basic categories: acute airway obstruction, excessive pulmonary secretions or desire for pulmonary toilet, loss of protective reflexes and inability to protect the airway, and respiratory failure. (*See textbook page* 6.)

5. **C.**   If oral intubation is needed by a patient with suspected injury to the cervical spine, an assistant should maintain the neck in the neutral position by ensuring axial stabilization of the head and neck as the patient is intubated. Any patient with multiple trauma who needs intubation should be treated as if cervical spinal injury is present. In the absence of maxillofacial trauma or cerebrospinal fluid rhinorrhea, nasal intubation may be the preferable technique. However, orotracheal intubation is more commonly performed, even in the setting of a cervical spinal injury. (*See textbook page* 13.)

6. **A.**   The most serious complication of extubation is laryngeal spasm. This is much more likely to occur if the patient is not fully conscious. If laryngeal spasm occurs, the application of positive pressure can sometimes relieve the problem. Succinylcholine can be administered intravenously or intramuscularly, if it is borne in mind that severe hyperkalemia can occur in a variety of clinical settings. Mechanical ventilation is needed until the patient has recovered from the effects of succinylcholine. The decision to extubate a patient is based on favorable clinical response to a carefully planned regimen of weaning, recovery of consciousness after anesthesia, or sufficient resolution of the initial indications for intubation. (*See textbook page* 15.)

7. **C.**   Although it is desirable to visualize the vocal cords during intubation, it is occasionally impossible to do so. When this is true, it is helpful to insert the soft metal stylet into the endotracheal tube and bend it into a "hockey-stick" configuration. Alternatively, a control-tip endotracheal tube may be used, which has a nylon cord running the length of the tube and attached to a ring at the proximal end. This allows the tip of the tube to be directed in an anterior direction. A stylet with a light or light wand also can be used. When the room lights are dimmed, the endotracheal tube containing the lighted stylet is inserted into the oropharynx and advanced into the midline. When the stylet is just superior to the larynx, a glow is seen over the anterior neck. The stylet is then advanced into the trachea, and the tube is threaded over it. The light intensity is diminished if the wand enters the esophagus. (*See textbook page* 10.)

8. **C.**   Proper positioning of the patient's head, especially with the head-tilt and jaw-thrust maneuvers, often may allow the patient to resume spontaneous breathing. If proper positioning of the head and neck or clearance of foreign bodies fails to establish an adequate airway, alternative approaches may be used. These include an oropharyngeal or nasopharyngeal airway, laryngeal mask airway, esophageal obturator, and various approaches to intubation. Facial trauma and cerebrospinal rhinorrhea are contraindications to the use of a nasopharyngeal airway. The laryngeal mask airway, which has recently been evaluated, can be positioned without direct visualization of vocal cords and conforms to the shape of the laryngeal inlet. Nasotracheal intubation should not be used in the care of a patient with extensive facial trauma. Nasotracheal intubation often is more comfortable than orotracheal intubation and therefore is most useful in the care of a conscious patient. (*See textbook page* 10.)

Chapter 2

1. **True.**   Catheter tip location is an important and often ignored consideration in central venous catheterization. The ideal location of the catheter tip is in the dis-

tal innominate vein or proximal superior vena cava 3 to 5 cm proximal to the caval atrial junction. Positioning of the catheter tip within the right atrium or right ventricle must be avoided. (*See textbook page* 18.)

2. **False.**   Migration of catheter tips can be impressive. Migration of 5 to 10 cm has been reported with antecubital catheters, as has migration of 1 to 5 cm with internal jugular vein or subclavian vein catheters. (*See textbook page* 18.)

3. **False.**   Using an adapter while inserting the catheter and using lead II on a standard ECG to monitor advancement of the catheter tip into the right atrium can aid in proper catheter placement. Whether or not this technique is used, a chest radiograph should be obtained after every initial central line catheter insertion to ascertain catheter tip location and to detect complications. Withdrawal of the catheter tip 3 to 5 cm after ECG monitoring with verification of P waves usually ensures correct positioning. (*See textbook pages* 18, 19.)

4. **True.**   Although phlebitis is more common with antecubital central venous catheterization, thrombosis, infection, limb edema, and pericardial tamponade can occur. Phlebitis is more common with antecubital central venous catheters, probably because of impaired blood flow and the proximity of the venous puncture site to the skin. There is a risk for pericardial tamponade, and the risk may increase because of the greater catheter tip migration that occurs during arm movement. (*See textbook page* 21.)

5. **E.**   Technical advances and a better understanding of anatomy have made insertion of central venous catheters safer, but there still is a high risk-to-benefit ratio, and some locations are more logical for certain therapeutic and diagnostic indications. Although subclavian vein cannulation can be achieved most easily during cardiopulmonary resuscitation, internal jugular vein cannulation requires less interruption of chest compressions. Volume resuscitation alone is not an indication for central venous catheterization. A 16-gauge catheter in a peripheral vein can infuse two times the amount of fluid as a longer 16-gauge central venous catheter. However, peripheral vein cannulation can be impossible if the patient has hypovolemia. In this case, the subclavian vein may be more reliable because of its attachments to the clavicle, which allow cannulation even in a hypovolemic state. The femoral vein also is a reasonable alternative. Central venous access often is required for the infusion of irritant medications or vasoactive medications, for diagnostic or therapeutic radiologic procedures, and in the care of a patient for whom peripheral access is impossible. (*See textbook pages* 18, 19.)

6. **D.**   Emergency transvenous pacemakers are best inserted through the right internal jugular vein because of the direct path to the right ventricle. This route is associated with the fewest instances of catheter tip malposition and the fewest complications of catheter and sheath introduction. With an indication for transvenous pacemaker insertion in a patient who has a coagulopathy, the external jugular vein, if readily apparent on the surface, may be a good alternative. When the subclavian vein is used for pulmonary arterial catheterization, the left subclavian vein is appropriate because a catheter inserted from the left subclavian vein follows a natural curve that traverses the right ventricle into the right pulmonary artery. This also avoids placement of an abrupt bend in the catheter, as occurs when the catheter is inserted in the right subclavian site. (*See textbook page* 17.)

7. **B.**   Knowledge of the structures neighboring the internal jugular vein is essential for avoidance of complications during central venous catheterization. The internal carotid artery has a course medial to that of the internal jugular vein and in rare instances may be directly posterior to the vein. Behind the internal carotid artery, just outside the carotid sheath, lie the stellate ganglion and the cervical sympathetic trunk. The dome of the pleura, which is high on the left, lies caudad to the junction of the internal jugular vein and the subclavian vein. Posteriorly through the neck, the cholinergic and vagus nerves course, and the thoracic duct

lies behind the internal jugular vein and enters the superior margin of the sub-clavian vein near the jugulosubclavian junction. (*See textbook page* 21.)

Chapter 3

1. **False.**   The technique of diagnosing occlusive arterial disease of the hand was described by Allen as an easily understood and performed test to document the intact nature of the collateral circulation of the hand. It consists of compression of both radial and ulnar arteries as the patient is asked to clench and unclench the fist repeatedly until pallor of the palm is produced. One artery is then released, and the amount of time until blushing of the palm is recorded. Normal palmar blushing is completed before 7 seconds; 8 to 14 seconds is considered an equivocal result, and 15 seconds or more is considered abnormal. This test is not an ideal screening pro-cedure; the sensitivity is 87% and the negative predictive value only 18%. In other words, only 18% of patients with no collateral flow according to the Allen test have this finding confirmed at Doppler study. (*See textbook pages* 39, 40.)

2. **False.**   Brachial artery catheterization is infrequently performed in large medical centers, because of concern about a lack of effective collateral circulation at that location in the arm and the fear of median nerve palsy due to bleeding into fascial planes, and compression of the median nerve. For this reason, coagulopathy is con-sidered a contraindication to brachial artery cannulation. (*See textbook page* 41.)

3. **D.**   *Staphylococcus* species are the most common cause of intraarterial catheter infections. *Candida* species also pose a risk in prolonged catheterization of glu-cose-intolerant patients taking systemic broad-spectrum antibiotics. Thrombosis is common in radial and dorsalis pedis artery catheters but less common in femoral or axillary catheters. Although infection is the most important compli-cation, thrombosis is more common. Air and fluid emboli have been reported to travel retrograde from an intraarterial catheter to the cerebral circulation. Heparin-induced thrombocytopenia may occur even with the small dose of heparin used for catheter flushing. (*See textbook pages* 42–44.)

Chapter 4

1. **False.**   A balloon guides the catheter by virtue of fluid dynamic drag from the greater intrathoracic veins through the right heart chambers into the pulmonary artery. The balloon when fully inflated in vessels of sufficiently large caliber is designed to protrude above the catheter tip. Progression of the catheter stops when the balloon encounters a pulmonary artery slightly smaller in diameter than the fully inflated balloon. From this position, pulmonary artery wedge pres-sure is obtained. The usual balloon inflation medium is air, but filtered carbon dioxide should be used in any situation in which balloon rupture might result in access to the arterial system. Periodic deflation and reinflation may be necessary, because carbon dioxide diffuses through the latex balloon. Liquids never should be used as the inflation medium because they can be difficult to retrieve and their presence prevents balloon deflation. (*See textbook pages* 47, 55.)

2. **False.**   In general, patients should have normal coagulation values before cen-tral venous access is attempted. However, in the care of some patients it is not possible to discontinue heparin for 3 hours to allow partial thromboplastin time to normalize. Although techniques for normalization of prothrombin time for patients receiving warfarin can be accomplished with infusion of fresh frozen plasma, it may be imprudent or impossible to correct these coagulation profiles before pulmonary arterial catheterization. In the care of these patients, techniques

can be used to minimize hemorrhagic risk, including cannulation of the basilic vein or the internal or external jugular veins as a secondary approach. The subclavian approach should be avoided in the care of patients with coagulopathies, because this site is inaccessible to direct pressure. (*See textbook page* 56.)

3. **False.**   Pleural pressure can exceed normal resting value even at end expiration with active expiratory muscle contraction or with the use of PEEP. How much PEEP is transmitted to the pleural space cannot be estimated with simplicity; however, it is believed that when normal lungs deflate passively, end-expiratory pleural pressure increases by approximately one half of the applied PEEP. Among patients with reduced lung compliance, the transmitted fraction is believed to be less, on the order of one fourth or less. Although it is difficult to estimate precisely true transmitted vascular pressure for a patient undergoing PEEP, temporarily disconnecting the PEEP to measure pulmonary arterial wedge pressure is not recommended. The abrupt removal of PEEP causes hypoxia, which may not reverse quickly on reinstitution of PEEP. (*See textbook page* 58.)

4. **False.**   Acute mitral regurgitation should be considered when a systolic murmur develops in the setting of acute ischemia or severe left ventricular failure of any origin. Left ventricular blood floods a normal-sized, noncompliant left atrium during ventricular asystole, causing giant V waves in the wedge pressure tracing. The giant V wave may be transmitted to the pulmonary artery tracing, yielding a bifid pulmonary artery waveform composed of a pulmonary artery systolic wave and the V wave. As the catheter is wedged, the pulmonary arterial systolic wave is lost, but the V wave remains. Prominent V waves may occur whenever the left atrium is distended and noncompliant because of left ventricular failure of any cause. (*See textbook page* 62.)

5. **False.**   A mean pulmonary arterial pressure greater than 20 mm Hg defines pulmonary hypertension. Pulmonary hypertension can be classified as passive (increases in left atrial or left ventricular end-diastolic pressure), active, or reactive. (*See textbook page* 63.)

6. **D.**   With the catheter in the right pulmonary arterial position, a chest radiograph should be obtained to confirm catheter position. Whatever the placement, catheter position should be documented and confirmed with daily chest radiographs. This monitors migration of the catheter tip. The balloon remains inflated until a wedge position has been achieved or a decision has been made to pull the catheter backward. Catheter passage into and through the right ventricle is the most risky time in terms of generation of arrhythmias during this procedure. Maintaining the balloon inflated minimizes ventricular irritation, although electrocardiographic monitoring is important throughout the procedure. (*See textbook page* 55.)

7. **C.**   With the tip of the pulmonary arterial catheter in the right atrium, normal resting right atrial pressure should be 0 to 6 mm Hg. Two main positive atrial pressure waves, the A wave and the V wave, usually can be recorded. The A wave is caused by atrial contraction, and the V wave represents the pressure generated by venous filling of the right atrium while the tricuspid valve is closed. It is possible to sample right atrial blood and monitor right atrial pressure through the proximal lumen once the pulmonary arterial catheter is placed. (*See textbook pages* 56, 57.)

8. **C.**   Right ventricular monitoring is being used increasingly in the surgical critical care setting. Normal resting right ventricular pressure is between 17 and 30 mm Hg over 0 to 6 mm Hg, recorded when the pulmonary arterial catheter crosses the tricuspid valve. Right ventricular systolic pressure should equal pulmonary arterial systolic pressure, except in cases of pulmonic valve stenosis or right ventricular outflow tract obstruction. Right ventricular pressure should equal mean right atrial pressure during diastole, when the tricuspid valve is open. (*See textbook page* 57.)

9. **A.**   Normal resting pulmonary arterial pressure is 15 to 30 mm Hg over 5 to 13 mm Hg with a normal mean pressure of 10 to 18 mm Hg. The pulmonary arterial waveform is characterized by systolic peak and diastolic trough with a

dicrotic notch caused by closure of the pulmonic valve. The peak pulmonary arterial systolic pressure occurs within the T wave of a simultaneously recorded electrocardiogram. The pulmonary vasculature is normally a low-resistance circuit, and pulmonary diastolic pressure is closely related to mean pulmonary arterial wedge pressure and can be used as an index of left ventricular filling pressure when wedge pressure cannot be obtained. However, if pulmonary vascular resistance is increased, as with pulmonary embolism, pulmonary fibrosis, or reactive pulmonary hypertension, pulmonary arterial diastolic pressure may markedly exceed mean pulmonary arterial wedge pressure and thus be rendered an unreliable index of left heart function. (*See textbook page* 57.)

10. D.   Pulmonary arterial wedge pressure is obtained when the inflated balloon impacts into a slightly smaller branch of the pulmonary artery. In this position, the balloon stops the forward flow, and the catheter tip senses pressure transmitted backward through the column of blood from the pulmonary venous circulatory bed. The lung is divided into physiologic zones depending on the relations between pulmonary arterial, pulmonary venous, and alveolar pressures. An appropriately positioned catheter is in zone 3, where pulmonary arterial and pulmonary venous pressures exceed the alveolar pressure to ensure an uninterrupted column of blood between the catheter tip and pulmonary veins. If on a lateral radiograph of the chest the catheter tip is below the level of the left atrium, in the posterior position if the patient is supine, it can be assumed to be in zone 3. With a few exceptions, estimated capillary hydrostatic filtration pressure from pulmonary arterial wedge pressure is acceptable, but the measurement does not take into account capillary permeability, serum colloid osmotic pressure, interstitial pressure, or actual pulmonary capillary resistance. These factors all play a role in the formation of pulmonary edema and should be interpreted in context. End expiration provides the most consistent, readily identifiable reference point for interpretation of pulmonary arterial wedge pressure because pleural pressure returns to baseline at the end of passive deflation, which is approximately equal to atmospheric pressure. (*See textbook pages* 57, 58.)

Chapter 5

1. A.   Temporary pacing may be used therapeutically or prophylactically in acute myocardial infarction. Bradyarrhythmias unresponsive to medical treatment that result in hemodynamic compromise may be such arrhythmias. Patients with anterior infarction and bifascicular block or type II second degree atrioventricular block, although in hemodynamically stable condition, may need a temporary pacemaker because they are at risk for development of complete heart block. Coordinated atrial contraction may be essential for preservation and maintenance of effective stroke volume, and therefore atrioventricular sequential pacing may be the modality of choice for these patients. For example, when right ventricular involvement complicates an inferior and posterior infarction, transvenous atrioventricular sequential pacing may be necessary to ensure adequate cardiac output. Prophylactic temporary cardiac pacing is an area of considerable controversy. The administration of thrombolytic therapy should take precedence over placement of prophylactic cardiac pacing. Transthoracic cardiac pacing is a safe and usually effective alternative for patients who are to undergo thrombolytic therapy. (*See textbook page* 57.)

2. A.   Left ventricular perforation. The procedure gains access through the venous system into the right ventricle. The right ventricle may be perforated, and the perforation can cause tamponade. It would be extremely unusual, however, for the left ventricle to sustain perforation. As in any venous access procedure, the patient may have complications such as infection and pneumothorax. Irritation of the right ventricle may cause arrhythmias. (*See textbook page* 76.)

Chapter 6

1. **False.** The term *cardioversion* is used to describe electrical countershock to terminate cardiac arrhythmias other than ventricular fibrillation. (*See textbook page* 78.)
2. **True.** Defibrillation is the process of electric depolarization of a critical mass of myocardium to terminate ventricular fibrillation. Cardioversion differs from defibrillation in that in cardioversion the electrical shock is synchronized. Synchronization is a process whereby the electrical unit recognizes the R or S wave to avoid shock during the period of electrical activity in the myocardium when it is vulnerable to generation of malignant tachyarrhythmias. (*See textbook page 78.*)
3. **False.** Synchronized direct current cardioversion has been performed successfully in all trimesters of pregnancy without apparent adverse effects on the fetus. Cardioversion of paroxysmal supraventricular tachycardia with 100 J and of atrial fibrillation with 300 J has been reported with effective results and without substantial risk to either fetus or mother. Multiple studies have shown that electric countershock does not induce premature labor, although in one instance a cesarean section was performed for fetal distress. Fetal rhythms should be monitored during cardioversion to ensure safety. Defibrillation of unstable tachyarrhythmias in a pregnant woman poses no ethical dilemma, because the procedure is life-saving to both mother and fetus. Current recommendations are that if the maternal arrhythmia is serious and refractory to other nonteratogenic treatments, synchronized direct current cardioversion should be performed with fetal monitoring. (*See textbook page* 83.)
4. **A.** 200 J. In the mid 1970s it was suggested that the 270 to 330 J delivered by most defibrillators that store 400 J was inadequate to successfully defibrillate 35% of persons weighing more than than 50 kg. Subsequent studies proved that 95% to 98% of persons with ventricular fibrillation can undergo successful defibrillation with 200 J of stored energy. Countershocks that provide higher than necessary levels of energy have an increased potential to cause myocardial damage. (*See textbook page* 86.)

Chapter 7

1. **False.** Although TTE has limitations in the ICU, it is still the initial screening procedure of choice for consideration of pericardial tamponade and to assess ventricular function in the ICU. The widespread use of TEE has extended the capabilities of echocardiography in the ICU, by allowing acquisition of high-quality diagnostic images for consideration of valvular vegetation in a patient with a fever, and for other considerations in which a high-quality diagnostic image is desired. (*See textbook pages* 90, 93.)
2. **False.** Recent studies suggest that simple visual estimation of ejection by an experienced physician compares favorably with results of more labor-intensive off-line computed calculation of ejection fraction from the same images. (*See textbook page* 97.)
3. **A.** Left ventricular analysis by means of echocardiography is commonly used in the ICU, because left ventricular chamber dimensions and volumes may be estimated visually or by means of quantitative analysis. Echocardiography can be used

to diagnose hypovolemia. In this setting, the echocardiogram demonstrates small end-diastolic and end-systolic left ventricular volumes and a normal or elevated ejection fraction. In general, reduction of coronary flow of 20% or more is needed to produce an abnormality in wall motion detectable by echocardiography. In general findings at echocardiographic examination of patients who become hypotensive in the ICU suggest the presence of marked ventricular hypertrophy, small chamber volumes, and an elevated ejection fraction. These findings can have a dramatic effect on management decisions. (*See textbook pages* 97–99.)

4. D.   In clinical congestive heart failure, it has been demonstrated that Doppler transmitral flow profile correlates with the presence of clinical heart failure in patients with acute myocardial infarction. These findings occur because the restrictive inflow pattern indicates abnormally elevated left ventricular diastolic pressures. Therefore, in clinical congestive heart failure, diastolic filling variables complement systolic function and allow comprehensive assessment of ventricular function. In studies by Echeverria, 50 patients were referred consecutively for echocardiography for congestive heart failure. Among patients with ejection fraction less than 50%, echocardiography revealed findings that were worse than clinically expected for 40% of patients. Echocardiography led to changes in the clinical care of these patients. The clinical influence of echocardiography was greater among the 40% of patients with congestive heart failure and normal ejection fraction. Most of these patients had hypertensive heart disease, and an unexpected finding among 90% of these patients was a normal ejection fraction. For these patients, echocardiographic findings led to changes in the clinical care of 90% of the patients. (*See textbook pages* 98, 99.)

5. D.   TTE and TEE are complementary diagnostic techniques in evaluations for infective endocarditis. Normal high-quality TTE images provide strong evidence against the diagnosis of bacterial endocarditis, particularly when valvular regurgitation is minimal. TEE offers an important increase in diagnostic sensitivity and specificity when TTE images are of poor quality, or when the findings at TTE are normal or equivocal in the setting of high clinical suspicion. TTE also appears to help ascertain whether a patient with endocarditis is at increased risk for complications. Patients with maximal vegetation diameters exceeding 10 mm are at a higher risk for development of emboli, congestive heart failure, the need for surgical intervention, and death than those with smaller vegetation diameters. Besides improving sensitivity of cardiac ultrasonography in the diagnosis of infective endocarditis, TEE may demonstrate clinically unsuspected intracardiac disease such as intracardiac abscess or infective endocarditis of both native and prosthetic valves. (*See textbook pages* 101, 102.)

Chapter 8

1. False.   The patient should be in a supine position with the head of the bed elevated to approximately 45 degrees from the horizontal plane. Elevation of the thorax allows free-flowing effusions to collect inferiorly and anteriorly, which are the sites that are easiest and safest to access with a subxiphoid approach. (*See textbook page* 109.)

2. A.   An understanding of the anatomy and anatomic relations of the pericardium begins with the visceral pericardium, which is closely but loosely adherent to the epicardial surface. The parietal pericardium is a fibrous structure that defines the outer membrane. Anatomic, physiologic, and pathophysiologic definition of a pathophysiologic condition of the pericardium is derived from the multiple attachments of the parietal pericardium within the thorax. At the posterior margin of the parietal pericardium above the esophagus and pleural sacs where the visceral pericardium is absent, the parietal pericardium attaches directly to the epicardium at the borders of the entrance of the inferior and superior venae cavae and pulmonary veins. These multiple attachments limit the inherent elasticity and distensibility of the pericardium. This complex anatomic arrangement provides an anchor for the contracting myocardium and results in a small space between the visceral and parietal layers. This space usually contains a small volume of clear, serous fluid, chemically similar to a plasma ultrafiltrate. Pericardial effusions that collect rapidly, over minutes to hours, may cause hemodynamic compromise with volumes of less than 250 mL. In contrast, effusions that develop slowly, over days to weeks, allow for both hypertrophy and distention of the fibrous parietal membrane. Volumes of 2 L may accumulate without marked hemodynamic compromise. (*See textbook page* 108.)

3. **C.** Factors associated with increased risk for complications after pericardiocentesis include small effusion, less than 250 mL, posteriorly located effusion, localized effusion, and a maximum clear space at echocardiography of less than 10 mm in an unguided approach. All patients undergoing pericardiocentesis should have a portable chest radiograph obtained immediately after the procedure to exclude pneumothorax. A second transthoracic, two-dimensional echocardiogram should be obtained within several hours to evaluate the adequacy of pericardial drainage and to confirm catheter placement. Close monitoring is required on a constant basis after pericardiocentesis to detect evidence of recurrent tamponade and to detect procedure-related complications. (*See textbook page* 111.)

4. **E.** Long-term treatment of patients with substantial pericardial fluid collection is dictated by ease of drainage and the underlying pathophysiologic condition. The indications for surgical intervention are established and include pericardial disease with constrictive physiologic characteristics, known loculated or posteriorly located effusions not amenable to pericardiocentesis, suspected purulent pericarditis, and effusions not successfully drained by means of pericardiocentesis. Nonsurgical management of chronically debilitated patients with metastatic disease of the pericardium may be indicated. Even in busy tertiary care and intensive care units, unguided pericardiocentesis is rarely indicated, and surgical drainage may be the preferred approach to pericardial drainage after initial pericardial decompression. (*See textbook page* 112.)

Chapter 9

1. **False.** Intraaortic balloon counterpulsation improves left ventricular performance with an increase in coronary perfusion and a decrease in myocardial oxygen consumption. Unlike other types of circulatory assist devices, the intraaortic balloon pump requires a minimum cardiac index of 1.2 to 1.4 L/min/m^2 to be effective. Thus, the intraaortic balloon pump cannot assist a patient who is asystolic or in ventricular fibrillation. (*See textbook page* 113.)

2. **True.** Intraaortic balloon counterpulsation is highly effective in the initial stabilization of the condition of patients with mechanical intracardiac defects that complicate myocardial infarction, such as acute mitral regurgitation, ventricular septal perforation, and pathway muscle rupture. Counterpulsation reduces pulmonary arterial pressure and increases cardiac output. It also has been seen to decrease the regurgitant V waves associated with mitral insufficiency. (*See textbook page* 113.)

3. **True.** Commonly accepted indications for intraaortic balloon pump use include unstable angina. Centers that use counterpulsation liberally for the management of unstable angina, report surgical mortalities approaching those for chronic stable angina (range 2% to 6%). One of the most useful indications for intraaortic balloon pump counterpulsation is to aid in weaning those patients from cardiopulmonary

bypass who have sustained perioperative myocardial injury. Myocardial dysfunction often is reversible if the patient's circulation can be assisted for 24 to 48 hours. The preoperative use of intraaortic counterpulsation has been advocated for certain patients at high risk—those with hemodynamically significant stenosis of the left main coronary artery and those with marked impairment of left ventricular function as indicated by an injection fraction less than 0.35. Although these indications have been advocated by some groups, most centers use intraaortic balloon counterpulsation selectively rather than routinely to treat patients with left coronary stenosis or diminished ejection fractions. Counterpulsation has been used to provide mechanical support for patients with heart failure while they await cardiac transplantation. Many centers now use counterpulsation to control unstable angina before and during coronary angioplasty. (*See textbook page* 114.)

4. **B.**   Aortic valvular insufficiency is an absolute contraindication to intraaortic balloon pump counterpulsation. Other absolute contraindications are severe aortoiliac disease and aortic dissection. The use of intraaortic balloon pumping for the management of refractory ventricular arrhythmias is receding with the advent of more potent antiarrhythmic drugs. (*See textbook pages* 114, 115.)

5. **D.**   Cessation of counterpulsation involves two steps—weaning and intraaortic balloon pump removal. The intraaortic balloon pump console can provide counterpulsation ratios of 1:1, 1:2, 1:3, 1:4, and 1:8. Some consoles also allow weaning by means of a gradual reduction in balloon volume. A patient may be progressively weaned by means of reducing the assist ratio or the intraaortic balloon volume and checking the cardiac index and filling pressures at each level. Once the patient has been weaned to a 1:3 ratio and his or her condition has been stable, the intraaortic balloon pump may be removed. The heparin infusion should be stopped 2 hours before removal of the percutaneous intraaortic balloon. The prothrombin and partial thromboplastin times should be near normal and the platelet count greater than 60,000 before percutaneous removal of an intraaortic balloon pump. During removal, arterial bleeding should be allowed for 1 to 2 seconds to flush any residual thrombus. Pressure firm enough to obliterate the femoral pulse for 45 minutes should be applied before the operator checks for bleeding. Local pressure occasionally does not control bleeding from the puncture site, and a hematoma occurs that necessitates surgical closure. Further, distal perfusion of the limb should be monitored to avoid complications of femoral artery thrombosis or distal embolization. (*See textbook pages* 120, 121.)

Chapter 10

1. **True.**   When these conditions exist for more than a few hours, there is an 85% mortality. In addition to hemodynamic criteria, other conditions must exist to make a patient a candidate for a ventricular assist device. There must be no surgically correctable lesions, and metabolic abnormalities should be absent. Other conditions that must exist before a left ventricular assist device is placed include optimizing preload and placement of an intraaortic balloon counterpulsation device. It is also assumed that the heart possesses some degree of possibility for future recovery, which allows removal of the device. (*See textbook page* 124.)

2. **D.**   Contraindications at this time include massive myocardial infarction, sepsis, bleeding disorders, or active bleeding from the gastrointestinal tract or central nervous system. Other contraindications include the presence of a chronic debilitating disease such as metastatic cancer, severe pulmonary hypertension, severe peripheral vascular disease, and neurologic impairment. Although overt sepsis is a contraindication, infections that respond to antibiotic therapy should not absolutely pre-

clude mechanical ventricular support. Although the presence of chronic end-stage renal failure has served as a deterrent, it is considered a relative contraindication at this time. The presence of single-organ dysfunction should not preclude placement of a ventricular assist device because improvement in end-organ perfusion may improve dysfunction when irreversible failure is not yet present. Survival rates among children supported with ventricular assist devices after cardiac operations have been greater than those among adults. (*See textbook page* 125.)

3. **E.**   Early signs of potential success and indications for left ventricular assist device weaning include less than 75 hours of pump support, no evidence of post-operative myocardial infarction according to electrocardiographic or physiologic criteria, some evidence of left ventricular recovery, mild or absent right ventricular failure, control of bleeding diathesis, and maintenance of renal function. (*See textbook page* 127.)

Chapter 11

1. **True.**   The pleural space is a closed serous sac surrounded by two layers—the parietal pleura and the visceral pleura. The lung fills all but approximately 10 mL of the hemithorax in the normal physiologic state. (*See textbook page* 131.)

2. **False.**   Although 500 mL of fluid may enter the pleural space each day under normal conditions, less than 3 mL of fluid is normally present within the space at any given time. This normal equilibrium may be disrupted by increased fluid entry caused by alterations in hydrostatic or oncotic pressures or by changes in the parietal pleura itself, such as in an inflammatory situation. A derangement in lymphatic drainage, as with lymphatic destruction, also may produce fluid accumulation. (*See textbook page* 131.)

3. **D.**   Accumulation of blood in the pleural space, or hemothorax, may be classified into two broad categories—spontaneous and traumatic. A hemothorax also may occur after attempts at thoracentesis or chest tube placement. In trauma, a pulmonary parenchymal source of hemorrhage often is self-limiting because of the low pressure of the pulmonary vascular system. However, if a systemic source of arterial bleeding is present from the intercostal, internal mammary, or subclavian arteries or from the aorta or heart, the bleeding may be potentially life threatening. Placement of a large-bore chest tube (36 to 40 F) assists in ventilation and helps in assessment of the need for immediate thoracotomy. In general, indications for open thoracotomy include initial blood loss of 1 to 1.5 L, more than 500 mL in the first hour, more than 200 mL/h after 2 to 4 hours, or more than 100 mL/h after 6 to 8 hours or lack of response to volume resuscitation on the part of a patient in unstable condition. (*See textbook page* 132.)

4. **C.**   The appearance of chyle in the pleural space may be delayed for 7 to 10 days after injury. The primary causes of chylothorax are trauma (including iatrogenic injury from surgical intervention), malignant tumor, congenital factors, and miscellaneous conditions, such as filariasis invasion or subclavian vein obstruction. Surgical procedures most often implicated in iatrogenic injury include those in which mobilization of the aortic arch is performed and esophageal resection. The fluid may collect in the posterior mediastinum before rupturing into the pleural space, sometimes on the right side. In a nontraumatic setting, malignant disease always must be suspected. Leaks can be caused by direct invasion of the thoracic duct or by obstruction by external compression or tumor embolus. Sarcoma, lymphoma, and primary lung carcinoma are most frequently implicated. Treatment consists of tube drainage and aggressive maintenance of fluid and nutritional status. Hyperalimentation and intestinal rest are recommended to limit flow through

the duct. Approximately 50% of instances of chylothorax resolve with this approach. A minimum of 2 weeks' observation usually is recommended. If this management fails, open thoracotomy is recommended to ligate the duct and close the fistula. Identification of the site is aided by preoperative oral administration of cream or olive oil or by injection of Evans blue dye. (*See textbook pages* 132, 133.)

Chapter 12

1. **False.**   Although transient bacteremia occurs among 15.4% to 33% of patients after rigid bronchoscopy, it does not occur predictably after transnasal flexible fiberoptic bronchoscopy. Therefore, the American Heart Association has recommended endocarditis prophylaxis for rigid but not for flexible bronchoscopy. (*See textbook pages* 141, 142.)

2. **False.**   In a retrospective study, flexible bronchoscopy was shown to be safe in the period immediately after acute myocardial infarction as long as there is no active ischemia at the time of the procedure. (*See textbook page* 142.)

3. **B.**   Bronchoalveolar lavage and transbronchial lung biopsy have a sensitivity of 94% to 100% for the detection of *Pneumocystis carinii* pneumonia. Bronchoalveolar lavage alone may have a sensitivity as high as 97%. The site and cause of bleeding are determined for approximately 90% of patients when bronchoscopy is performed before bleeding ceases. This yield drops to 50% when the procedure is performed after bleeding has stopped. Bronchoscopy performed with a standard-size bronchoscope through an endotracheal tube requires a tube size of at least 8 mm in internal diameter. If a smaller tube is used it is not possible to ventilate the patient during the procedure unless a helium-oxygen mixture is used. An alternative is use of a smaller bronchoscope, such as a pediatric version or an intubation endoscope. Pneumothorax occurs among approximately 0.2% of patients, whereas fever (1.2% to 16%), pneumonia (0.6% to 6%), vasovagal reactions (2.4%), hypotension, and cardiac arrhythmia (0.9%) all occur more frequently. (*See textbook page* 141.)

Chapter 13

1. **True.**   Sputum Gram stain may have a moderate degree of reliability if the specimen contains fewer than 10 squamous epithelial cells and more than 25 polymorphonuclear cells per low-power field. (*See textbook pages* 145, 146.)

2. **False.**   Transtracheal aspiration, although the standard with which multiple studies are compared, is not routinely used to treat adults. Serious complications of the procedure, such as bleeding, paratracheal and cutaneous infection, and subcutaneous or mediastinal emphysema have limited use of this procedure. (*See textbook page* 141.)

3. **False.**   The protective brush method of sampling lower respiratory tract secretions involves a closed brush system within a bronchoscope, whereas bronchoalveolar lavage samples a larger and more representative amount of lower respiratory tract secretions than does protected brush catheterization, and provides a large enough sample for smears for rapid identification and culture. When quantitative cultures are performed, 10^3 colony-forming units per milliliter (CFU/mL) usually are needed for a positive result with the protected brush method, whereas

10^4 CFU/mL usually are needed for a positive result with bronchoalveolar lavage. (*See textbook pages* 147, 148.)

4. **C.** Potassium chloride wet mount may be useful in the diagnosis of infection with certain gram-negative bacteria such as *Klebsiella pneumoniae*. Overall, only 40% of patients can produce a sputum sample when requested, and only 50% of the samples are suitable for analysis. Direct immunofluorescence for *Legionella* species has a high specificity (94%) but a low sensitivity (50%). Routinely processed expectorated sputum samples are neither sensitive nor specific in the diagnosis of bacterial pneumonia. (*See textbook pages* 145, 146.)

Chapter 14

1. **D.** Regarding thoracentesis and a bloody effusion, grossly bloody effusions with a red blood cell count of 5,000 to 10,000 cells per cubic millimeter must be present for fluid to appear pink. Effusions containing more than 100,000 red blood cells per cubic millimeter are consistent with trauma, malignant tumor, or pulmonary infarction. To differentiate traumatic thoracentesis from preexisting hemothorax, several observations may be helpful. Preexisting hemothorax has been defibrinated so it does not form a clot after it stands. Traumatic thoracentesis is suggested when pleural and blood hematocrit values match. (*See textbook page* 156.)

2. **C.** Cytologic examination of pleural fluid should be performed for an exudative effusion of unknown cause; between 100 and 200 mL of fluid is needed. Malignant tumors can produce pleural effusions by means of two basic mechanisms—implantation of malignant cells on the pleura or impairment of lymphatic drainage by tumor obstruction. The most common tumors that cause pleural effusions are lung cancer, breast cancer, and lymphoma. Heparin should be added to the container to prevent clotting of the fluid. In addition to malignant disease, cytologic examination can help diagnose rheumatoid pleuritis in which there is the presence of slender, elongated macrophages; giant, round, multinucleated macrophages, and amorphous granular background material. (*See textbook page* 156.)

Chapter 15

1. **True.** It is impossible to predict the level of PaO_2 and $PaCO_2$ reliably from physical signs and symptoms. Therefore, arterial blood gas analysis is indicated whenever there is a reason to rule in or out the presence of a respiratory or metabolic disturbance and to assess the nature, progression, or severity of a respiratory or metabolic disorder. (*See textbook page* 158.)

2. **False.** After puncture of the radial artery, pressure should be applied to the puncture site for a full 5 minutes. (*See textbook page* 159.)

3. **False.** A PO_2 greater than 50 mm Hg can be obtained from a vein. (*See textbook page* 159.)

4. **B.** Thirty-five seconds of breath holding has been associated with a fall in PaO_2 of 50 mm Hg and in pH of 0.07 and a rise in $PaCO_2$ of 10 mm Hg. This is one reason why local anesthesia is suggested for routine use with this procedure. The procedure is quite safe; complications occur in approximately 0.58% of cases. Normal value for the PaO_2 of a nonsmoking adult is defined with the equation $108.75 - (0.39 \times$ age in years). In cases of total occlusion of the radial artery, the

ulnar artery provides adequate blood flow to the hand 92% of the time. (*See textbook pages* 158, 159.)

Chapter 16

1. **False.**   The transport of critically ill patients to the operating room for elective or semielective tracheotomy is not without potential complications. As many as 33% of intensive care unit patients moved to other departments of the hospital for diagnostic tests and surgical procedures have marked and possibly dangerous physiologic changes. This is especially true of patients undergoing specialized ventilatory support in which the ventilator must travel with the patient or may not be available in the other setting. Tracheotomy can be performed at the bedside in one of two ways: (a) by having the operating room personnel bring the sterile supplies to the intensive care unit and having the procedure performed as a surgical procedure, and (b) as a percutaneous bronchoscopy-assisted technique. (*See textbook pages* 162, 169.)

2. **False.**   The cricothyroid space is 7 to 9 mm in vertical dimension, which is smaller than the outside diameter of most tracheotomy tubes. The no. 6, or small Shiley, has an outside diameter of 10 mm. (*See textbook page* 168.)

3. **B.**   Late hemorrhage after tracheotomy is usually caused by bleeding granulation tissue or a minor cause. However, it was previously reported that 50% of all tracheotomy bleeding occurring more than 48 hours after the procedure was caused by rupture of the innominate artery from erosion of the tracheotomy tube. Although less common since the advent of the low-pressure cuff, trachea–innominate artery fistulas still occur within the first month after tracheotomy. Infection and other factors, such as position of the tube, contribute to this potential complication. The mortality is higher than 50%. (*See textbook page* 166.)

4. **C.**   The advantages of percutaneous guide-wire dilational elective tracheotomy, most often described by Ciaglia in the literature, include no need for an operating room, a faster overall performance time than for conventional tracheotomy, relatively less expense, and decreased dissection. However, it is not a technique for emergency cricothyroidotomy, nor should it be performed in a completely blind manner. It is currently recommended in the literature that upper airway endoscopy may help to identify intratracheal placement of the needle and J guide-wire along with selection of the proper intratracheal ring membrane. The risk for posterior perforation of the trachea into the esophagus is decreased in comparison with that of surgical tracheotomy. (*See textbook page* 169.)

Chapter 17

1. **B.**   ECLS is a critical care technique that has made considerable technologic advances in recent years. ECLS is standard therapy for neonatal respiratory failure. Key factors to success in pediatric, infant, and adult populations is early intervention before the appearance of irreversible organ damage. Early trials in the 1970s comparing ECMO with conventional mechanical ventilation showed no survival advantage for ECMO; however, these trials were severely flawed in design. To date, almost 16,000 patients have been treated with ECLS at 90 centers across the United States and overseas. (*See textbook pages* 174, 179, 180.)

2. **D.**   It is thought that patients do better with ECLS if it is started early, preferably within 5 days of initiation of mechanical ventilation when the process remains reversible. Patients with the potential for severe bleeding are unlikely to

tolerate the necessary anticoagulation. At present ECLS is limited to care of persons younger than 60 years. Nonnecrotizing pneumonia may be managed with ECLS. (*See textbook page* 177.)

Chapter 18

1. **C.**   Lower gastrointestinal endoscopy can be performed for acute lower gastrointestinal bleeding. This procedure is technically difficult in an intensive care unit and on unprepared intestine. For these reasons, and because of the relative lack of sensitivity of endoscopy in this setting, erythrocyte scanning, angiography, or both are indicated for diagnosis. Endoscopic colonic decompression is advocated for patients in the intensive care unit. Results of uncontrolled studies suggest that when the diameter of the right colon exceeds 12 cm, perforation is imminent, and decompression is indicated. The placement of nasogastric suction, rectal tube placement, and position changes should be initiated before attempts at endoscopic decompression. Placement of a decompression tube into the colon is recommended because relapse is common. (*See textbook pages* 182–184.)

Chapter 19

1. **True.**   Root et al. reported 100% accuracy in identification of hemoperitoneum using 1 L of lavage fluid. Many subsequent studies confirmed these results. The largest of these studies was reported by Fischer et al. They showed a false-positive rate of 0.2%, a false-negative rate of 1.2%, and overall accuracy of 98.5%. For penetrating trauma a false-negative rate of 4.9% has been reported. (*See textbook pages* 187, 188.)

2. **False.**   The most common complications of abdominal paracentesis are bleeding and persistent fluid leak. Therefore, it is important to correct coagulopathy before performing this procedure. The Z-track technique is helpful in preventing fluid leak. This technique is performed by means of pulling the skin taut inferiorly after the skin has been punctured but before the peritoneal cavity has been entered. This allows the needle to enter the peritoneal cavity at a site different from the skin entrance site. Other complications of paracentesis include perforation of the intestinal or urinary bladder, peritonitis, and infection. Hypotension may occur when a large volume of fluid is removed. (*See textbook pages* 186, 187.)

3. **A.**   A red blood cell count of 1,000/mL is below the standard of 100,000/mL generally accepted as a positive result after nonpenetrating abdominal trauma. Any white blood cell count greater than 500/mL also is considered positive, as is an amylase value greater than 175 units/mL, return of food particles or intestinal content, immediate return of gross blood, aspiration of 10 mL blood through the catheter, and return of fluid through a chest tube or urinary bladder catheter. (*See textbook page* 190.)

Chapter 20

1. **C.**   Aspiration pneumonia is the most common complication of use of balloon tamponade for control of variceal hemorrhage. The incidence ranges from zero to 12%. Acute laryngeal obstruction is the most severe complication. Migration of the tube is the cause of this potentially fatal complication and occurs when the

gastric balloon is not inflated properly after adequate positioning in the stomach or when extensive traction of greater than 1.5 kg is used. Mucosal ulceration of the gastroesophageal junction is common and is directly related to prolonged traction time, greater than 36 hours. (*See textbook page* 195.)

2. **A.**   Endotracheal intubation should be performed before tube insertion. The incidence of pulmonary complications has been shown to be lower when endotracheal intubation is routinely performed. The esophageal balloon must be deflated for 30 minutes every 8 hours, but the gastric balloon may remain inflated continuously for up to 48 hours. After confirmation of tube position by means of auscultation in the epigastrium while a flush of air is injected through the gastric lumen, a chest radiograph must be obtained before the balloon inflation procedure continues. The esophageal balloon should ultimately be inflated with a bedside manometer to approximately 45 mm Hg. (*See textbook pages* 192, 193.)

Chapter 21

1. **True.**   Precipitation of proteins when exposed to an acid pH may be an important factor leading to the clogging of feeding tubes. Medications also are frequent causes of clogging, as is inadequate interval and volume of flushing between administrations of enteral feeding formulas. Several maneuvers are used for clearing clogged feeding tubes. These include irrigation with warm saline solution, with carbonated liquid, with cranberry juice, or with an enzyme solution. Pancrease—a mixture of lipase, amylase, and protease dissolved in a sodium bicarbonate solution—has been found to be useful. This mixture is instilled into the tube with a syringe and clamped for 30 minutes to allow enzymatic degradation of precipitated enteral feeding formula. (*See textbook page* 202.)

2. **C.**   Erythromycin, 200 mg administered intravenously 30 minutes before tube insertion, has been shown to improve the success of postpyloric tube placement. A tube 30 to 36 inches (76 to 91 cm) long is needed for placement of the tip in the stomach. A tube 43 inches (108 cm) long normally is used when access to the duodenum is desired. The combination of metoclopramide and a tapered, unweighted feeding tube with a stylet has been shown to achieve a transpyloric position in 84% of patients at 4 hours, in comparison with a 36% success rate with weighted tubes. After confirmation of tube position by means of auscultation in the epigastrium while a flush of air is injected through the tube, a chest radiograph must be obtained before infusion of a feeding formula is begun. Placement of a tube into a jejunal location reduces but does not eliminate risk for aspiration. (*See textbook pages* 197, 198.)

Chapter 22

1. **True.**   Hemapheresis involves separation and removal of a blood component with reinfusion of the remaining blood. Blood components of different specific gravities usually are separated by means of centrifugation. The plasma also can be separated from whole blood by means of a parallel plate membrane plasma exchange system of filtration. The centrifugation method is most popular in the United States, and the filtration method is popular in Japan and western Europe. (*See textbook page* 203.)

2. **B.**   The following are indications for treatment with therapeutic plasma exchange in the intensive care unit: acute Guillain-Barré syndrome, myasthenia gravis, thrombotic thrombocytopenic purpura, hyperviscosity syndrome, hemolytic ure-

mic syndrome, posttransfusion purpura, chronic idiopathic demyelinating poly-neuropathy, Goodpasture's syndrome, Refsum's disease, cold agglutinin disease, cryoglobulinemia, circulating anticoagulants, HELLP syndrome, renal failure with myeloma, systemic vasculitis due to systemic lupus erythematosus or rheumatoid arthritis, familial hyperlipoproteinemia, pemphigus vulgaris, drug overdose, and poisoning. (*See textbook page* 206.)

Chapter 23

1. **True.**   Conservative treatment consists of bed rest, hydration, and analgesics. Nonphenothiazine antiemetic agents are prescribed if nausea occurs. Methyl-xanthines (caffeine or theophylline) are used if the headache is severe or un-responsive to conservative measures. (*See textbook page* 213.)
2. **True.**   The conus medullaris is more caudal in children than in adults and requires more caudal needle insertion than the typical L3-4 location used for most adult procedures. (*See textbook page* 212.)
3. **C.**   Spinal fluid accelerates red blood cell hemolysis, and hemoglobin products are released within 2 hours of the initial hemorrhage. This causes slight discol-oration of the cerebrospinal fluid, also called *xanthochromia*. Mild degrees of xan-thochromia may be detectable only with a spectrophotometer. A decreasing red blood cell count in tubes collected serially during lumbar puncture, presence of a fibrinous clot in the collected specimen, and leukocyte to erythrocyte ratio of 1 : 700 are characteristics of a traumatic spinal tap. (*See textbook pages* 209, 210.)

Chapter 24

1. **C.**   The Glasgow Coma Scale score was originally developed as a prognostic tool for traumatic brain injury but became popular as a quick, reproducible estimate of level of consciousness. Three findings at physical examination are used to deter-mine the score—eye opening, motor response, and verbal response. For the patient described, the important findings are opens eyes to painful stimulus, 2 points; speaks isolated inappropriate words, 3 points; extremity movements attempt to push away painful stimulus, 5 points; the score is 10. (*See textbook page* 220.)
2. **False.**   Retrograde cannulation of the jugular bulb is a low-risk, technically sim-ple procedure. The jugular venous bulb is an appropriate site for measurement of cerebral oxygen consumption. The internal jugular vein can be located in relation to external anatomic landmarks, and the catheter is directed toward the mastoid, over which lies the jugular venous bulb. Continuous monitoring of venous satu-ration is feasible with commercially available oximetry catheters. (*See textbook page* 223.)

Chapter 25

1. **False.**   Percutaneous cystostomy also may be complicated by intestinal perforation, hypotension, and loss of a portion of the catheter in the bladder. Bladder spasms are the most common complication, and can be avoided by means of pulling the cys-tostomy tube against the bladder wall, immediately after placement and then advanc-ing the tube 2 cm into the bladder to allow for movement. Oxybutynin 5 mg two to four times a day also may be used for severe spasms. (*See textbook page* 236.)

2. **B.**   Prostate cancer may be an indication if the tumor leads to unsuccessful ure-thral cannulation. In addition to bladder cancer, nonpalpable bladder, coagulopathy, and clot retention, previous lower abdominal operation is a relative contraindication. Ultrasound is often useful in the setting of a previous lower abdominal operation to identify adhesions that may hold a loop of intestine in the planned insertion area. (*See textbook pages* 234, 235.)

Chapter 26

1. **False.**   The viscosity of synovial fluid is a measure of the hyaluronic acid content of the fluid. Hyaluronic acid is one of the main substances in the synovial fluid that gives it its viscous quality. Enzymes such as hyaluronidase are released in inflammatory conditions and destroy hyaluronic acid in other proteinaceous material. This produces a thinner, less viscous fluid. (*See textbook page* 240.)
2. **B.**   Bursitis, tendinitis, and cellulitis all may mimic true joint arthritis. Before arthrocentesis, a physical examination must be performed to ascertain that the true joint is inflamed and that an effusion is present. If a large effusion is suspected, a patellar tap is performed. Arthrocentesis also is used for therapeutic purposes. (*See textbook page* 237.)

Chapter 27

1. **True.**   Investigators have noticed that a return of consciousness can take minutes after termination of up to 8 hours of propofol infusion even though the elimination half-life of propofol is 5 hours. This suggests that the initial fall in drug concentration after termination of the infusion is a function of redistribution more than of elimination half-life. (*See textbook page* 242.)
2. **True.**   Recent data suggest that reversal of opioids with an opioid combination agonist-antagonist such as nalbuphine may be safer than with naloxone. Antagonists with some intrinsic analgesic properties produce more gradual reversal than does naloxone. A mixed agonist-antagonist can either increase or decrease opioid effect depending on the dose administered, the particular agonist already in the bloodstream, and the amount of drug to be reversed. (*See textbook page* 244.)
3. **False.**   Barbiturates are used to facilitate endotracheal intubation, and they reduce cerebral oxygen utilization. However, cardiovascular side effects include hypotension with possible cardiac arrest, myocardial depression, and an increase in venous capacitance. Etomidate has the same beneficial effect on cerebral oxygen kinetics as barbiturates yet is virtually devoid of cardiovascular side effects. (*See textbook page* 244.)
4. **False.**   Depending on the level of discomfort of the procedure and the requirements of the ICU, a combination of analgesia and sedation is critical. Analgesic agents such as alfentanil, sufentanil, and ketamine and sedative agents such as propofol and midazolam are used in combination in the ICU and are effective in combination. It should be emphasized that use of sedative agents without analgesic agents is to be avoided for any procedures in the ICU. Sedative agents alone may be appropriate for ventilator weaning and anxiety, in which there are no pain considerations. (*See textbook pages* 241, 242, 247.)
5. **C.**   The practice of administering small doses of naloxone (0.04 mg) to patients to reverse the respiratory depression of narcotic administration is inadvisable in the ICU. Many anecdotal reports indicate that naloxone has serious side effects

on cardiovascular function with or without prior narcotic administration. Naloxone levels also decline rapidly, whereas narcotic levels may be persistently elevated for a longer time. Side effects such as vomiting, delirium, arrhythmias, pulmonary edema, cardiac arrest, and sudden death occur after administration of naloxone in this setting. Recurring respiratory depression therefore remains a distinct possibility for an unintubated patient with potential morbidity and even mortality. (*See textbook page* 244.)

6. **A.** Midazolam provides more complete anterograde amnesia than diazepam or lorazepam and produces less pain on intravenous injection than diazepam or lorazepam. Midazolam is highly protein bound, approaching 95% to albumin, and has a comparatively short half-life of 2 hours versus 36 hours for diazepam and 12 hours for lorazepam. However, the half-life can be notably prolonged among ICU patients, obese patients, and elderly patients and among about 6% of normal patients for unknown reasons. (*See textbook pages* 244, 245.)

Chapter 28

1. **False.** Indirect methods of blood pressure monitoring have a role in following trends of pressure change; for frequent pressure checks among patients in stable condition; in patient transport situations; in minimizing risk for infection for a severely burned patient; and when group averages are most important. They are of little value in situations in which pressure is likely to fluctuate rapidly. In general, they exhibit such divergence from directly measured values that critical management decisions should not be based on the results of indirect blood pressure monitoring unless confirmation from a more reliable method is not available. (*See textbook pages* 254, 255.)

2. **A.** Intramucosal pH monitoring is used to monitor changes in tissue pH in response to changes in local oxygen delivery and metabolism. These trends can be used to identify organ tissue dysfunction and predict multiple organ failure. The technique is used to measure PCO_2 and pH in saline solution within a gas-permeable balloon placed in the lumen of a hollow viscus. The most common site monitored in the intensive care unit is the stomach. Although intramucosal pH monitoring may predict complications among patients who have undergone cardiac operations, a survival advantage has not been well demonstrated. (*See textbook pages* 264, 265.)

3. **B.** Perforation of the tympanic membrane has been reported after tympanic temperature measurement. Bleeding from the external ear canal also has been reported. Sublingual temperatures are affected by ingestion of hot or cold beverages and tachypnea. Measurement of mixed venous temperature can be performed with a thermistor-equipped pulmonary arterial catheter. All critically ill patients should have their temperature measured at least every 4 hours. (*See textbook pages* 252, 253.)

Chapter 29

1. **C.** Exhaled minute ventilation. The essential measurements of indirect calorimetry are inspired and expired oxygen fractions, carbon dioxide fractions, and minute ventilation. Oxygen consumption and carbon dioxide production are calculated from those values. Inhaled minute ventilation is calculated with a formula called the *Haldane transformation*. Energy expenditure usually is calculated from these

values with the modified Weir equation, which is a mathematically derived formula based on the series of equations describing foodstuff combustion. (*See textbook pages* 271, 272.)

Chapter 30

1. **False.**   The presence of infection with any fluid accumulation in the abdomen is almost always an absolute indication for drainage. (*See textbook page* 276.)
2. **False.**   The care after catheter insertion requires frequent flushing starting a few hours after insertion. Normal saline solution is injected every 4 hours to flush the catheter and prevent clogging of the side holes. After 24 hours, the purpose of flushing is to agitate dependent debris in the collection so that sediment eventually can be aspirated into the catheter. Flushing is performed every 4 hours until the drainage fluid clears. (*See textbook page* 279.)
3. **False.**   Cholestasis is a common condition in the intensive care unit and actually occurs among most patients. Distention of the gallbladder is a common finding. For a patient with sepsis of unknown source, cholecystostomy is indicated in the presence of a distended gallbladder and especially with findings of pericholecystic fluid or thickened gallbladder wall at ultrasonography. (*See textbook page* 279.)

II. Cardiovascular Problems in the Intensive Care Unit

31. Cardiopulmonary Resuscitation

True or False

1. Most infants and children who need resuscitation in an intensive care setting have had a primary myocardial dysrhythmia or other pump failure as the cause of the need for cardiopulmonary resuscitation (CPR).
2. The proper use of defibrillator devices in an intensive care setting requires special attention to selection of proper energy levels.

Select the best answer

3. Which of the following is *not true*?

   A. The depth of sternal compression in adult CPR is 1.5 to 2.0 inches (3.75 to 5.0 cm).
   B. The appropriate rate for rescue breathing for an adult during CPR is 12 breaths per minute.
   C. The appropriate rate for rescue breathing for an infant during CPR is 20 breaths per minute.
   D. Adult CPR techniques are appropriate for children who appear to be at least 12 years old.
   E. The frequency of sternal compressions for infants and children is 100 per minute.

4. Which of the following statements is *true*?

   A. The administration of calcium can be through use of its two available salts—calcium chloride and calcium gluconate.
   B. Each form of calcium is degraded in the plasma, and each provides the same bioavailability of calcium.
   C. Calcium chloride salt provides the least direct source of calcium ion and produces the slowest effect.
   D. Calcium gluconate salt is unstable. Calcium gluceptate and gluconate salts require renal degradation to release the free calcium ion.

32. Critical Aortic Stenosis and Hypertrophic Cardiomyopathy

True or False

1. The most common symptom occurring in left ventricular outflow obstruction is angina pectoris.
2. An auscultatory finding that is common to all forms of left ventricular outflow obstruction is the systolic (crescendo-decrescendo type) murmur.
3. A chest radiograph of a patient with left ventricular outflow obstruction shows a dilated heart silhouette most of the time.

Select the best answer

4. Which of the following statements regarding aortic stenosis is *true*?

   A. Cardiac catheterization has the sole objective of corroborating Doppler findings in the setting of severe aortic stenosis.
   B. Because of the sensitivity of Doppler echocardiography and other noninvasive tests, cardiac catheterization for coronary arteriography is used to evaluate only patients at highest risk before surgical intervention.
   C. Accurate measurement of cardiac output with the Fick method or dye dilution technique can be performed during measurement of the gradient across a diseased valve.
   D. A gradient of 50 mm Hg or more is found in healthy persons.

5. Which of the following should not be considered standard intensive care management of severe aortic stenosis?

   A. Nitroglycerin ointment 0.5 to 1.0 inch (1.25 to 2.5 cm) applied topically every 4 hours
   B. Nitroglycerin intravenous drip
   C. Referral for aortic valve replacement
   D. Captopril 6.25 to 25 mg three times a day
   E. Metoprolol 25 to 50 mg twice a day

33. Critical Care for Pericardial Disease

True or False

1. Acute pericarditis might be asymptomatic but usually is symptomatic with a pleuritic chest component. Symptoms frequently are of sudden onset.
2. Pericardial friction rubs have traditionally been described as having a "to-and-fro" description, although the classic pericardial rub has three components.
3. Three potential electrocardiographic (ECG) stages are recognizable in the evolution of pericarditis.

Select the best answer

4. Regarding pericarditis:

   A. The optimal management of pericarditis is indomethacin over a 2- to 3-day period.

B. Initial and optimal management of pericarditis is to begin with 600 mg ibuprofen by mouth every 6 hours.

C. Effective initial management of pericarditis can lead to relief of pain within 15 minutes.

D. Azathioprine (Imuran) should never be used for management of pericarditis.

E. Steroid therapy in high doses is often indicated in management of pericarditis.

5. Which of the following statements is *true*?

   A. Any pericardial effusion greater in volume than 250 mL will cause symptomatic compromise of myocardial function.

   B. The configuration of the cardiac silhouette on a radiograph allows easy differentiation of cardiomegaly, large pericardial cyst, and pericardial effusion.

   C. Rapid accumulation of as little as 200 mL of intrapericardial fluid can cause acute hemodynamic compromise and circulatory collapse.

   D. If pericardial fluid is of an inflammatory nature, it is unlikely that a pericardial rub will be audible.

34. Sudden Cardiac Death

True or False

1. Sudden cardiac death occurs among 400,000 patients per year in the United States.

2. Cardiac causes of ventricular tachycardia and ventricular fibrillation in the absence of acute myocardial infarction include prior myocardial infarction, cardiomyopathy, and electrical disorders.

Select the best answer

3. Regarding the management of sudden cardiac death:

   A. Prevention has no role.

   B. Amiodarone and sotalol have been demonstrated to improve survival when used in the treatment of survivors of sudden cardiac death.

   C. Implantable cardioverter-defibrillator devices have become obsolete in the management of ventricular fibrillation.

   D. None of the above.

35. Dissection of the Aorta

True or False

1. Aortic dissection is much more common than acute myocardial infarction.

2. The process of aortic dissection begins with an intimal tear.

3. Hypertension is the most important disease associated with the development of aortic dissection.

4. The original classification of DeBakey divides aortic dissection into five types.

Select the best answer

5. Regarding the diagnosis of aortic dissection:

    A. The electrocardiogram is very useful in the diagnosis of acute aortic dissection.

    B. The most common plain chest radiographic finding (seen among more than 80% of patients with aortic dissection) is widening of the superior mediastinum.

    C. Echocardiography is not useful in the diagnosis of aortic dissection.

    D. The chief limitation of computed tomography in the diagnosis of aortic dissection is limited visualization of the descending aorta.

6. Regarding acute aortic dissection:

    A. Untreated acute aortic dissection has a nearly uniformly fatal outcome.

    B. Because of its superior antihypertensive effect, nifedipine is the preferred calcium channel blocker when β-blockade is contraindicated.

    C. Maintenance of a supranormal mean arterial blood pressure is critical in the management of acute aortic dissection.

    D. Adequate β-blockade is occasionally necessary after the use of sodium nitroprusside in the medical management of acute aortic dissection.

36. Acute Aortic Insufficiency

True or False

1. Acute aortic insufficiency is generally the result of myocardial infarction.

2. It is uncommon for acute bacterial endocarditis to be caused by *Staphylococcus aureus.*

3. The presence of large valvular vegetations of the aortic valve is consistent with fungal endocarditis.

Select the best answer

4. Regarding acute infective endocarditis with aortic insufficiency:

    A. It is most common for an infection of the aortic valve to affect a previously normal valve.

    B. Infective endocarditis of an aortic valve rarely involves an anatomically bicuspid aortic valve.

    C. Usually there is no marked aortic stenosis or aortic insufficiency before the onset of infective endocarditis.

    D. Infective endocarditis resulting in acute severe aortic insufficiency rarely causes life-threatening cardiac complications.

5. Hemodynamic findings associated with acute severe aortic sufficiency include:

    A. Decreased arterial pulse pressure

    B. Equilibration of left ventricular end-diastolic and aortic diastolic pressures

    C. A marked decrease in left ventricular end-diastolic pressure

    D. Decreased pulmonary artery wedge pressure

6. Regarding acute endocarditis of the aortic valve, which statement is *false?*

    A. Patients with a congenital bicuspid aortic valve are at increased risk for aortic valve endocarditis.

    B. A bicuspid aortic valve is associated with turbulent flow.

   C. Bicuspid aortic valve is commonly symptomatic and if not symptomatic, usually is found during a routine physical examination in childhood.
   D. Antibiotic prophylaxis is indicated for dental or other surgical procedures on patients with known bicuspid aortic valve.

7. Which of the following medication effects is least likely to be beneficial in the management of acute aortic insufficiency?

   A. Increased impedance to forward blood flow out of the heart (increased afterload)
   B. Reduced left ventricular end-diastolic volume (preload)
   C. Increased myocardial contractility
   D. Reduction of anxiety

37. Acute Mitral Regurgitation

True or False

   1. Life-threatening acute mitral regurgitation caused by papillary muscle rupture in the setting of myocardial infarction occurs among less than 1% of patients with acute myocardial infarction.
   2. The presence of moderately severe or severe mitral regurgitation in the setting of acute myocardial infarction is associated with a higher mortality rate than that among patients with acute myocardial infarction who have no evidence of mitral regurgitation.
   3. The anterolateral papillary muscle is more vulnerable to ischemia than the posteromedial papillary muscle.

Select the best answer

   4. Regarding intensive care management of mitral regurgitation:

   A. Afterload reduction is imperative in the management of mitral regurgitation.
   B. Intraaortic balloon pumping is not indicated in cases of severe mitral regurgitation.
   C. Inotropic support with high-dose dopamine is highly effective in the management of mitral regurgitation.
   D. Pulmonary arterial catheterization should be used only in severe cases of mitral regurgitation.

38. Syncope

True or False

   1. Syncope is classified as cardiovascular and noncardiovascular.
   2. Syncope due to obstructive disorders of the heart typically occurs during exercise.
   3. Hypertrophic cardiomyopathy is a particularly frequent cause of syncope among younger patients and athletes.

Select the best answer

4. Regarding causes of syncope:

    A. Tachycardia rarely results in syncope.
    B. Pulmonary hypertension may lead to recurrent syncope.
    C. Pulmonary embolism is a rare cause of syncope.
    D. Acute myocardial ischemia rarely presents itself with syncope.

5. Regarding the sick sinus syndrome:

    A. The sick sinus syndrome is characterized by impaired sinoatrial impulse formation or propagation.
    B. Sinus node dysfunction is frequently masked by low concentrations of drugs such as digoxin, β-blockers, and calcium channel blockers.
    C. A decreased sensitivity to endogenous adenosine appears closely related to the development of the sick sinus syndrome.
    D. Patients with sick sinus syndrome who have syncope usually need surgical correction of this syndrome.

39. Systemic Embolism

True or False

1. Embolism to the systemic circulation nearly always originates as a thrombus within the left heart.
2. Systemic emboli do not originate in the venous circulation.

Select the best answer

3. Regarding the source of systemic emboli:

    A. Atrial fibrillation is a rare cause of systemic embolization.
    B. Coronary artery disease with left ventricular dysfunction is a rare cause of systemic embolization.
    C. Valvular heart disease is a common cause of systemic embolization.
    D. Coronary artery disease and valvular heart disease are most likely to be complicated by systemic embolism when low ejection fraction and normal sinus rhythm are present.

4. Regarding arterial emboli:

    A. Most noncerebral emboli lodge in the upper extremities.
    B. It is important to differentiate arterial thrombosis superimposed on atherosclerotic disease of the lower extremities and systemic embolization to the lower extremities.
    C. Embolic arterial occlusion to the lower extremities rarely is life threatening.
    D. Use of the Fogarty catheter has markedly reduced the high mortality among patients with embolization to the lower extremities.
    E. Limb salvage rate with or without embolectomy is poorly related to the severity of ischemia at presentation.

5. Regarding the treatment of patients with suspected systemic embolism:

    A. Intravenous heparin is contraindicated because of the need for surgical intervention.

B. For acute systemic embolism to the lower extremities, embolectomy is often performed with a Fogarty catheter.

C. Patients with systemic embolism are rarely subject to recurrent embolization.

D. Long-term management after embolectomy is achieved with 325 mg aspirin every day by mouth.

40. Supraventricular Tachycardias

True or False

1. By definition, the atrioventricular (AV) junction cannot participate in the generation of a supraventricular tachycardia.

2. The three general mechanisms that account for the generation of supraventricular tachyarrhythmias are increased automaticity, reentry, and suppression of triggered activity.

3. A telemetry reading is of no value in the diagnosis of a tachyarrhythmia. A 12-lead electrocardiogram (ECG) is the only way in which proper diagnosis can be made.

4. Treatment of a supraventricular tachycardia is geared toward treatment of the myocardial dysfunction.

Select the best answer

5. Regarding adenosine in the management of supraventricular tachycardias:

   A. Adenosine is an exogenous nucleoside that causes adenosine receptor stimulation with a resultant hyperpolarization of cells.

   B. Adenosine is given by means of slow intravenous infusion.

   C. Smaller doses of adenosine may be used in the presence of methylxanthines.

   D. Adenosine has a rapid metabolism, and its effects resolve within several seconds.

6. Regarding the use of digoxin in the treatment of supraventricular tachycardia:

   A. The mechanism of action is conduction slowing and increased refractoriness of the sinoatrial (SA) and AV nodes through hypersensitization of the carotid baroreceptor.

   B. Digoxin is administered by the intravenous route only. Its onset of action usually is within 10 minutes.

   C. Oral absorption is completely predictable.

   D. Digoxin is excreted primarily by the liver, and therefore the maintenance dose must be adjusted for patients with hepatic failure.

Select the best answer

7. Regarding digoxin toxicity:

   A. Digoxin toxicity is uncommon given its broad therapeutic window. Toxic levels of digoxin rarely lead to arrhythmia.

   B. If digoxin administration leads to an arrhythmia, it is a solitary type.

   C. The increased vagal tone from digoxin toxicity can produce sinus bradycardia or AV block.

   D. Therapy for digoxin toxicity is immediate intravenous administration of digoxin-specific Fab antibody fragments.

8. Regarding atrial fibrillation:

   A. Atrial fibrillation is a reentry arrhythmia with multiple wavelets of depolarization traveling in random sequence.
   B. On an ECG, the atrial depolarizations are irregular and discharge at a rate of 130 to 150 beats/min.
   C. The most serious consequence of atrial fibrillation is pulmonary edema.
   D. Among untreated patients with normal AV node function, the discharge rate usually is 80 to 90 beats/min.

9. Regarding atrial flutter:

   A. Atrial flutter usually exists in patients without underlying structural heart disease.
   B. Atrial flutter is an unstable rhythm.
   C. Atrial conduction rate during flutter usually is the same as atrial fibrillation.
   D. There is a lack of constancy to the conducted atrial beats.

Answers

Chapter 31

1. **False.**   Most infants and children who need resuscitation have had a primary respiratory arrest. Cardiac arrest results from the ensuing hypoxia and acidosis. The focus of pediatric resuscitation should be airway maintenance and ventilation. Among children cessation of cardiac activity usually is the manifestation of prolonged hypoxia. (*See textbook page* 291.)
2. **True.**   The selection of proper energy levels for defibrillation in an intensive care setting lessens myocardial damage and the induction of arrhythmias that are brought about by an unnecessarily high delivery of energy. Inadequate energies do not terminate an arrhythmia. (*See textbook page* 296.)
3. **D.**   Adult CPR techniques are appropriate for children who appear to be at least 8 years old. The decision often has to be based on the appearance of the child without specific knowledge of chronologic age. Appropriate breathing rates are 12 breaths per minute for adults, 15 breaths per minute for children, and 20 breaths per minute for infants. The appropriate depth of sternal compression is 1.5 to 2.0 inches (3.75 to 5.0 cm) for adults, 1.0 to 1.5 inches (2.5 to 3.75 cm) for children, and 0.5 to 1.0 inches (1.25 to 2.5 cm) for infants. The frequency of chest compressions is 80 to 100 per minute for adults and 100 per minute for infants and children. (*See textbook pages* 288–293.)
4. **D.**   Administration of calcium may be in the form of any of its three available salts—calcium chloride, calcium gluceptate, and calcium gluconate. The gluconate salt is unstable. Chloride salt provides the most direct source of calcium and produces the most rapid effect. The gluceptate and gluconate salts require hepatic degradation to release free calcium ion. Calcium chloride is highly irritating to the tissues and must be injected into a large vein. (*See textbook pages* 303, 304.)

Chapter 32

1. **True.**   Angina pectoris is the most commonly encountered symptom associated with outflow obstruction. In the absence of epicardial coronary disease, myocardial ischemia is presumed to be caused by exaggerated oxygen requirements from left ventricular hypertrophy. (*See textbook page* 315.)

2. **True.**   The crescendo-decrescendo systolic ejection murmur is common to all forms of left ventricular outflow obstruction. This murmur is often accompanied by a palpable thrill. The intensity of the murmur is related poorly to the severity of stenosis. The duration of the murmur is a better index of severity of obstruction. (*See textbook page* 316.)

3. **False.**   In most patients, the heart is not dilated, and the cardiothoracic ratio is normal on a posteroanterior chest radiograph. (*See textbook page* 315.)

4. **C.**   Cardiac catheterization is warranted in the care of any patient with suspected severe symptomatic aortic stenosis. Catheterization has two principal objectives—to corroborate Doppler findings and to define substantial coronary arterial stenosis. Accurate measurement of cardiac output by means of the Fick method or dye dilution technique should be performed with gradient measurement across a diseased valve. The cross-sectional valve area can then be estimated. A mean systolic gradient of 50 mm Hg or more is consistent with severe aortic stenosis. In such severe cases, the calculated valve area usually is less than 0.8 cm². However, as cardiac output drops because of systolic pump dysfunction, mean systolic gradients less than 50 mm Hg can be recorded with critical stenosis. (*See textbook page* 318.)

5. **E.**   Metoprolol 25 to 50 mg twice a day. β-Blockers, calcium channel blockers, and most antiarrhythmic agents should be used with extreme caution to treat patients with severe aortic stenosis. Nitroglycerin in either topical or intravenous form is standard therapy to reduce preload. Afterload reduction with angiotensin-converting enzyme inhibitors such as captopril has met with some success. Definitive treatment rests with surgical correction. (*See textbook page* 319.)

Chapter 33

1. **True.**   Acute pericarditis may be asymptomatic, but more often there is central chest pain, usually very sharp, often with a pleuritic component. There may be a sensation of pressure. The onset is often sudden and may interrupt sleep. (*See textbook page* 327.)

2. **True.**   The pericardial rub or friction sound is pathognomonic of pericarditis. A fully developed rub has three components—an atrial rub, a ventricular systolic rub, and an early diastolic rub. The diastolic rub follows the second heart sound, usually is the faintest of the three components, and often is not audible. This accounts for the "to-and-fro" description of the pericardial friction rub. (*See textbook page* 327.)

3. **False.**   There are four potential ECG stages. *Stage I*: An entirely typical ECG is diagnostic of pericarditis. Concave ST-segment changes occur with elevation in most leads, particularly leads I, II, aVL, aVF, and V3 through V6. *Stage II*: This evolutionary stage shows all ST junctions returning to baseline. *Stage III*: Widespread T-wave inversions appear that cannot be differentiated from those of diffuse myocardial injury or myocarditis. *Stage IV*: T waves return to their prepericarditic condition. The entire ECG evolution occurs in days or weeks. Transition from stage III usually is relatively slow. Stage I evolves into stage II relatively quickly. Some patients continue with some degree of T-wave inversion for long periods of time. (*See textbook page* 327.)

4. **C.**   The initial optimal management of pericarditis is to begin with 600 mg ibuprofen by mouth every 6 hours, which often gives relief of pain within 15 minutes to 2 hours. The dose can then be reduced to 400 mg or increased to 800 mg. Should this fail, aspirin or indomethacin can be used. Symptomatic pericarditis occasionally calls for drastic treatment, as with phenylbutazone. Corticosteroid

therapy should be avoided if at all possible because patients may become steroid dependent. If it must be given, corticosteroid therapy should be administered at the lowest effective dose only with appropriate tapering. Although it may have to be performed in an extreme case of treatment failure, pericardiectomy may not be successful in relieving pain and must be considered a final therapeutic maneuver. (*See textbook page* 329.)

5. **C.**   The pericardium is a nondistensible membrane encircling the heart. As little as 200 mL of fluid accumulation in an acute setting can cause hemodynamic collapse. Rather large effusions, however, may not clinically embarrass the heart as long as the rate of exudation is slow enough to prevent the pericardium from stretching. The configuration of the cardiac silhouette cannot help one differentiate cardiomegaly, large pericardial cyst, and pericardial effusions. This must be done by means of contrast radiography, radioisotope scanning, computed tomography, or, most often, echocardiography. As many as 70% of patients in whom pericardial fluid is an inflammatory exudate have an audible pericardial rub. (*See textbook page* 330.)

Chapter 34

1. **True.**   Sudden cardiac death occurs among 400,000 patients per year in the United States, accounting for approximately 50% of all cardiovascular mortality. Sudden cardiac death is defined as loss of consciousness within 1 hour of the onset of symptoms for a person who has known or unknown preexisting heart disease. (*See textbook page* 338.)

2. **True.**   Cardiac causes of ventricular tachycardia and ventricular fibrillation in the absence of acute myocardial infarction include prior myocardial infarction and cardiomyopathy, including idiopathic dilated, valvular, hypertrophic, arrhythmogenic right ventricular dysplasia, congenital heart disease, and infiltrative diseases. Electric disorders also can cause ventricular tachycardia and ventricular fibrillation. They include long QT syndrome, preexcitation syndromes (e.g., Wolff-Parkinson-White), conduction disorders, and primary idiopathic ventricular fibrillation. (*See textbook page* 338.)

3. **D.**   None of the above. Ongoing trials are comparing therapy with amiodarone or sotalol and use of implantable cardioverter-defibrillator devices for protection against sudden cardiac death among survivors of sudden cardiac death and patients at risk for sudden cardiac death. Several noncontrolled, nonrandomized studies involving patients who have received implantable devices appear to demonstrate that the devices can decrease the recurrence rate of sudden cardiac death to 1% or less per year. The overall approach to the treatment of patients at risk or who have sustained sudden cardiac arrest can be divided into the following phases: (a) Adequate prevention of coronary artery disease among those at high risk. This includes modification of risk factors, and treatment with aspirin, β-blockers, and other agents. (b) Stabilization after cardiac arrest. (c) Identification of reversible causes, such as medications, electrolyte imbalances, and myocardial infarction. (d) Definition of the coronary anatomy and the functional status of the left ventricle with echocardiography, stress testing, or cardiac catheterization. (e) Definition of conduction abnormalities and tachyarrhythmias with Holter monitoring, exercise testing, signal-averaged electrocardiography, or electrophysiologic studies. (f) Select therapies including implantation of a defibrillator, guided or empiric drug therapy, and coronary artery bypass grafting possibly with implantation of a defibrillator. (*See textbook pages* 340, 341.)

Chapter 35

1. **False.** The severe chest pain associated with aortic dissection usually leads to a mistaken initial diagnosis of acute myocardial infarction. However, acute aortic dissection is much less common than acute myocardial infarction. Estimates indicate that 1 in 10,000 patients admitted to the hospital have aortic dissection. (*See textbook page* 343.)

2. **True.** It is generally accepted that the process of aortic dissection begins with an intimal tear that most often occurs in the proximal ascending aorta. However, most reported series of aortic dissection indicate that less than 5% to 20% of patients with acute dissection do not have an identifiable intimal tear at autopsy. It has been postulated that for those patients the dissection begins with hemorrhage of the vasa vasorum within the media and subsequent rupture into the intima. (*See textbook pages* 343, 344.)

3. **True.** Hypertension is by far the most important disease associated with development of aortic dissection. Clinical evidence or a history of hypertension was present in 92% of 463 autopsy cases reviewed in Hirst's classic article. After hypertension, congenitally malformed aortic valves are the most common pathologic state predisposing to aortic dissection. Other conditions associated with aortic dissection include Marfan's syndrome, Ehlers-Danlos syndrome, coarctation of the aorta, aortic stenosis, Turner's syndrome, relapsing polychondritis, and pregnancy. The importance of pregnancy as an independent risk factor has recently been disputed. (*See textbook page* 344.)

4. **False.** The original classification of DeBakey divides aortic dissection into three types, as follows: (a) Type I dissection begins in the ascending aorta and extends distally to the arch and descending aorta. (b) Type II dissection begins in and is limited to the ascending aorta. (c) Type III dissection begins in and is limited to the descending aorta. Daley et al. in 1970 changed the classification to involve cases involving the ascending aorta (type A) and those in which the dissection was limited to the descending aorta (type B). Dissection is considered acute if it is of less than 2 weeks' and chronic if it is of more than 2 weeks' duration. (*See textbook pages* 344, 345.)

5. **B.** The most common plain chest radiographic finding, occurring among more than 80% of patients with aortic dissection, is widening of the superior mediastinum. This finding is nonspecific and may occur with hypertension, aortic aneurysm, and aging. Electrocardiography is more useful in ruling out myocardial infarction in the setting of acute onset of chest pains. Echocardiography is especially useful if it is multiplane transesophageal echocardiography, which allows visualization of the ascending aorta, aortic arch, and descending aorta. Computed tomography can be useful, but its chief limitation is an inability to visualize aortic valve disruption and aortic valvular insufficiency and an inability to adequately visualize the ascending aorta. (*See textbook pages* 347–349.)

6. **A.** Untreated acute aortic dissection has an extremely rapid, usually fatal clinical course. In Jamieson's series, the time from presentation to death was less than 24 hours among 72% of untreated patients. Initial treatment of patients with suspected acute aortic dissection includes establishing venous access and continuous blood pressure monitoring. The goals of medical therapy are to stop the spread of intramural hematoma and to prevent rupture. Sodium nitroprusside is one of the most valuable agents for lowering blood pressure, but it also increases myocardial contractility and thereby may cause progression of dissection. To avoid this, adequate β-blockade is essential and should be initiated before infusion of sodium nitroprusside, not after. Intravenous propranolol, labetalol, or esmolol may be administered to achieve β-blockade. In the rare cases when β-blockade is contraindicated, some authors advocate the use of calcium channel blockers. In those

cases, the goal of calcium channel blockade is to provide a negative inotropic effect. In that case, diltiazem and verapamil are more effective than nifedipine. Immediate surgical treatment is recommended for all patients with ascending aortic dissection in the absence of contraindications. Patients with uncomplicated dissection limited to the descending aorta should be treated with intensive parenteral drug therapy for 48 to 72 hours, after which they should be treated with an oral regimen or other antihypertensive medications. Even if the dissection is asymptomatic, patients with evidence of expansion, complications, or continued dissection should undergo immediate surgical intervention. (*See textbook pages* 350, 351.)

Chapter 36

1. **False.** Acute aortic insufficiency usually is the result of infective endocarditis, dissection of the ascending aorta, trauma, or spontaneous rupture of the valve itself. (*See textbook page* 355.)
2. **False.** Acute bacterial endocarditis is commonly the result of *S. aureus* infection. It often produces necrosis and perforation or detachment of one or more aortic valve leaflets. Infection of the aortic annulus with necrosis and abscess formation can cause weakening and progressive dilatation of the aortic root so that the aortic valve leaflets fail to coapt properly during diastole. This leads to aortic insufficiency. (*See textbook pages* 355, 356.)
3. **True.** Large valvular vegetations may prevent proper diastolic coaptation of the aortic valve leaflets. Although present in staphylococcal endocarditis, such bulky vegetations are more characteristic of fungal endocarditis caused by aspergillosis, histoplasmosis, or other such fungal diseases. (*See textbook page* 356.)
4. **C.** It is possible for acute endocarditis with an organism of sufficient severity to cause valve destruction to affect a previously normal valve. More commonly, however, acute endocarditis resulting in aortic insufficiency involves an anatomically bicuspid aortic valve. This is more common among persons addicted to narcotics who administer the drugs intravenously. Usually there is no marked aortic stenosis or aortic insufficiency before the onset of infective endocarditis. Infective endocarditis resulting in acute severe aortic insufficiency may cause several life-threatening cardiac complications. (*See textbook page* 356.)
5. **B.** Hemodynamic findings associated with acute severe aortic insufficiency include slightly increased arterial pulse pressure, equilibration of left ventricular and aortic pressures, and marked elevation in left ventricular end-diastolic pressure. Other hemodynamic findings in aortic insufficiency are indicative of left ventricular failure. It is important to differentiate acute and chronic aortic insufficiency. (*See textbook pages* 357, 358.)
6. **C.** Patients with a congenitally bicuspid aortic valve are at increased risk for aortic valve endocarditis. This bicuspid valve is associated with turbulent flow, and this may contribute to the increased incidence of endocarditis. The valve lesion is commonly asymptomatic and may escape detection into adulthood. The asymptomatic nature of a congenital bicuspid aortic valve means that antibiotic prophylaxis may not have been prescribed for dental or other procedures throughout the patient's life. (*See textbook page* 356.)
7. **A.** The goals of initial therapy are maintenance of blood pressure, improvement of forward flow, and resolution of pulmonary edema. These are accomplished by reducing preload and afterload, improving myocardial contractility, and alleviating the patient's anxiety. Medications that are useful in this context are diuretics, morphine, vasodilators such as sodium nitroprusside, and inotropic agents such as

dobutamine. Definitive therapy requires correction of the cause of the problem with antibiotics or frequently with surgical intervention. (*See textbook pages* 362, 363.)

Chapter 37

1. **False.**   In the prethrombolytic era, life-threatening acute myocardial infarction with mitral regurgitation was estimated to occur in 1% of acute myocardial infarctions. More recently, an analysis at Duke University Medical Center of 1,480 patients undergoing acute cardiac catheterization within 6 hours of myocardial infarction reported a 17.9% incidence of mitral regurgitation with a 3.4% incidence of moderately severe or severe mitral regurgitation. (*See textbook page* 365.)

2. **True.**   The presence of moderately severe or severe mitral regurgitation is associated with a higher mortality rate (24% at 30 days, 42% at 6 months, and 52% at 1 year). When the presence of mitral regurgitation is added to the regression model, it approaches statistical significance as an independent predictor of mortality after acute myocardial infarction. (*See textbook page* 365.)

3. **False.**   The pathophysiologic mechanism of papillary muscle rupture and mitral regurgitation depends on the amount of tissue infarcted. The papillary muscles are supplied by the most distal portions of the coronary arterial tree, and therefore they are vulnerable to transient ischemia and infarction as well as trauma and catastrophic acute coronary artery occlusion. Because its entire blood supply comes from the posterior descending artery, the posteromedial papillary muscle is more vulnerable to ischemia than the anterolateral papillary muscle. In a recent report by Sharma et al. of 50 patients with severe ischemic mitral regurgitation, 14 of 15 patients who needed operations for valve repair or replacement had pathologic documentation of posteromedial papillary muscle dysfunction. (*See textbook pages* 367, 368.)

4. **A.**   The mainstays of medical therapy for mitral regurgitation are vasodilating drugs and an intraaortic balloon pump. Sodium nitroprusside is the therapy of choice for afterload reduction. This agent improves hemodynamic values in acute mitral regurgitation by lowering systemic vascular resistance and impedance to left ventricular ejection with a resultant decrease in left ventricular volume. These agents also decrease the size of the regurgitant mitral valve orifice. In cases of mitral regurgitation, systemic arterial pressures and pulmonary arterial pressures should be continuously monitored with an indwelling arterial catheter and pulmonary arterial catheter. For patients who have low systemic arterial pressures, the judicious use of an inotropic agent such as dopamine or dobutamine can be useful. High-dose dopamine, however, carries the disadvantage of elevating systemic vascular resistance and may therefore increase mitral regurgitation and myocardial ischemia. Patients with low systemic arterial pressures are probably best treated with a combination of vasodilator drugs and intraaortic balloon pump therapy. (*See textbook page* 373.)

Chapter 38

1. **True.**   Syncope can be cardiovascular or noncardiovascular. Cardiovascular syncope accounts for 85% or more of cases of syncope. Cardiovascular syncope may further be divided into neurally mediated and neurally independent mechanisms. (*See textbook pages* 377, 378.)

2. **True.** Syncope due to obstructive disorders of the heart typically occurs during exercise. This is because limited cardiac output is unable to meet the increased oxygen demand and overcome peripheral vasodilatation. Syncope is one of the classic presenting signs of aortic stenosis and usually suggests that valve replacement is needed because of critical reduction in valvular cross-sectional area. (*See textbook page* 378.)

3. **True.** Hypertrophic cardiomyopathy is a particularly important cause of syncope to consider. The physical signs may be subtle, and the disorder frequently involves young patients and athletes. The evaluation of syncope for a young patient is particularly important to consider, because many patients with hypertrophic cardiomyopathy and syncope are at increased risk for sudden death. (*See textbook page* 380.)

4. **B.** Pulmonary hypertension with acute arterial spasm and marked increase in left ventricular preload may lead to recurrent syncope and sudden death. Any form of tachycardia, including sinus tachycardia, can lead to a sudden fall in cardiac output. Pulmonary emboli also can present itself with syncope; however, in animal studies, it was found that more than half of the pulmonary artery vasculature must be occluded to cause hemodynamic compromise. Acute myocardial ischemia also can present with syncope from various mechanisms such as global ischemia, ventricular arrhythmia, conduction system disease, or mechanical complications. (*See textbook page* 380.)

5. **A.** Sick sinus syndrome is characterized by impaired sinoatrial impulse formation or propagation manifesting as sinus pause or sinus arrest resulting in syncope. If this syndrome is accompanied by supraventricular tachyarrhythmia, most commonly atrial fibrillation, the term *bradycardia-tachycardia syndrome* is used. Sinus node dysfunction frequently is unmasked by a relatively low concentration of drugs such as digoxin, β-blockers, and calcium channel blockers. Patients with sick sinus syndrome exhibit enhanced sensitivity to endogenous adenosine. Therefore theophylline, which is an adenosine antagonist, has been tried as therapy. However, almost all patients with syncope caused by sick sinus syndrome need a permanent pacemaker. (*See textbook page* 381.)

Chapter 39

1. **True.** Embolism to the systemic circulation nearly always originates as a thrombus within the left heart. In a large series of 1,575 patients with systemic emboli, it was found that 89% of emboli originated as thrombi within the heart. Other sources include a diseased aorta with or without aneurysm and a paradoxic venous source. (*See textbook pages* 386, 387.)

2. **False.** Systemic embolization may occur with its source in the venous circulation. This is called *paradoxic embolism.* It may occur among patients with an intracardiac defect, such as an atrial or ventricular septal defect, patent ductus arteriosus, or pulmonary arteriovenous fistula. Most cases of paradoxic embolism occur among patients who have a patent foramen ovale. (*See textbook page* 387.)

3. **C.** Valvular heart disease is a common cause of systemic embolization. The three disorders that most frequently cause thrombi in the left heart that may predispose to systemic embolization are atrial fibrillation, coronary artery disease with infarction, and valvular heart disease, including prosthetic heart valves. Of these disorders, atrial fibrillation is most commonly associated with systemic embolism. Among patients with coronary artery disease and valvular heart disease, systemic embolization is most likely associated with atrial fibrillation. (*See textbook page* 387.)

4. **B.**   The principal differential diagnosis of arterial embolism to the lower extremities is arterial thrombosis superimposed on atherosclerotic disease and arterial embolization. Most arterial emboli that enter the circulation, will lodge in the lower extremities. Embolic occlusion of arteries in the lower extremities may lead to irreversible ischemia with tissue necrosis. This tissue necrosis can lead to acidosis, myonecrosis, hypokalemia, and possible renal failure. Embolectomy is performed with local anesthesia and a Fogarty thrombectomy catheter. The high mortality among patients with emboli to the lower extremities who undergo embolectomy has not changed greatly since the introduction of the Fogarty catheter in 1963. Although the mortality is the same, the limb salvage rate with or without embolectomy is clearly related to the severity of ischemia at presentation. Thrombectomy may lead to the systemic release of toxic material from the involved limb on reperfusion if the degree of ischemia is irreversible. (*See textbook page* 391.)

5. **B.**   Embolectomy through the femoral artery approach with a Fogarty technique offers the best option for limb salvage after systemic embolization to the lower extremities. Once the diagnosis of systemic embolism is suspected, therapy with intravenous heparin should be initiated. Patients with systemic embolization are likely to have recurrent embolism. All series show a low recurrence rate among patients who undergo anticoagulation. For most patients, the underlying condition predisposing to systemic embolization is evident at baseline evaluation. Warfarin is used to maintain an international normalized ratio of 2.0 to 3.0. (*See textbook page* 391.)

Chapter 40

1. **False.**   Tachycardia is considered to be supraventricular in origin if the atrium or AV junction participates in the arrhythmia either as the origin of the abnormal impulse or as an essential part of a reentry circuit. (*See textbook pages* 394, 395.)

2. **False.**   Two general mechanisms account for the generation of supraventricular tachyarrhythmias. The first mechanism is abnormal impulse formation, including increased automaticity and triggered activity. Increased automaticity tachyarrhythmia can be generated when an area of myocardium other than the SA node exhibits an enhanced rate of spontaneous depolarization. An example of this is multifocal atrial tachycardia. Triggered activity occurs as a result of a preceding impulse or series of impulses. This is in contrast to automaticity, which occurs spontaneously. The impulse that initiates triggered activity is an afterdepolarization and is classified as early or late. An example of this is digoxin toxicity. The second mechanism of supraventricular tachyarrhythmia is reentry. Reentry tachycardia classically has been described as requiring areas of slow conduction and a unidirectional block. If the relation between these two factors is appropriate, a perpetuating reentry loop is established. An example of this is atrial flutter. (*See textbook page* 395.)

3. **False.**   A direct recording of the arrhythmia is the most important initial information for diagnosis. For a patient in hemodynamically stable condition, a 12-lead ECG is optimal. However, if the arrhythmia is of a transient nature, the patient is in hemodynamically unstable condition, or a 12-lead ECG is not readily available, a telemetry tracing can be used to gather valuable information. The P waves can be identified, and their structure, regularity, rate, and relation to the QRS or ventricular depolarization should be documented. The size of the QRS complex also is suggested at telemetry. (*See textbook pages* 395, 397.)

4. **False.**   Therapy for supraventricular tachycardia is geared toward identifying and managing the underlying cause. In general, the primary management of arrhyth-

mias produced by enhanced automaticity is to remove the stimulus or manage the underlying process. The ectopic automaticity can sometimes be diminished with agents that slow depolarization. Ventricular rate can be controlled with agents to increase the degree of AV block. Arrhythmias with reentry circuits that involve the SA or AV nodes may terminate in response to agents that change the refractoriness or slow conduction in these regions. (*See textbook page* 397.)

5. **D.**   Adenosine is an endogenous nucleoside that causes adenosine receptor stimulation, which results in hyperpolarization of cells. It is administered as therapy for supraventricular tachycardia by means of rapid intravenous bolus. Methylxanthines are competitive inhibitors. Therefore, larger doses may be needed in their presence. The injection often is associated with symptoms of dyspnea and flushing. The symptoms last for 15 to 20 seconds, and the effect of the drug itself lasts only seconds. (*See textbook pages* 397–399.)

6. **A.**   Cardiac glycosides such as digoxin have been used in the management of supraventricular tachycardias for many years. These drugs slow conduction and increase refractoriness of the SA and AV nodes mainly in an indirect manner by means of hypersensitization of the carotid baroreceptors. Digoxin may be given orally or intravenously. Its onset of action after an intravenous dose is 30 minutes to 1 hour. It must be loaded regardless of route of administration. Digoxin is excreted primarily by the kidneys; therefore the maintenance dose must be adjusted for patients with renal failure. (*See textbook page* 399.)

7. **C.**   Digoxin toxicity is not uncommon because the drug has a narrow therapeutic window. Signs of toxicity include fatigue, nausea, visual disturbances, and confusion. Digoxin toxicity also can cause multiple types of arrhythmia. They arise primarily from the increased vagal tone and can lead to sinus bradycardia or AV block. This can lead to increased atrial and ventricular excitability, resulting in premature atrial and ventricular beats, ectopic atrial tachycardia, ventricular tachycardia, or ventricular fibrillation. Therapy of a patient with digoxin toxicity depends on the arrhythmia and the underlying clinical condition. Stopping the digitalis and correcting any underlying hypokalemia often are sufficient treatment. A temporary pacemaker may be needed, and digoxin-specific Fab antibody fragments can be used in life-threatening cases not responsive to conservative measures. (*See textbook page* 399.)

8. **A.**   Atrial fibrillation is a reentry arrhythmia with multiple wavelets of depolarization traveling in a random sequence. This results in disorganized atrial depolarization with ineffective atrial contraction. Electrographically, the atrial depolarizations are irregular at the rate of 400 to 600 beats/min. The ventricular response is irregularly irregular with a variable rate depending on conduction time through the AV node. Among untreated patients this rate usually is 120 to 180 beats/min. The most serious consequence is cerebral embolization, which occurs among patients older than 65 years at a rate of 4.5% per year when anticoagulation is not achieved. (*See textbook page* 402.)

9. **B.**   Atrial flutter is believed to be caused by a reentry mechanism that occurs among patients with underlying structural heart disease in the setting of pulmonary embolism, pericarditis, ethanol abuse, or thyroid toxicosis. It is an unstable rhythm that reverts to sinus rhythm or degenerates into atrial fibrillation. The atrial rate during atrial flutter is 250 to 350 beats/min. Usually a 2:1 block at the AV node level results in a ventricular rate of 150 beats/min. With a 2:1 AV block, it can be difficult to differentiate atrial flutter from other regular narrow QRS complex supraventricular tachycardias. Vagal maneuvers or intravenous adenosine can be used to increase the degree of AV block, thus unmasking the characteristic "sawtooth" flutter waves. They are normally inverted in the inferior leads on an ECG. (*See textbook page* 403.)

III. Coronary Care

41. Acute Heart Failure

Select the best answer

1. Which of the following is not a major classification of the mechanism of heart failure?

   A. Abnormalities of the heart valves, pericardium, endocardium, great vessels, and other structures
   B. Primary myocyte dysfunction
   C. Alterations in organization or signaling of cardioelectric activity
   D. Deranged response to sepsis and infection

2. Regarding computed tomography (CT):

   A. CT is limited by ineffective assessment of myocardial wall thickness.
   B. CT is effective in estimating left ventricular volumes and ejection fraction.
   C. CT is the most effective means of assessing myocardial perfusion.
   D. CT is effective and is more sensitive than other modalities in the assessment of aortic abnormalities, specifically proximal aortic dissection.

3. Regarding magnetic resonance imaging (MRI):

   A. MRI is superior to all other modalities for the diagnosis of myocardial abnormalities in areas of wall thickness, wall motion, regional perfusion, ejection fraction, and proximal coronary anatomy.
   B. The diagnosis of aortic dissection is more sensitive and specific with MRI than with CT scan.
   C. MRI is more sensitive than transthoracic echocardiography for the diagnosis of prosthetic valve insufficiency.
   D. The diagnosis of aortic dissection by MRI requires demonstration of an intraluminal flap and flow equivalence between the true and false lumens.

4. Which of the following describe the hemodynamic effects of dobutamine infusion on acute congestive heart failure?

   A. Increased cardiac output, increased pulmonary capillary wedge pressure, decreased systemic vascular resistance, and increased stroke volume.
   B. Increased cardiac output, increased pulmonary capillary wedge pressure, increased systemic vascular resistance, and increased stroke volume.
   C. Decreased pulmonary capillary wedge pressure, increased cardiac output, decreased systemic vascular resistance, and increased stroke volume.

    D. Increased cardiac output, decreased pulmonary capillary wedge pressure, increased systemic vascular resistance, increased pulmonary vascular resistance.

5. Regarding dysfunction of a prosthetic valve:

    A. In the intensive care unit, the syndrome of thrombosed prosthetic aortic valve with thromboemboli is relatively common.

    B. Patients with dysfunction of a prosthetic mitral valve seek medical attention with chronic heart failure that has been present in a progressive manner over several months.

    C. The diagnosis should be confirmed with arteriography.

    D. When the diagnosis is made, immediate surgical repair is indicated.

42. Clinical Approach to the Diagnosis and Management of Thrombotic Disorders of the Arterial and Venous Circulatory Systems

True or False

1. Distal arterial embolization to the lower extremity is the most common arterial thrombotic event in clinical practice.

2. The term *non-Q-wave myocardial infarction* is reserved for myocardial infarctions that involve small portions of the left ventricle.

3. The presence of hard, collagenous material determines whether an arterial plaque is vulnerable to rupture.

Select the best answer

4. Regarding vascular thromboresistance:

    A. The vascular endothelium is a bilayer of simple squamous cells approximately 0.5 mm thick that are joined by intercellular junctions.

    B. Vascular endothelial cells are polygonal and are elongated in the long axis of the vessel (in the direction of blood flow).

    C. The endothelium has four surfaces—the luminal or nonthrombogenic, subluminal, adhesive, and cohesive.

    D. The luminal surface under normal circumstances is entirely nonthrombogenic because of its abundant electron-dense connective tissue.

5. Regarding heparin:

    A. Physician-guided heparin titration has been proved to achieve therapeutic levels of anticoagulation for most patients.

    B. Intravenous nitroglycerin given in high doses increases the anticoagulant activity of heparin.

    C. The anticoagulant effect of heparin may be modified by circulating plasma proteins.

    D. Other adverse effects associated with heparin use include thrombocytosis.

6. Regarding the complication of hemorrhage in the setting of anticoagulation:

    A. For patients receiving warfarin, the international normalized ratio (INR) should be monitored, whereas patients receiving heparin should have the activated partial thromboplastin time checked.

    B. The platelet count should be checked at least once a week for patients receiving intravenous heparin.

C. For hemorrhage in the setting of oral anticoagulation with warfarin, administration of 1 mg vitamin K intravenously or 10 mg vitamin K subcutaneously can reduce the INR within 4 hours.

D. Larger doses of 10 mg intravenous vitamin K do not reduce the time to reversal of the INR.

7. Which of the following is included among the interventions recommended for unstable angina and non-ST-segment elevation myocardial infarction?

   A. Thrombolytic therapy with tissue plasminogen activator
   B. Oral warfarin sodium titrated to an INR of 2.0 to 3.0
   C. Non-enteric-coated aspirin, 160 to 325 mg by mouth
   D. Heparin, 5000 units administered subcutaneously twice a day)

43. Unstable Angina

True or False

1. Unstable angina is caused by thrombus formation on a complicated atherosclerotic plaque.
2. Unstable angina is classified as new onset or crescendo angina when chest pain occurs at rest or at a progressively lower threshold of exercise or when prolonged chest pain is poorly relieved with nitroglycerin.

Select the best answer

3. Regarding the differential diagnosis of chest pain:

   A. Chest pain of cardiac origin should be considered after all other possible sources of pain have been considered and ruled out.
   B. Chest pain from different causes may coexist in the same patient.
   C. Noncardiac pain is most often pulmonary in origin.
   D. The differential diagnosis for esophageal spasm is straightforward.

4. Regarding the laboratory diagnosis of unstable angina:

   A. An electrocardiogram (ECG) obtained during an episode of chest pain is less informative than an ECG obtained at rest.
   B. Deep T-wave inversions occurring during an episode of angina involving the anterior and lateral leads are characteristic of substantial narrowing in the proximal right coronary artery.
   C. Myocardial scintigraphy obtained during an episode of chest pain can help detect transient myocardial ischemia.
   D. Echocardiographic imaging should not be used during an episode of myocardial ischemia.

5. Regarding therapy for unstable angina and non-ST-segment elevation myocardial infarction:

   A. The clinical benefits of thrombolytic therapy have been well documented in the three largest trials completed to date.
   B. Enoxaparin has been shown to reduce acute ischemic events in comparison with unfractionated heparin.
   C. The goal of treatment in Q-wave myocardial infarction is to open the artery in question.
   D. In unstable angina and non-ST-segment myocardial infarction, the goal of therapy is to stent the occluded artery open to improve blood flow.

44. Complicated Myocardial Infarction

True or False

1. After acute myocardial infarction, a leading cause of morbidity and mortality is recurrent ischemia and recurrent ischemic events.
2. Effective prevention of recurrent ischemic events has been shown to consist of three components—antiplatelet therapy, antithrombotic therapy, and β-blockade.
3. Patients who have Q waves on an electrocardiogram (ECG) have been found to have peak enzyme levels and ejection fractions similar to those of patients who do not have Q waves on an ECG after myocardial infarction.

Select the best answer

4. Regarding right ventricular infarctions:

   A. The management of right ventricular myocardial infarction is the same as the management for left ventricular myocardial infarction.
   B. The coincidence of right ventricular infarction with inferior wall myocardial infarction is low.
   C. The simplest test to determine the presence of right ventricular infarction is echocardiography.
   D. The differential diagnosis of right ventricular infarction includes hypotension due to left ventricular infarction, pericardial tamponade, constrictive pericarditis, and pulmonary embolism.

5. Regarding clinical manifestations and complications of right ventricular infarction:

   A. Systemic hypotension is a frequent complication of right ventricular infarction.
   B. The incidence of atrioventricular (AV) or sinoatrial nodal block is less than that of left ventricular infarction.
   C. The incidence of cardiogenic shock is considerably less than that of left ventricular infarction.
   D. The prognosis of right ventricular infarction is considerably better than that of isolated left ventricular infarction.

6. Regarding diastolic dysfunction:

   A. Clinically significant diastolic dysfunction occurs almost uniformly among patients with acute myocardial infarction.
   B. Diastolic dysfunction is a common cause of late congestive heart failure in the setting of myocardial infarction.
   C. The pathophysiologic mechanism of diastolic dysfunction begins with decreased myocardial wall compliance from ischemia and infarction.
   D. The heart sound associated with diastolic dysfunction usually is S_3.

7. Regarding the management of diastolic dysfunction:

   A. The use of diuretics is contraindicated.
   B. Intravenous nitroglycerin and nitroprusside are contraindicated.
   C. Administration of a β-blocker is contraindicated.
   D. The prognosis is good compared with that among patients with systolic dysfunction.

8. Regarding myocardial infarction:

   A. Rupture of the papillary muscles occurs among 6% to 8% of patients after acute myocardial infarction.

B. Ventricular septal rupture occurring in the setting of new inferior myocardial infarction is associated with a mortality of approximately 20%.

C. The development of thromboembolism can occur among 5% to 10% of patients after acute myocardial infarction.

D. Pericardial irritation occurs among approximately 40% of patients with acute myocardial infarction.

9. Regarding cardiogenic shock:

A. Congestive heart failure from systolic dysfunction is the most serious complication after acute myocardial infarction.

B. Cardiogenic shock is related to diastolic dysfunction.

C. Afterload reduction is contraindicated in systolic dysfunction and cardiogenic shock.

D. Cyclic adenosine monophosphate agents are contraindicated in the management of cardiogenic shock.

10. Regarding intraventricular conduction blocks:

A. The blood supply to the distal conducting system makes conduction disturbances an infrequent complication of anterior wall myocardial infarction.

B. Intraventricular conduction disturbances carry a low in-hospital mortality if recognized early.

C. β-Blockade should be administered to high-risk patients with intraventricular conduction block pending placement of a temporary pacemaker.

D. Patients with a permanent bundle branch block and transient Mobitz II second-degree AV block may benefit from permanent pacemaker implantation.

45. Reperfusion Therapy for Acute Myocardial Infarction

True or False

1. Thrombolytic therapy in the management of acute myocardial infarction has been shown to reduce mortality.

2. Thrombolytic therapy in the setting of acute myocardial infarction is associated with improved left ventricular function.

3. Patients brought to medical attention within the first 12 hours of symptom onset should be treated with thrombolytic therapy.

4. The GUSTO trial established that routine late percutaneous transluminal coronary angioplasty is indicated as a mechanical method to achieve coronary reperfusion.

Select the best answer

5. Regarding contraindications to thrombolytic therapy:

A. Hypertension is not a contraindication to thrombolytic therapy.

B. Pregnancy is a contraindication to thrombolytic therapy.

C. Recent surgical intervention or trauma is not a contraindication to thrombolytic therapy.

D. Reports indicate no increased rate of intracranial bleeding among patients with a history of hypertension or poorly controlled blood pressure when given thrombolytic therapy.

6. Regarding time intervals for reperfusion therapy:

    A. After administration of the drug, the difference in time to therapeutic action between various thrombolytic medications is clinically insignificant.
    B. The window for administration of thrombolytic agents is the first 6 hours after onset of chest pain.
    C. The National Heart Attack Alert Program has set a goal of administering thrombolytic agents within 30 minutes after arrival at a hospital.
    D. To reduce the delay in arrival at a medical facility, patients at high risk should be advised to use the first available transportation once symptoms of coronary ischemia are detected.

46. Secondary Prevention After Acute Myocardial Infarction: A Coronary Care Unit Perspective

True or False

1. Admission to a coronary care unit offers a unique opportunity to assist patients with smoking cessation; these patients achieve higher success rates than do outpatients.
2. Magnesium and calcium have a synergistic effect at the cellular level and cause both systemic and coronary vasodilatation.
3. One of the most powerful predictors of death after myocardial infarction is the extent of left ventricular systolic dysfunction.
4. Angiotensin-converting enzyme (ACE) inhibitors are a preferred agent for preventing long-term mortality among most patients with acute myocardial infarction.
5. Nitrates have favorable hemodynamic effects and a small but statistically significant favorable effect on mortality.

Select the best answer

6. Regarding calcium channel blockers:

    A. Nifedipine and the dihydropyridines have been shown to have consistent benefit in acute or threatened myocardial infarction.
    B. Verapamil and diltiazem are considered to have adverse effects because of their potent peripheral vasodilatory properties.
    C. Verapamil and diltiazem have a more profound negative inotropic effect than do dihydropyridines.
    D. The benefit of administration of calcium channel blockers after myocardial infarction is best seen among patients with atrioventricular block.

47. Diagnostic Testing in the Coronary Care Unit

True or False

1. Electrocardiogram (ECG) changes of 1 mm or greater ST-segment elevation in a single lead establish the diagnosis of acute myocardial infarction.
2. The normal pericardium is evident on plain chest radiographs.
3. Thallium stress test imaging is useful for diagnosis but is of no utility in predicting morbidity in a preoperative setting.

Select the best answer

4. Regarding cardiac performance:

    A. Left ventricular ejection fraction is the only measurement that can be obtained with radionuclide techniques.
    B. First-pass radionuclide studies are used to measure the initial transit of radio-tracer through the heart.
    C. Equilibrium studies such as radionuclide ventriculography or radionuclide angiography rely on counts of tracer present within the ventricles during multiple cardiac cycles.
    D. Right ventricular function is the most important noninvasive predictor of rein-farction and sudden death after myocardial infarction.
    E. Ejection fraction is determined by means of dividing the difference in count rates at end systole and end diastole by the count rate at end systole.

5. Which of the following is the correct formula for calculation of corrected QT interval (QTc)?

    A. QTc = QT/RR interval
    B. QTc = QT/(square root of RR interval)
    C. QTc = QT/(RR interval)^2
    D. QTc = QT/0.41

48. Clinical Management of Cardiac Arrhythmias in the Coronary Care Unit

True or False

1. In the first 48 hours after myocardial infarction, the incidence of ventricular arrhythmias ranges from 10% to 12%.
2. Enhanced automaticity can lead to tachyarrhythmia after myocardial infarction.

Select the best answer

3. Regarding ventricular tachycardia:

    A. Ventricular tachycardia is defined as six or more consecutive ventricular depolarizations at a rate of more than 100 beats/min.
    B. Sustained ventricular tachycardia lasts for more than 10 seconds.
    C. Unsustained ventricular tachycardia lasts from three beats to less than 30 seconds and terminates with treatment.
    D. Ventricular tachycardia can be described as uniform or polymorphic.

4. Regarding supraventricular tachycardia:

    A. The presence of atrial fibrillation after myocardial infarction is an indicator of worse prognosis.
    B. β-Blockade should be undertaken for all patients who have an episode of supraventricular tachycardia.
    C. The supraventricular tachycardia most frequently associated with unstable coronary syndromes is sinus tachycardia.
    D. Atrial fibrillation and atrial flutter are infrequent among patients treated in a critical care unit.

5. Regarding the management of tachyarrhythmias:

   A. Supraventricular and ventricular tachyarrhythmias show the same basic physiologic mechanism and therefore have a common treatment pattern.
   B. Supraventricular tachycardias usually are associated with hemodynamic compromise.
   C. Ventricular tachyarrhythmias may be associated with hemodynamic compromise.
   D. The diagnosis of supraventricular tachycardia usually shows a QRS complex distinct from the sinus rhythm.

6. Initial therapy for wide complex tachycardia that does not cause hemodynamic compromise and cannot be specifically diagnosed with a 12-lead electrocardiogram involves:

   A. Cardioversion at 200 J
   B. Lidocaine 1.5 mg/kg intravenous bolus followed by an intravenous drip
   C. Adenosine 6.0 mg intravenously
   D. Verapamil 5.0 mg intravenously

49. Mechanisms of Acute Myocardial Ischemia and Infarction

True or False

1. With increasing myocardial oxygen demands, oxygen extraction and coronary blood flow can increase three-to fourfold.
2. Coronary arterial blood flow is determined by the pressure gradient between the aorta in diastole and the coronary sinus.
3. There is no known interaction between coronary artery thrombosis and coronary artery spasm.
4. Penetrating and blunt trauma each can cause myocardial infarction.

50. Nonischemic Chest Pain

True or False

1. In studies of acute myocardial infarction, the electrocardiogram (ECG) usually shows ST-segment and Q-wave changes.

Select the best answer

2. From the following, select potential noncardiac causes of chest pain:

   A. Pulmonary hypertension
   B. Pneumonia
   C. Pneumothorax
   D. Herpes zoster
   E. All of the above

51. Evaluation and Management of Hypertension in the Intensive Care Unit

True or False

1. The management of hypertension in the intensive care unit (ICU) usually involves one of four situations—hypertensive emergencies, chronic hypertension, new onset of hypertension, and hypertension unique to the perioperative setting.
2. The differentiation between hypertensive emergencies and urgencies is made on the basis of mean arterial pressure.
3. The management of malignant hypertension or emergency hypertension in the ICU should involve initiation of treatment before diagnosis of the underlying cause.

Select the best answer

4. Regarding the management of hypertensive crisis:

   A. The goal of initial therapy is to return blood pressure to normal levels.
   B. The lower limit of cerebral autoregulation determines the initial target of therapies.
   C. A reasonable target for blood pressure reduction is to decrease systolic blood pressure 50%, taking into consideration the patient's medical history.
   D. For most patients with hypertensive emergencies, the pathophysiologic condition is a decrease in systemic vascular resistance.

5. Regarding perioperative hypertension:

   A. In the setting of perioperative care, blood pressure greater than 160/100 mm Hg for a previously normotensive patient or an increase of more than 30 mm Hg over preoperative levels necessitates treatment.
   B. In the period from 36 to 72 hours after a major surgical procedure, volume expansion due to mobilization of fluids may cause hypertension.
   C. Routine blood pressure therapy should be discontinued on the morning of an operation.
   D. Oral therapy is indicated for control of perioperative hypertension.

6. Regarding labetalol:

   A. Labetalol is a racemic mixture of a selective β-blocker and a selective α_1-antagonist.
   B. Labetalol produces prompt reduction in peripheral vascular resistance and blood pressure.
   C. Myocardial oxygen consumption is increased and coronary hemodynamics are improved among patients with coronary disease.
   D. The side effects of labetalol administration are related to β-blockade effects and are manifested by orthostatic hypotension.

Answers

Chapter 41

1. **D.** Heart failure can be acute or chronic failure. Acute heart failure is dramatic decompensation, whereas chronic congestive heart failure is a gradual process that allows for adaptation. There are three mechanisms by which the heart may

fail: (a) abnormalities of the heart valves, pericardium, endocardium, great vessels, and other structures that impair cardiac filling and emptying (e.g., aortic stenosis, pulmonary embolism, extreme hypertension); (b) pathologic situations of primary myocyte dysfunction (e.g., myocarditis, ischemic disease, cardiomyopathy); (c) alterations in the organization or signaling of cardiac contraction (e.g., tachy- or bradydysrhythmias). Sepsis causes circulatory failure that affects many parts of the circulatory system, including myocardial abnormalities that usually would be included in category (b). (*See textbook page* 413.)

2. **D.**   Computed tomography, including ultrafast CT and gated CT, has been studied to determine its usefulness in cardiac diagnostics. Although CT is effective in assessment of wall thickness, myocardial mass, left ventricular volumes, and ejection fraction, other tests are superior in these areas of diagnostics. In the setting of acute heart failure, the only valid indication for CT is assessment of acute aortic abnormalities, most specifically proximal aortic dissection. (*See textbook pages* 415, 416.)

3. **B.**   Magnetic resonance imaging is rapidly evolving as an important tool for the diagnosis of cardiac disease. Although wall thickness, wall motion, regional perfusion, ejection fraction, and proximal coronary anatomy can be assessed with MRI, other modalities are superior. Currently, the main indications for MRI are the diagnosis of pericardial disease and effusion, cardiac masses, and aortic abnormalities. In a clinical situation of acute heart failure, MRI is considered superior to CT for the diagnosis of aortic dissection and for demonstration of an intraluminal aortic flap. A flow differential, not equivalent flow, is expected between the true and false lumens. The limitation of MRI as a diagnostic modality is related to the contraindication to use in the presence of magnetic objects. Any patient with a metal prosthesis or embedded metallic foreign body, including some cardiac valves and pacemakers and intravenous infusion pumps cannot undergo MRI. (*See textbook page* 416.)

4. **C.**   Dobutamine improves myocardial contractility and causes vasodilation. This leads to improvement in forward flow. Therefore decreased pulmonary capillary wedge pressure, increased cardiac output, decreased systemic vascular resistance, and increased stroke volume are seen. (*See textbook page* 418.)

5. **D.**   The syndrome of a thrombosed prosthetic aortic valve is extremely rare, whereas thrombosis of the mitral valve is more common. The incidence of thrombosed mitral valve is related to the model of valve, the Bjork-Shiley valve having a considerably higher incidence than other models. Patients with mitral valve failure come to medical attention with acute heart failure, syncope, altered prosthetic heart sounds. The diagnosis should be immediately suspected and confirmed with echocardiography. Cardiac catheterization usually is not necessary. Immediate surgical therapy is indicated. (*See textbook page* 422.)

Chapter 42

1. **False.**   Myocardial infarction occurs among more than 1 million persons per year in the United States. It is the arterial thrombotic event most commonly seen in clinical practice. (*See textbook page* 431.)

2. **False.**   Non-Q-wave myocardial infarction (also called unstable angina with non-ST-segment elevation myocardial infarction) is the term used to describe myocardial infarction that presents no Q waves on an electrocardiogram. Mounting evidence suggests that chronic recurrent plaque rupture of mild to moderate severity may be responsible. Over time this leads to plaque growth and ultimate obstruction of the arterial lumen. Some patients may have clinical features rem-

iniscent of acute Q wave myocardial infarction. These patients frequently have multivessel coronary disease. (*See textbook page* 432.)

3. **False.** Although dense collagenous sclerosis contributes the most voluminous amount to coronary arterial plaque, the soft, lipid-rich component or atheromatous portion determines the vulnerability of a plaque to rupture. (*See textbook page* 432.)

4. **B.** The vascular endothelium is essential for normal vessel responsiveness and thromboresistance. In most vertebrates, vascular endothelial cells form a single layer, with the cells 0.1 to 0.5 μm in thickness. The cells are polygonal and are elongated in the long axis of the vessel in the direction of blood flow. The endothelial layer has three surfaces: nonthrombogenic (luminal), adhesive (subluminal), and cohesive (abluminal). The luminal surface is nonthrombogenic because it is devoid of electron-dense connective tissue. (*See textbook page* 431.)

5. **C.** Histidine-rich glycoprotein, platelet factor 4, and vitronectin, also called "acute phase proteins," may alter the anticoagulant effect of heparin. This explains the state of relative heparin resistance that occurs among some patients with acute thrombotic conditions. Physician-guided heparin titration has been shown to achieve subtherapeutic levels of anticoagulation for many patients. Nitroglycerin given intravenously in high doses decreases the anticoagulant activity of heparin. Heparin also may cause thrombocytopenia. (*See textbook page* 434.)

6. **A.** For patients receiving heparin, activated partial thromboplastin time should be monitored. INR should be monitored for patients receiving warfarin. Platelet count should be assessed daily for patients receiving heparin. When a patient receiving heparin has bleeding, the site of bleeding must be identified and appropriate measures taken. This may include simple observation while antithrombotic therapy is continued, or it may involve stopping the heparin infusion or neutralizing residual heparin with protamine sulfate. The anticoagulation effect of warfarin can be reversed by means of replacing coagulation factors that depend on vitamin K. Administration of 0.5 to 1 mg intravenous vitamin K or 10 mg subcutaneous vitamin K can reduce the INR within 12 to 24 hours. A larger dose of 10 mg intravenous vitamin K can reduce the INR within 6 hours. Caution is recommended with high doses of intravenous vitamin K. More rapid reversal can be achieved with administration of fresh frozen plasma. (*See textbook pages* 441, 442.)

7. **C.** It is strongly recommended that all patients with myocardial infarction receive 160 to 325 mg non-enteric-coated aspirin to chew and swallow as soon as the clinical impression of myocardial infarction is being formed. This dose should be repeated daily and indefinitely. Thrombolytic therapy is not recommended for unstable angina with non-ST-segment elevation myocardial infarction. The minimum dose of heparin to be administered is 7,500 units twice a day although more heparin often is used. Long-term maintenance oral anticoagulation is not recommended unless a patient is at high risk for the development of mural thrombosis. (*See textbook pages* 438, 439, 443.)

Chapter 43

1. **True.** Unstable angina is a well-defined clinical entity with specific causes, pathophysiologic mechanisms, symptoms, laboratory findings, and treatment. In the mid-1980s, thrombus formation on a complicated atherosclerotic plaque was recognized as the cause of unstable angina. (*See textbook page* 449.)

2. **True.** The essential diagnostic feature of unstable angina is recognition that the symptoms are becoming more severe and departing from the usual pattern of

angina for a given patient. Unstable angina is routinely classified as (a) new-onset or crescendo angina with chest pain occurring at rest or at a progressively lower threshold of exercise or (b) prolonged chest pain poorly relieved with nitroglycerin, or (c) recurrence of anginal pain after myocardial infarction. (*See textbook pages* 450, 451.)

3. B. Pain of cardiac origin must first be suspected and differentiated from noncardiac pain. Noncardiac pain may be of various causes, and these different causes may coexist in the same patient. Most often noncardiac pain is of musculoskeletal, pulmonary, or gastrointestinal origin. The differential diagnosis of esophageal pain is difficult, as is the differentiation between symptoms of gastroesophageal reflux and cardiac pain. (*See textbook page* 451.)

4. C. Myocardial scintigraphy performed during an episode of chest pain can be used to detect transient myocardial ischemia with high sensitivity. Technetium Tc 99m sestamibi is the most valuable agent in these situations because it can be injected during an ischemic episode and the images read several hours later. However, an ECG remains the most useful tool for documentation of myocardial ischemia because it is available in all medical centers and it is relatively sensitive. The presence of ST-T wave changes on an admission ECG aids in the diagnosis of unstable angina. However, an ECG obtained during an episode of chest pain is far more informative. The ST-T changes can be used to evaluate the location and severity of the ischemic process. Deep T-wave inversions involving the anterior and lateral leads are characteristic of marked narrowing in the proximal left anterior descending coronary artery. Echocardiography can be useful in documenting the presence of transient wall motion abnormalities during an episode of myocardial ischemia and suggest the areas at risk for infarction. (*See textbook pages* 451, 452.)

5. C. The goal of management of Q-wave myocardial infarction is to open the artery in question. The goal of therapy for unstable angina and non-ST-segment elevation myocardial infarction is to prevent progression of blood clots and thrombotic occlusion. Aspirin and heparin are useful in this regard. Clinical benefits have been inconsistently seen with thrombolytic therapy. The three largest trials showed a trend toward increased risk for ischemic events with thrombolysis and suggested use of this modality could be harmful. These studies tested recombinant tissue plasminogen activator, anisoylated plasminogen streptokinase activator complex, and urokinase. Subset analysis of patients with non-ST-segment elevation myocardial infarction in the TIMI-3B, GISSI-1, and ISIS-2 trials has not documented a benefit. Low-molecular-weight heparins have not demonstrated superiority in ability to reduce rates of myocardial infarction, ischemic events, or mortality. However, they seem to be equivalent to unfractionated heparin in their effect on these outcomes. Low-molecular-weight heparins offer the advantages of being (a) easier to administer, (b) less likely to be associated with thrombocytopenia, and (c) more predictable in anticoagulant effect. The use of these agents is likely to increase in the near future. (*See textbook pages* 453, 454.)

Chapter 44

1. True. Recurrent ischemic events after acute myocardial infarction are a leading cause of mortality and morbidity. Recurrent ischemia may be caused by an unstable coronary plaque or thrombus that reoccludes the artery or by a stable, persistently stenotic lesion in the same artery or a in different coronary artery that may cause further ischemia with stress or increased oxygen demand by the myocardium. (*See textbook page* 460.)

2. False. The management of recurrent ischemic events falls into two categories—prevention and management of the acute event. Antithrombotic therapy and β-blockade are essential pharmacologic components of prevention. The first component of antithrombotic therapy is aspirin. Aspirin is administered to all patients with acute myocardial infarction unless there is a specific absolute contraindication to use of this medication. When thrombolysis with tissue plasminogen activator is used, heparin is a necessary adjunct. Heparin appears to be optional after thrombolysis with other approved agents. Warfarin has been used after the acute phase. However, at present warfarin alone or warfarin in combination with aspirin has not been shown to reduce reinfarction rate or mortality beyond those with aspirin alone. Regarding β-blockade in the setting of a myocardial infarction, studies have shown that early intravenous β-Blockade followed by oral β-blockade has the potential to reduce reinfarction rate, infarct size, and rate of recurrent ischemia. β-Blockade should be used in the care of all patients without contraindications such as bradycardia, AV block, hypotension, pulmonary edema, or history of bronchospasm. (*See textbook page* 461.)

3. False. The ECG is the most widely used tool in the evaluation of patients with acute myocardial infarction, and the presence or absence of Q waves provides valuable information regarding the extent of the infarction and an indication of prognosis. Patients with Q-wave infarction have been found to have higher peak creatine kinase levels and lower ejection fractions than those without Q waves. At autopsy, patients with Q-wave infarction have been found to have larger infarctions. Patients with Q-wave infarction have an in-hospital mortality twice that of patients with non-Q-wave infarction. On the other hand, after hospital discharge the mortality is greater among patients who did not have Q waves. (*See textbook page* 463.)

4. D. Although much attention is paid to the left ventricle during acute myocardial infarction, consideration of right ventricular infarction is critical. The incidence of right ventricular infarction is quite high. Between 35% and 50% of patients with inferior myocardial infarction have associated right ventricular infarction. The treatment of right ventricular infarction is different from the treatment of left ventricular infarction. Whereas early reperfusion is important regardless of which ventricle is affected, correction of hypotension due to right ventricular infarct depends mostly on achieving an adequate filling pressure of the right ventricle. Therefore a large amount of fluid may be necessary to fill the right ventricle. The simplest test to investigate the presence of right ventricular infarction involves use of the right precordial ECG leads. Other modalities include thallium or sestamibi perfusion scanning, coronary arteriography, echocardiography, or hemodynamic measurement with a pulmonary arterial catheter. The presence of an elevated right atrial pressure equal or nearly equal to pulmonary capillary wedge pressure indicates the presence of right ventricular dysfunction. Thus the differential diagnosis of right ventricular infarction includes hypotension due to left ventricular infarction, pericardial tamponade, constrictive pericarditis, and pulmonary embolism. (*See textbook pages* 464, 465.)

5. A. Right ventricular infarction carries a high morbidity and mortality when associated with left ventricular infarction. Systemic hypotension is a serious complication of right ventricular infarction. Poor right ventricular output leads to decreased filling of the left ventricle. The overloaded right ventricle also may encroach on the left ventricle, further decreasing cardiac output. The second important complication is AV or sinoatrial nodal block. Nodal dysfunction occurs among 10% to 15% of patients with inferior wall myocardial infarction but occurs among nearly 25% of patients with right ventricular infarction. The need for temporary pacing parallels the incidence of complete AV block, as does the occurrence of ventricular fibrillation, ventricular tachycardia, and cardiogenic shock.

Coexisting right ventricular infarction increases the mortality of inferior wall myocardial infarction from 5% to 31%. (*See textbook pages 464, 465.*)

6. **C.** Diastolic dysfunction occurs almost uniformly among patients with acute myocardial infarction but becomes clinically significant for one fourth to one third of patients. It is the most common cause of early congestive heart failure. The pathophysiologic process of diastolic dysfunction begins with increased wall stiffness from ischemia and infarction. This decreased left ventricular compliance causes clinical signs of elevated pulmonary venous congestion such as shortness of breath, dyspnea, orthopnea, rales at physical examination, or pulmonary vascular redistribution on a chest radiograph. The heart sound associated with diastolic dysfunction usually is S_4, which indicates decreased compliance of the left ventricle. Systolic function may be entirely normal among these patients. (*See textbook page 465.*)

7. **D.** The management of diastolic dysfunction includes diuresis and therapy for ischemia. Furosemide is commonly used as a diuretic, although it is important to guard against overdiuresis. Intravenous nitroglycerin and nitroprusside are widely used. Nitroglycerin is the vasodilator most active in producing venous dilation, whereas nitroprusside is a balanced vasodilator. Administration of a β-blocker may be invaluable in the care of patients whose pulmonary congestion is caused by isolated diastolic dysfunction, because these agents reduce ischemia and improve left ventricular compliance. Left ventricular systolic function often is preserved among patients with isolated diastolic dysfunction, rendering a prognosis that is relatively good compared with that among patients with systolic dysfunction. However, patients with systolic or diastolic dysfunction have a worse long-term outcome than those without either of those manifestations. (*See textbook pages 465, 466.*)

8. **C.** The development of thromboembolism is a recognized complication of acute myocardial infarction that occurs among 5% to 10% of patients. Both arterial and venous emboli can occur with left ventricular mural thrombi. Ventricular septal rupture occurs among 2% to 4% of patients with acute myocardial infarction but is associated with a mortality of 75%, whereas infarction and rupture of the papillary muscles occurs in 1% of cases. Pericardial irritation occurs among approximately one fourth of patients with acute myocardial infarction, and it usually begins 2 to 4 days after myocardial infarction. There are three types of presentation—asymptomatic pericardial effusion, early symptomatic pericarditis with or without effusion, and late pericarditis. (*See textbook pages 470–472.*)

9. **A.** Congestive heart failure from systolic dysfunction is the most serious complication after acute myocardial infarction. The most malignant end of the spectrum of congestive heart failure after acute myocardial infarction is cardiogenic shock. The hemodynamic characteristics of cardiogenic shock include an elevated pulmonary capillary wedge pressure and reduced cardiac index. The initial treatment goals are to ensure adequate oxygenation and to maintain systolic blood pressure. Preload and afterload reduction and inotropic support may be necessary for patients with marked systolic dysfunction and cardiogenic shock. Dopamine and dobutamine often are used as agents in this setting. In addition to these agents, phosphodiesterase inhibitors such as milrinone and amrinone can be used to increase intracellular cyclic adenosine monophosphate by reducing its metabolism. This improves contractility and causes vasodilation. Because the β-agonists and phosphodiesterase inhibitors act through different pathways, their beneficial effects in this setting are additive when proper attention is paid to volume status. (*See textbook pages 466–468.*)

10. **D.** Patients with complete heart block as a result of acute myocardial infarction should receive a permanent pacemaker before discharge. Because of the blood supply to the distal conducting system, intraventricular conduction disturbances frequently accompany anterior wall myocardial infarction. This usually reflects

a large infarct and carries a high in-hospital mortality. β-Blockers should be avoided in high-risk patients with complete heart block unless placement of a temporary pacemaker is undertaken. (*See textbook pages* 466, 467.)

Chapter 45

1. **True.** When administered to select patients with acute myocardial infarction, thrombolytic therapy reduces infarct mortality. This has been demonstrated with several different thrombolytic regimens. However, comparative trials of tissue plasminogen activator (tPA) and streptokinase indicate a statistically significant difference in mortality in favor of tPA. Mortality reduction occurs only among patients who exhibit restoration of normal antegrade blood flow in the infarction-related artery. (*See textbook pages* 484, 485.)

2. **True.** In addition to its positive influence on mortality, thrombolytic therapy limits infarct size and is associated with improved left ventricular function. This occurs both globally and regionally at the infarct zone. Improved left ventricular function has been demonstrated to occur after treatment with streptokinase and tPA, although tPA-treated patients seem to demonstrate a larger benefit. (*See textbook pages* 483–485.)

3. **True.** Survival after myocardial infarction can be improved by means of reperfusion therapy through both myocardial salvage and prevention of infarct expansion and ventricular remodeling. The time available for myocardial salvage varies depending on the type of arterial occlusion and the availability of collateral circulation to the infarcted area. However, the benefits associated with prevention of infarct expansion extend to at least 12 hours among most patients and longer among patients with persistent chest pain and electrocardiographic ST-segment elevation. (*See textbook pages* 487, 488.)

4. **False.** Several studies have demonstrated that there is no improvement in mortality or nonfatal reinfarction rate when routine cardiac catheterization and subsequent percutaneous transluminal coronary angioplasty are performed on patients treated with thrombolytic therapy who do not have recurrent symptoms of angina or ischemia during exercise stress testing. (*See textbook pages* 499, 500.)

5. **B.** The absolute contraindications to thrombolytic therapy include instances in which active bleeding or potential hemorrhage exists. Patients with aortic dissection, ongoing internal bleeding, recent intracranial operation, intracranial neoplasm, head trauma, or history of hemorrhagic stroke should not be treated with thrombolytic therapy. Sustained uncontrolled hypertension also is an absolute contraindication to thrombolytic therapy. Blood pressure greater than 200/120 mm Hg is an absolute contraindication. Other contraindications include pregnancy, recent operation, or trauma. Previous allergic reaction to streptokinase or APSAC suggests a contraindication to use of those agents. However, patients who have a reaction to recent treatment with APSAC or streptokinase can be treated with tPA or urokinase. (*See textbook page* 491.)

6. **C.** The National Heart Attack Alert Program has set a goal of administering thrombolytic agents within 30 minutes after arrival at a hospital. Differences to action of the medications can cause substantial additional delay before reperfusion, and this should be taken into account in selecting agents for thrombolysis. Thrombolytic therapy may be administered for 12 hours after the onset of symptoms. Patients should be encouraged to use emergency medical systems when available for transport in all medical emergencies, including acute myocardial infarction. This reduces transport time and may accelerate the delivery of care on arrival. (*See textbook pages* 486, 487.)

Chapter 46

1. **True.** There is evidence that an organized approach to assist those who wish to stop smoking after admission to the coronary care unit offers a unique opportunity for success. The cessation rate is 40% to 70%. Many patients cite the advice of their physicians as the most important factor in the decision to stop smoking. (*See textbook page* 506.)

2. **False.** Magnesium has several effects on the myocardium that may be protective after myocardial infarction. Magnesium antagonizes the effect of calcium at the cellular level and causes both systemic and coronary vasodilation. Platelet aggregation and adhesion may be reduced. Magnesium also suppresses some types of ventricular arrhythmias and may limit ischemic injury to the myocardium after reperfusion. (*See textbook page* 506.)

3. **True.** One of the most powerful predictors of death after myocardial infarction is the extent of left ventricular systolic dysfunction. Ejection fraction is commonly used to measure left ventricular performance. The 1-year mortality rises precipitously as left ventricular ejection fraction falls below 40%. A more powerful predictor of death is the extent of left ventricular dilatation at echocardiography or cardiac catheterization. (*See textbook page* 507.)

4. **False.** Trials suggest that ACE inhibitors are a safe but only modestly effective intervention among unselected populations of patients with myocardial infarction. ACE inhibitors are preferred in the care of patients with extensive myocardial infarction, heart failure, or left ventricular dysfunction and are most effective when continued long term. (*See textbook pages* 507, 508.)

5. **False.** Nitrates have been used for more than a century in the management of angina. Hemodynamic benefits include a reduction in preload and ventricular filling pressure and coronary vasodilation. However, two large studies failed to demonstrate any effect on mortality after acute myocardial infarction. (*See textbook pages* 508, 509.)

6. **C.** Cellular calcium overload has been identified as a final common pathway of cellular injury in myocardial infarction. This observation led to the widespread administration of calcium channel blockers to reduce infarct size, decrease mortality, and reduce reinfarction rate. The available agents are grouped according to chemical structure. Verapamil and diltiazem tend to depress atrioventricular nodal conduction and sinus node activity to a greater degree and are considered rate slowing. Most investigators have found that at recommended doses verapamil and diltiazem have a more potent negative inotropic effect. Nifedipine and dihydropyridines have been found to have an overall lack of benefit, and in some instances, there has been evidence of harm after acute myocardial infarction. The leading hypothesis to explain the adverse effects of dihydropyridines is that their potent peripheral vasodilatory action reduces coronary perfusion pressure and triggers reflex catecholamine release. (*See textbook page* 509 and 510.)

Chapter 47

1. **False.** The ECG is critical for early confirmation of acute myocardial infarction. When a patient comes to medical attention because of typical chest pain and characteristic ECG changes of 1 mm or greater ST segment elevation in two or more contiguous leads, the diagnosis of acute myocardial infarction is established. (*See textbook page* 518.)

2. **False.** Normal pericardium is seldom evident on plain chest radiographs. A pericardial stripe greater than 2 mm along the inferior heart border seen on the lateral projection suggests pericardial effusion. (*See textbook page* 520.)

3. **False.** In addition to its diagnostic utility, thallium stress test imaging is helpful in determining the prognosis for coronary artery disease among unselected patients, patients with recent myocardial infarction, or patients undergoing pre-operative evaluation for vascular operations. Thallium is a cationic potassium analogue, the myocardial uptake of which depends on cell membrane integrity and is proportional to blood flow. Thallium scintigraphy after infusion of dipyridamole has been shown to have independent and significant prognostic utility among unselected patients referred for diagnostic evaluation. (*See textbook page 524.*)

4. **B.** Right and left ventricular ejection fractions and regional wall motion may be safely and reproducibly determined with noninvasive radionuclide techniques. First-pass radionuclide studies measure the initial transit of radiotracer through the heart. Equilibrium studies such as gated blood pool scanning (MUGA), radionuclide ventriculography, and radionuclide angiography rely on counts of tracer within the intravascular space, not only the heart, during multiple cardiac cycles. Left ventricular function is the most important noninvasive predictor of reinfarction and sudden death after myocardial infarction. Ejection fraction is determined by means of dividing the difference in count rates at end diastole and end systole by the count rate at end diastole [EF = (ED − ES)/ED]. (*See textbook page 524.*)

5. **B.** QTc = QT/(square root of RR interval) (*See textbook page 516.*)

Chapter 48

1. **False.** In the first 48 hours after myocardial infarction, the incidence of ventricular arrhythmia ranges from 34% to 100%. (*See textbook page 531.*)

2. **True.** Mechanisms of generation of tachyarrhythmia include disorders of impulse propagation, such as reentry, and disorders of impulse generation, such as enhanced automaticity and triggered activity. The most common result of enhanced automaticity is sinus tachycardia. (*See textbook page 530.*)

3. **D.** Ventricular tachycardia is defined as three or more consecutive ventricular depolarizations at a rate greater than 100 beats/min. Sustained ventricular tachycardia lasts for more than 30 seconds. Unsustained ventricular tachycardia lasts from 3 beats to less than 30 seconds and terminates spontaneously. Ventricular tachycardia also can be differentiated as uniform or of constant morphologic features or as polymorphic. (*See textbook page 532.*)

4. **C.** The most frequent tachycardia associated with unstable coronary syndromes is sinus tachycardia. This usually is an appropriate physiologic response related to pain, anxiety, the presence of metabolites of tissue injury, and use of medications. Management of the primary disorder is recommended as is management of the sinus tachycardia with β-blocking agents to decrease myocardial oxygen consumption. β-Blockade should only be undertaken for patients without signs of congestive heart failure or bronchospasm. Although the presence of atrial fibrillation may make the management of acute myocardial infarction more difficult, it does not appear to affect prognosis. (*See textbook page 530.*)

5. **C.** Although supraventricular and ventricular tachyarrhythmias derive from the same physiologic mechanism, management of these tachyarrhythmias may vary considerably. Supraventricular arrhythmias usually are not associated with hemodynamic compromise and rarely necessitate emergency intervention. Ventricular arrhythmias may lead to hemodynamic compromise and death and may necessitate emergency intervention. Appropriate treatment of a patient with tachyarrhythmia involves accurate identification of the arrhythmia and its underlying mechanism. The diagnosis of supraventricular tachycardia is almost always cer-

tain when the QRS complex of the tachycardia is identical to that of the sinus rhythm. Proper identification of the mechanism underlying wide QRS tachycardia may be very difficult. (*See textbook pages* 529, 532, 533, 535.)

6. **C.**   Intravenous administration of 6.0 mg adenosine may be useful in differentiating supraventricular from ventricular tachycardia. Synchronized cardioversion is appropriate in the care of a patient in unstable condition but not necessary initially in the situation described. Lidocaine is the treatment of choice when tachycardia is known to be ventricular in origin. Verapamil may be harmful if a bypass tract cannot be excluded as it may cause a paradoxic tachycardic effect. (*See textbook page* 537.)

Chapter 49

1. **False.**   With increasing myocardial oxygen demands, oxygen consumption may increase three- to fourfold. Myocardial oxygen extraction cannot increase substantially. Therefore coronary blood flow must increase to meet the demands placed on the heart. (*See textbook pages* 542, 543.)

2. **True.**   The pressure gradient between the aorta in diastole and the coronary sinus is referred to as the *perfusion pressure.* This relation is influenced by atherosclerotic narrowings and elevations in left ventricular and diastolic pressure and right atrial pressure. Coronary blood flow is maintained when mean arterial pressure exceeds 65 mm Hg. (*See textbook page* 543.)

3. **False.**   An interaction between coronary thrombosis and coronary spasm is possible whereby spasm may induce stasis and lead to enhanced thrombin activity and fibrin production. Diseased coronary artery endothelium also may exhibit impaired production of endogenous plasminogen activators such as tPA. The combination of the thrombogenic potential of diseased endothelium with coronary stasis can produce a vicious circle that includes ischemia or frank myocardial necrosis. (*See textbook page* 545.)

4. **True.**   Both penetrating and blunt trauma can cause myocardial infarction. Penetrating trauma such as stab or gunshot wounds can cause coronary laceration or pericardial tamponade. Blunt trauma can cause myocardial infarction even in the absence of preexisting atherosclerotic disease. This infarction is possibly related to intimal coronary tear, coronary artery rupture, myocardial contusion, or a combination of those factors. (*See textbook pages* 545, 546.)

Chapter 50

1. **False.**   Only 13% of patients with acute myocardial infarction have ST-segment elevation and Q waves on their initial ECG. In one study of acute myocardial infarction, 62% of patients discharged from the emergency ward had a normal ECG on careful review. Serial ECGs, however, are abnormal in 80% to 90% of cases of acute myocardial infarction. (*See textbook page* 552.)

2. **E.**   A more complete listing of the differential diagnosis of chest pain is found in the full text in Table 50-1. Some pulmonary causes of chest pain are pulmonary hypertension, pleuritic chest pain from pleural effusion, pneumonia, pneumothorax, and pulmonary embolism. Vascular causes of chest pain include aortic dissection and aortic aneurysm. Herpes zoster (shingles) can affect the anterior chest and mimic angina pectoris. However, the pain is dermatomal and does not cross the midline. Pleurodynia is associated with coxsackievirus B infection and

causes pleuritic chest pain. Usually there is a viral prodrome. The discomfort experienced by patients with pulmonary hypertension may be identical to that described for typical angina. The pain may be caused by underlying right ventricular ischemia or dilatation of the pulmonary arteries. (*See textbook page* 551.)

Chapter 51

1. **False.** In the intensive care unit, evaluation and treatment of patients with elevated blood pressure involve two general scenarios. Patients may have a hypertensive crisis that necessitates urgent or emergency therapy, or may have a transient, more benign elevation in blood pressure that is of a less critical nature. (*See textbook page* 559.)

2. **False.** Differentiation between a hypertensive urgency and an emergency is based on the presence of target-organ damage. According to this definition, *hypertensive emergency* refers to blood pressure elevation associated with ongoing target-organ damage. *Hypertensive urgency* means that the potential for target-organ damage is great and damage is likely to occur if blood pressure is not controlled soon. (*See textbook page* 560.)

3. **False.** A brief history and physical examination should be initiated to assess the degree of target-organ damage and rule out secondary causes of hypertension. Important historical data include symptoms attributable to changes in target-organ perfusion and function. The history should include inquiries about prior hypertension, other diseases, neurologic symptoms, cardiac symptoms, or urinary symptoms. This history may be obtained from the patient but also should be obtained from family members and the medical record. The evaluation should involve intraarterial monitoring if necessary. Ophthalmologic examination should follow, with examination for hemorrhage, exudates, and papilledema. Auscultation of the lungs and heart includes determination of the presence of rales and S_3 gallop. (*See textbook pages* 560, 561.)

4. **B.** The goal of initial therapy is to terminate ongoing target-organ damage not to return blood pressure to normal levels. The lower limit of cerebral autoregulation determines targets for initial therapy. Among hypertensive and normotensive patients, this target is approximately 25% below the initial mean arterial pressure or a diastolic pressure between 100 and 110 mm Hg. A reasonable target for blood pressure reduction is to decrease mean arterial pressure by 20% to 25%. For most patients with hypertensive emergencies, the pathophysiologic mechanism is an increase in systemic vascular resistance, not a change in cardiac output. It is the increase in systemic vascular resistance that overrides autoregulation within the end organs and leads to ischemia and organ damage. (*See textbook page* 561.)

5. **B.** In the ICU, concern exists when blood pressure is higher than 160/100 mm Hg for a previously normotensive patient or increases more than 30 mm Hg above preoperative levels for a patient known to have hypertension. Any routine blood pressure therapy should be continued up to the morning of the operation as regularly scheduled. Induction of anesthesia represents a challenge to circulatory stability. Pain, hypothermia with shivering, hypoxia, or reflex excitement after anesthesia can lead to changes in blood pressure that necessitate subtle minute-to-minute adjustment. Because hypertension in this setting is neither severe nor long lasting, small doses of intravenous antihypertensive medications are indicated. Sodium nitroprusside is effective in most situations. For a patient with fixed coronary lesions, nitroglycerin can be used to improve poststenotic collateral flow. Labetalol as minibolus or infusion therapy can provide longer duration of action. In the first 36 to 72 hours after a surgical procedure, many patients

experience intravascular volume expansion because of extravascular fluid mobilization and intraoperative fluid administration. An increase in blood pressure in this period may respond well to intravenous loop diuretics, such as furosemide, and to fluid restriction. (*See textbook page 564.*)

6. B.   Labetalol is a racemic mixture of a nonselective β-blocker and a selective α_1-antagonist. It produces prompt reduction in peripheral vascular resistance and blood pressure. The β-blockade component prevents reflex tachycardia or changes in cardiac output. Myocardial oxygen consumption is reduced, and coronary hemodynamics are improved among patients with coronary artery disease. The disadvantages relate to several factors; usually the α-blocking effects are cited. The α-blocking effects can cause orthostatic hypotension. Other side effects are nausea, vomiting, flushing, and tingling. The ratio of β-blocking effects to α-blocking effects is approximately 7 : 1. For this reason, any contraindication to use of β-blockade also applies to the use of labetalol. (*See textbook page 565.*)

IV. Pulmonary Problems in the Intensive Care Unit

52. A Physiologic Approach to Managing Respiratory Failure

Select the best answer

1. An 80-year-old woman needs medical care because of respiratory distress and stupor. She is found to have the following arterial blood gas values at sea level on a true source of FIO_2 1.0: pH 7.24, $PaCO_2$ 60 mm Hg, PaO_2 550 mm Hg, SaO_2 100%, HCO_3^- 26 mmol/L. The most likely physiologic mechanism to explain her hypoxemia is:

   A. Pure hypoventilation
   B. Diffusion impairment
   C. Severe ventilation-perfusion mismatch
   D. Right to left shunt
   E. Low-inspired oxygen tension

53. Pulmonary Edema Etiology and Pathogenesis

Select the best answer

1. Development of noncardiogenic edema is characterized by:

   A. Increases in interstitial oncotic pressure compared with changes that occur with hydrostatic edema.
   B. An increased reflection coefficient for protein in the Starling equation.
   C. Changes in pulmonary venous pressure that do not affect extravascular lung water.
   D. Low protein content of alveolar fluid compared with findings during hydrostatic edema.

54. Acute Respiratory Distress Syndrome

Select the best answer

1. Improved survival in acute respiratory distress syndrome (ARDS) has been proved with which of the following interventions?

    A. Early (days 1 through 7) intravenous corticosteroids
    B. Nebulized artificial surfactant
    C. Inhaled nitric oxide
    D. Intravenous *N*-acetylcysteine
    E. None of the above

2. The alveolar capillary injury in ARDS:

    A. Always begins on the capillary side
    B. Results in a heterogeneous distribution of pulmonary edema
    C. Is dependent on normal neutrophil numbers or function
    D. Does not disturb surfactant levels or function
    E. None of the above

3. The typical hemodynamic pattern among patients with ARDS includes:

    A. Normal pulmonary capillary wedge pressure, increased cardiac output, reduced systemic vascular resistance
    B. Elevated pulmonary capillary wedge pressure, increased cardiac output, reduced systemic vascular resistance
    C. Reduced central venous pressure, reduced pulmonary capillary wedge pressure, reduced cardiac output, elevated systemic vascular resistance
    D. Elevated oxygen delivery, elevated oxygen consumption, increased extraction ratio
    E. None of the above

4. The condition associated with the highest percentage of cases of ARDS is:

    A. Sepsis syndrome–systemic inflammatory response syndrome
    B. Aspiration of gastric contents
    C. Viral pneumonia
    D. Toxic gas inhalation
    E. Illicit drug administration

55. *Status Asthmaticus*

Select the best answer

1. Administration of theophylline during an acute asthma exacerbation:

    A. Improves outcome during the emergency department management of asthma
    B. Is more effective than treatment with β-adrenergic agonists
    C. Is associated with more side effects than treatment with β-adrenergic agonists
    D. Should aim for a serum concentration of 20 to 30 μg/mL
    E. None of the above

2. A 38-year-old woman with severe asthma is admitted to the intensive care unit after emergency department management of asthma with β-adrenergic agonists and 125 mg intravenous methylprednisolone. Despite frequent albuterol nebulization, bronchospasm continues. Respiratory acidosis develops and necessitates endobronchial intubation and mechanical ventilation. On settings of an FiO_2 of 0.4, volume assist-control rate of 16 L/min, tidal volume of 750 mL, and applied positive end-expiratory pressure (PEEP) of 0, peak airway pressure is 62 cm H_2O, and an intrinsic PEEP of 14 cm H_2O is present. Arterial blood gas

values are pH 7.30, Po_2 72 mm Hg, and a Pco_2 of 52 mm Hg. The most appropriate management is:

   A. To decrease the tidal volume to 600 mL per breath
   B. To increase the mandatory rate to 20 breaths/min
   C. To paralyze the patient with pancuronium
   D. To add 10 cm applied PEEP to facilitate weaning

3. The following should *not* be administered in the management of status asthmaticus for a pregnant woman at 16 weeks' gestation.

   A. Methylprednisolone at doses greater than 120 mg per day
   B. Intravenous magnesium sulfate
   C. Inhaled albuterol
   D. Mechanical ventilation with controlled hypercapnia
   E. None of the above

56. *Chronic Obstructive Pulmonary Disease*

Select the best answer

1. A 68-year-old man with advanced chronic obstructive pulmonary disease (COPD; FEV_1 0.75 L) is admitted with a 3-day history of fever, cough with purulent sputum, and worsening dyspnea. A chest radiograph reveals hyperinflation. The respiratory rate is 25 breaths/min. Arterial blood gas analysis with administration of 4 L of oxygen through a nasal cannula shows a Po_2 of 52 mm Hg, a Pco_2 of 55 mm Hg, and a pH of 7.35. Sputum Gram stain reveals many neutrophils and predominant small gram-negative diplococci. Pending cultures, the most appropriate antibiotic choice is:

   A. Erythromycin
   B. Cefuroxime
   C. Penicillin G
   D. Ampicillin

2. Which of the following has not been shown to be a result of the use of supplemental oxygen in acute exacerbations of COPD?

   A. Decrease in the formation of pulmonary edema
   B. Improved survival
   C. Improvement in right-sided heart function
   D. Reduced hospital length of stay
   E. Decreased cardiac arrhythmias and ischemia

57. *Extrapulmonary Causes of Respiratory Failure*

Select the best answer

1. Factors associated with prolonged neuromuscular blockade or weakness after use of pancuronium to facilitate mechanical ventilation include all the following except

A. Concomitant renal failure
B. Corticosteroid use
C. Pseudocholinesterase deficiency
D. Prolonged administration

2. A 22-year-old woman is transferred to the intensive care unit because of worsening shortness of breath and a vital capacity of 700 mL determined at the bedside. She had been admitted to the neurology service 48 hours earlier with a 3-day history of distal lower extremity hypesthesia followed by progressive ascending muscle paralysis. Electromyography confirms the presence of demyelinating polyradiculopathy, and a diagnosis of Guillain-Barré syndrome is made. In the intensive care unit, respiratory rate increases to 40 breaths/min, and arterial blood gas analysis shows hypoventilation with respiratory acidosis. An endotracheal tube is inserted and mechanical ventilation is begun. The most appropriate next treatment is:

A. Plasmapheresis
B. Corticosteroids
C. Azathioprine
D. Pyridostigmine

58. Acute Respiratory Failure in Pregnancy

Select the best answer

1. A 36-year-old multiparous patient undergoes cesarean section at 35 weeks' gestation because of fetal distress. During delivery of the infant, the anesthesiologist finds that blood pressure is dropping, hypoxemia has developed, and blood is oozing from an upper extremity site of an insertion of an intravenous line. The obstetrician comments on increased bleeding in the operative field. Arterial blood gas values during administration of 100% oxygen show pH 7.27, P_{CO_2} 32 mm Hg, and P_{O_2} 63 mm Hg. Hemoglobin level is 10.2 g/dL. Prothrombin time is 16.2 seconds, and partial thromboplastin time is 82 seconds. The platelet count is 42,000/μL. Which of the following statements is true?

A. She probably has a venous thromboembolism.
B. She probably has noncardiogenic pulmonary edema.
C. She probably has aspirated gastric contents.
D. She probably has an air embolism.

2. A 32-year-old woman begins bed rest during her seventh month of pregnancy. Three weeks later, she awakens with shortness of breath and left-sided pleuritic chest pain. Evaluation in the emergency department shows normal blood pressure, although tachypnea and tachycardia are present. Fetal heart tones also are present. The patient's lower extremities exhibit mild bilateral pretibial edema. A chest radiograph shows minimal atelectasis at the left base. Arterial blood gas analysis with room air shows P_{O_2} 68 mm Hg, P_{CO_2} 28 mm Hg, and pH 7.50. Results at duplex ultrasonography suggest a nonocclusive clot in the right common femoral vein. A ventilation-perfusion ($\dot{V}/\dot{Q}$) lung scan shows two segmental mismatched defects in the left lung. Which of the following statements is true?

A. She should be treated with intravenous heparin, and warfarin can be started on day 2.
B. She should be considered for inferior vena caval filter placement.

C. Thrombolytic therapy is indicated because of proximal deep venous thrombosis.

D. She should be treated with intravenous heparin followed by subcutaneous heparin.

59. *Pulmonary Embolism and Deep Venous Thrombosis*

True or False

1. For patients with respiratory failure receiving mechanical ventilation, the appropriate first step in the diagnostic evaluation for pulmonary embolism is duplex ultrasonography of the legs.

Regarding patients with acute pulmonary embolism:
2. The chest radiograph is usually normal.
3. The alveolar-arterial oxygen tension gradient ($PaO_2 - PaO_2$) may be normal.
4. Most have high-probability lung scans.
5. Warfarin therapy should be titrated to an international normalized ratio (INR) of 2 to 3.
6. Thrombolytic therapy is indicated if the PO_2 is 50 mm Hg or less.

60. *Managing Hemoptysis*

Select the best answer

1. A 26-year-old man with advanced cystic fibrosis is hospitalized for worsening cough, fever, and sputum production. A chest radiograph shows bilateral, severe, upper lobe predominant bronchiectatic changes. The patient is treated with intravenous antipseudomonal antibiotics. On the second hospital day, he expectorates 500 mL of bright red blood and has increased shortness of breath. A chest radiograph demonstrates increased opacification in both upper lobes. The patient is taken to the intensive care unit, and an endotracheal tube is inserted because of continued large-volume hemoptysis. Follow-up bronchoscopy shows diffuse bilateral blood staining of all major bronchi. A definite bleeding source cannot be found, but blood clots are present in the right upper lobe orifice. The next procedure should be:

    A. Intubation of the left main stem bronchus
    B. Exploratory thoracotomy and probably right upper lobectomy
    C. Bronchial arteriography
    D. Pulmonary angiography
    E. Computed tomography of the chest

61. *Aspiration*

Select the best answer

1. Which of the following statements is true?

    A. *Streptococcus pneumoniae* infection is a common cause of aspiration pneumonia.

B. Aspiration of gastric material with a pH greater than 4.0 is unlikely to cause acute respiratory distress syndrome.

C. Cough is the primary defense mechanism against aspiration pneumonia.

D. The rate of aspiration among patients receiving nutrition through nasoenteric tubes can be reduced by 50% if the tip of the tube is placed in a postpyloric location.

E. All of the above.

62. Near-Drowning

Select the best answer

1. Which of the following is the most common risk factor for immersion accidents?

   A. Therapeutic and illegal drugs that act on the central nervous system
   B. Child abuse
   C. Inadequate adult supervision
   D. Aquatic sports
   E. Ethanol use

2. Which of the following statements about near-drowning is true?

   A. Freshwater near-drowning with aspiration inactivates surfactant.
   B. Freshwater near-drowning with aspiration stimulates type II pneumocyte function.
   C. Seawater near-drowning with aspiration inactivates surfactant.
   D. Seawater near-drowning with aspiration often results in severe hemoconcentration.

63. Pulmonary Hypertension

Select the best answer

1. Pulmonary arterial occlusion pressure is likely to be significantly less than pulmonary arterial diastolic pressure in all the following clinical conditions except:

   A. Left heart failure
   B. Primary pulmonary hypertension
   C. Pulmonary venoocclusive disease
   D. Severe chronic obstructive lung disease

64. Pleural Disease in the Critically Ill Patient

Select the best answer

1. A 19-year-old woman with type I diabetes mellitus, anorexia nervosa, and bulimia is admitted because of diabetic ketoacidosis. She had been vomiting repeatedly for 24 hours before admission. A chest radiograph at admission shows a hyperlucent stripe along the left mediastinal border. Physical examination does not

reveal chest wall crepitation. Computed tomography of the chest demonstrates pneumomediastinum. Barium swallow examination documents a distal esophageal rupture with extravasation of contrast medium into the left pleural space and mediastinum. The most appropriate management is:

A. Tube thoracostomy and parenteral antibiotics
B. Thoracotomy, drainage, and esophageal repair
C. Thoracentesis, no oral intake, and parenteral antibiotics
D. Immediate upper gastrointestinal endoscopy for confirmation of the diagnosis

2. A 42-year-old man is hospitalized because of severe pancreatitis. Over the first 48 hours of hospitalization, he has worsening dyspnea and hypoxemia with diffuse bilateral pulmonary infiltrates. Findings after pulmonary arterial catheterization confirm normal left ventricular filling pressures. The diagnosis is acute respiratory distress syndrome. With FIO_2 0.50, positive end-expiratory pressure (PEEP) 10 cm H_2O, pressure-controlled ventilation with peak inspiratory pressure of 40 cm H_2O, respiratory rate of 18 breaths/min, and inspiratory-expiratory (I:E) ratio of 1:1, arterial blood gas analysis shows PO_2 68 mm Hg, PCO_2 38 mm Hg, and pH 7.44. On morning rounds, examination reveals bilateral neck and anterior chest wall crepitations. There is no evidence of air trapping on pressure and flow graphics. A chest radiograph shows pneumomediastinum but no pneumothorax. Appropriate ventilator adjustments are:

A. Decrease PEEP, increase I:E ratio
B. Decrease pressure relief, decrease PEEP
C. Increase rate, decrease PEEP
D. Decrease rate, increase I:E ratio

3. Despite making the appropriate adjustments for the patient in question 2 and decreasing peak and mean airway pressures, he experienced sudden distress and hypotension, and a right tension pneumothorax was diagnosed. Emergency chest tube insertion was performed and set to 20 cm H_2O water suction. A large continuous air leak occurred and persisted without improvement for 5 days. Oxygenation did not change, and the acid-base balance remained stable. Despite the continued air leak, chest radiographs showed good lung reexpansion. The most appropriate management of the bronchopleural fistula would be:

A. Thoracotomy with oversewing of the pleural defect
B. Bleomycin pleurodesis
C. To increase chest tube suction to 40 cm H_2O
D. To continue current management
E. Bronchoscopy-directed occlusion of the offending bronchus

65. Mechanical Ventilation: Initiation

Select the best answer

1. In pressure-support mode of mechanical ventilation, the dependent variables include all the following except:

A. Pressure
B. Flow
C. Volume
D. Rate

2. Positive end-expiratory pressure (PEEP) for patients with noncardiogenic edema:

    A. Decreases intrapulmonary shunt
    B. Decreases extravascular lung water
    C. Decreases peak airway pressure
    D. Decreases mean airway pressure

3. The application of extrinsic PEEP to a ventilator-dependent patient with chronic obstructive pulmonary disease with evidence of substantial intrinsic PEEP or "auto PEEP":

    A. Decreases alveolar overdistention
    B. Improves lung compliance
    C. Decreases peak airway pressure
    D. Facilitates inspiratory triggering

66. Mechanical Ventilation: Weaning

Select the best answer

1. The most common reason for failure to wean patients after prolonged (>7 days) mechanical ventilation is:

    A. Inadequate respiratory drive
    B. Psychologic difficulties
    C. Respiratory muscle fatigue
    D. Persistent lung or cardiovascular disease

2. A 72-year-old man undergoes intubation and mechanical ventilation because of hypercapnic respiratory failure after exacerbation of bronchitis. After 4 days of mechanical ventilation, he is awake, alert, and afebrile. Ventilation is in pressure support mode with 18 cm H_2O inspiratory pressure. The patient is breathing 18 times per minute with an average tidal volume of 450 mL. With 35% oxygen, arterial blood gas analysis shows pH 7.42, P_{CO_2} 58 mm Hg, and P_{O_2} 69 mm Hg. Morning bedside mechanical evaluation with a hand-held spirometer reveals negative inspiratory force 26 cm H_2O, respiratory rate 26 breaths/min, and tidal volume 350 mL. Testing of vital capacity is attempted, but patient effort and cooperation are questionable. Which of the following statements is true?

    A. This patient can probably be weaned and extubated.
    B. This patient probably cannot be weaned and extubated at this time.
    C. There is insufficient information to decide about weaning and extubation.

67. Air Embolism and Decompression Sickness

Select the best answer

1. A 22-year-old amateur diver surfaces from a scuba dive to 40 feet (12 m). He immediately reports chest pain and shortness of breath. True statements concerning this diver include all the following except:

   A. Immediate recompression is needed.
   B. He should hold his breath while ascending.
   C. Air embolism is possible.
   D. Pneumothorax may occur.

68. Respiratory Adjunct Therapy

Select the best answer

1. Which of the following is the most appropriate initial pharmacologic therapy for a patient arriving in an emergency department with acute asthma?

   A. Ipratropium bromide aerosol 4 to 6 puffs (18 μg/puff) through a metered dose inhaler (MDI)
   B. Albuterol solution 2.5 mg (0.5 mL) in 2.5 mL saline solution through a jet nebulizer
   C. Albuterol aerosol 4 puffs (90 μg/puff) through an MDI with spacer
   D. Albuterol aerosol 2 puffs (90 μg/puff) through an MDI with spacer

2. A patient with difficult-to-control asthma comes to medical attention with acute dyspnea and inspiratory wheeze localized to the upper airway. At bronchoscopy, this patient is found to have paradoxic vocal cord movement during inspiration. Which of the following is likely to be the most effective treatment in the acute setting?

   A. 80% Helium, 20% oxygen
   B. Racemic epinephrine
   C. Speech therapy
   D. Albuterol solution through a jet nebulizer

69. The Chest Radiographic Examination

Select the best answer

1. How far can the tip of an orally placed endotracheal tube move when the position of the neck is moved from flexion to extension?

   A. 2 cm
   B. 4 cm
   C. 6 cm
   D. 8 cm

2. The syndrome of fat embolism is most often associated with which of the following chest radiographic findings?

   A. Diffuse alveolar filling pattern
   B. Patchy areas of airspace consolidation
   C. Normal chest radiograph
   D. Areas of oligemia
   E. Bilateral pleural effusion

---

70. Acute Inhalation Injury

Select the best answer

1. Carbon monoxide exposure and the formation of carboxyhemoglobin result in which of the following?

   A. Shift of the oxyhemoglobin dissociation curve to the left
   B. Increased total oxygen-carrying capacity in the blood
   C. Decreased affinity of hemoglobin for oxygen
   D. Increased oxidative metabolism at the cellular level

2. Silo-filler's disease is caused by extensive exposure to nitrogen dioxide (NO_2) and is characterized by:

   A. Nasal and oral mucous membrane edema
   B. Pulmonary edema
   C. Eosinophilia
   D. Laryngeal edema

3. Deaths of smoke inhalation are most often caused by:

   A. Pulmonary edema
   B. Heat injury to the lower airway
   C. Upper airway edema and obstruction
   D. Carbon monoxide poisoning

---

71. Disorders of Temperature Control: Hypothermia

True or False

Regarding the shivering phase of hypothermia:
1. Oxygen consumption rises two to five times.
2. Cardiac output increases dramatically.
3. Severe lactic acidosis may develop.
4. Mixed venous oxygen saturation decreases.

Characteristic changes in pulmonary mechanics and gas exchange during hypothermia include the following:

5. Increased minute ventilation during shivering
6. Widened alveolar-arterial oxygen tension gradient ($Pao_2 - Pao_2$)
7. Poor thoracic compliance
8. Increased airway resistance

Select the best answer

9. Hypothermic effects on organ system function can be characterized as follows:

   A. Glomerular filtration rate decreases, urine becomes concentrated, and oliguria occurs.
   B. A type of leukocytosis develops that is common in severe hypothermia and not necessarily associated with infection.

C. Hypoglycemia is a common finding because of the associated liver dysfunction and exaggerated insulin action at the tissue level.

D. Pancreatitis is common.

72. Disorders of Temperature Control: Hyperthermia

Matching

1. Excessive thermogenesis due to muscle contraction
2. Autosomal dominant pattern of inheritance
3. Allergic reaction
4. Rhabdomyolysis
5. Dantrolene is effective
6. Pancuronium is effective
7. Bromocriptine is effective
8. Extrapyramidal signs are common

A. Malignant hyperthermia
B. Neuroleptic malignant syndrome
C. Both
D. Neither

73. Severe Upper Airway Infections

Select the best answer

1. The most common cause of acute supraglottitis among adults is infection with

A. *Moraxella catarrhalis*
B. *Streptococcus pneumoniae*
C. *Staphylococcus aureus*
D. *Haemophilus influenzae*

2. A 42-year-old man with advanced dental caries arrives in the emergency department with a several-day history of fever, chills, mouth and neck pain, and dysphagia. Physical examination reveals swelling and tenderness over the lower right gingiva, with advanced caries and pyorrhea. There is diffuse submandibular swelling, erythema, and tenderness. The most appropriate empiric antibiotic regimen is:

A. Penicillin and metronidazole
B. Clindamycin and ceftazidime
C. Nafcillin and gentamicin
D. Vancomycin and sulfamethoxazole

74. Acute Infectious Pneumonia

Select the best answer

1. Risk factors for nosocomial pneumonia include all the following except:

A. Endotracheal intubation

  B. Sucralfate use
  C. Nasogastric tubes
  D. Altered consciousness

2. Bronchoalveolar lavage and protected-specimen brush specimens obtained bronchoscopically for a patient with suspected nosocomial pneumonia:

  A. Are less useful when antibiotics are already being given
  B. Are not useful in the diagnosis of a nonbacterial cause of infection
  C. Are consistent in differentiation between infection and colonization
  D. Decrease mortality

3. Enteral feeding through a nasogastric tube:

  A. Improves the outcome of nosocomial pneumonia by minimizing the effect of malnutrition on immune function
  B. Results in improved feeding efficiency compared with small-intestinal feeding
  C. Should be done only when the patient is supine
  D. May predispose to nosocomial pneumonia

4. Studies on selective decontamination of the digestive tract among critically ill patients have shown:

  A. Decreased rates of lower respiratory tract infection among treated patients
  B. Lower in-hospital mortality rates among treated patients
  C. No evidence of emergence of resistant bacteria
  D. Decreased length of stay in the intensive care unit (ICU) among treated patients

5. A 54-year-old male cigarette smoker arrives in the emergency department with a low-grade fever that has lasted 72 hours, fatigue, dyspnea, cough, and minimal yellow sputum production. He has a history of intermittent bouts of bronchitis in the winter months but no history of pneumonia. The physical examination findings are pertinent for tachypnea (32 breaths/min), fever of 38.4°C, and regular tachycardia at 120 beats/min. Chest examination reveals bibasilar crackles, left greater than right, and scattered expiratory wheezes. Pulse oximetry with room air is 84%. The white blood cell count is 12,400/mm^3 with 80% neutrophils and 10% band forms. A chest radiograph shows bilateral, lower lobe, patchy infiltrates compatible with pneumonia. Sputum Gram stain shows few neutrophils and no predominant organism. The most appropriate initial antibiotic regimen is:

  A. Ampicillin-sulbactam
  B. Cefuroxime-erythromycin
  C. Ceftazidime-tobramycin
  D. Clindamycin-ceftazidime

75. *Lung Biopsy*

Select the best answer

1. Which of the following is not an absolute contraindication to transbronchial lung biopsy?

  A. Suspected ecchinococcal lung disease
  B. Positive pressure ventilation
  C. Pulmonary hypertension
  D. Uncontrollable cough

Answers

Chapter 52

1. **C.**   The key is to calculate and understand the importance of the alveolar-arterial oxygen tension gradient ($PaO_2 - PaO_2$). To do this one must know the alveolar air equation:

PaO_2 = [(Barometric pressure − water vapor pressure) × FIO_2] − [PaO_2 ÷ respiratory quotient]

With FIO_2 1.0 at sea level this simplifies to

$[(760 - 47) \times 1.0] - PaCO_2 \div 0.8$

or

$713 \times PaCO_2 \div 0.8$

If $PaCO_2 = 60$, then

$(713 - 60) \div 0.8 = 638$

If the alveolar to arterial oxygen tension gradient is $PaO_2 - PaO_2$, then $638 - 550 = 88$ is the gradient. We know that $PAO_2 - PaO_2$ varies with age, and a normal $PaO_2 - PaO_2$ is calculated as follows:

$PaO_2 - PaO_2 = 2.5 + (0.21 \times$ age in years)

The maximum acceptable $PaO_2 - PaO_2$ for an 80-year-old person is 19.3 mm Hg. Therefore $PaO_2 - PaO_2$ is increased.

In response to the question, by finding an abnormal $PaO_2 - PaO_2$ we can exclude pure hypoventilation, which is characterized by a normal gradient. Diffusion impairment by itself is not considered to be a cause of hypoxemia in clinical situations. Right to left shunt almost never causes elevation of $PaCO_2$ and would not be expected to show such an elevation of PaO_2 in response to supplemental oxygen. We know that low-inspired oxygen tension is incorrect because the FIO_2 is given to us. In addition, low-inspired oxygen tension is a clinical problem only at high altitude. Severe ventilation-perfusion mismatching can cause hypoxemia, elevated $PaO_2 - PaO_2$, improvement with supplemental oxygen, and carbon dioxide retention. (*See textbook pages* 571–573.)

Chapter 53

1. **A.**   Noncardiogenic edema is also called *increased permeability pulmonary edema* and is caused by increased pulmonary vascular permeability. Fluid that accumulates in the interstitial compartment has a higher protein concentration than hydrostatic edema in which the endothelial surface is intact. Increased protein concentration raises oncotic pressure. A decrease in the reflection coefficient for protein in the Starling equation signifies increased pulmonary vascular permeability. Changes in pulmonary venous pressure in the setting of increased pulmonary capillary permeability can cause dramatic shifts in extravascular lung water. Protein concentration in alveolar fluid reflects the fluid in the interstitium, which has a

higher protein concentration in noncardiogenic edema than does hydrostatic edema. (*See textbook pages* 578, 579.)

Chapter 54

1. **E.**   In randomized, placebo-controlled trials, none of these agents demonstrated efficacy in reducing the mortality of ARDS. With the exception of nitric oxide, the interventions mentioned have all been tried in randomized, controlled trials and have been shown not to improve survival. To date, only early fluid restriction accompanied by diuresis and late administration of corticosteroids have shown statistically significant improvement in mortality when evaluated in a randomized, controlled manner. (*See* page 588 and Meduri GU, Headley S, Golden E, et al. Effect of prolonged methylprednisolone therapy in unresolving acute respiratory distress syndrome. *JAMA* 1998;280:159–165.)

2. **B.**   Although a chest radiograph characteristically shows diffuse abnormalities, computed tomographic scans of the chests of patients with ARDS show more heterogeneous distribution of pulmonary edema to dependent lung zones, possibly because of the effect of hydrostatic forces. Injury to the alveolar–capillary surface interface may begin on the vascular side (e.g., endotoxinemia) or the airway side (e.g., gastric acid aspiration). Although neutrophils are important in some animal models of ARDS, normal neutrophil number and function are not a prerequisite for ARDS among humans, presumably because of the presence of other tissue and circulating inflammatory and phagocytic cells and cytokines. The edema, inflammation, and hemorrhage in ARDS decrease and denature surfactant, resulting in worse alveolar collapse and shunt. (*See textbook pages* 582, 586, 589.)

3. **E.**   There is no hemodynamic pattern characteristic of ARDS. The hemodynamic pattern seen usually is associated with the disease that led to ARDS, such as septic or hypovolemic shock. Although pulmonary arterial hypertension often occurs, it usually is mild or moderate and its presence is not enough to confirm the diagnosis of ARDS. ARDS can occur in the presence or the absence of elevated hydrostatic pressure. (*See textbook pages* 584, 586.)

4. **A.**   Sepsis syndrome or systemic inflammatory response syndrome is associated with approximately one half of all cases of ARDS. On the other hand, one third of patients who aspirate gastric contents eventually have ARDS, but the total number of such cases of ARDS is believed to be lower than the number associated with systemic inflammatory response syndrome. Viral pneumonia, illicit drug use, and inhalation of toxic gases are common causes when ARDS develops in otherwise healthy persons, but these patients compose a minority of persons with ARDS. (*See textbook page* 581.)

Chapter 55

1. **C.**   Most studies do not support the use of theophylline in emergency department management of acute asthma. Theophylline is considered to have a greater profile of side effects than do inhaled bronchodilators. There is no evidence that theophylline affects the rate of clinical or spirometric improvement or emergency department outcome (admission to the hospital or discharge to home). It also is no more effective than is treatment with β-adrenergic agonists alone and do not have any less toxicity. When theophylline preparations are used, a serum concentration of 10 to 15 μg/mL is generally considered therapeutic. (*See textbook page* 597.)

2. **A.**   This patient has severe airway obstruction manifested by poor alveolar ventilation, high peak airway pressures, and severe gas trapping at end expiration. The most appropriate treatment is controlled hypoventilation to decrease peak airway pressure, air trapping, and alveolar distention, thereby decreasing risk for ventilator-associated lung injury while maintaining adequate oxygenation and acid-base balance. A reduction in tidal volume will decrease airway pressures and minute ventilation. Higher FIO_2 may be needed to compensate for decreased alveolar ventilation. Introducing applied PEEP to a patient with severe air trapping and intrinsic PEEP may facilitate machine triggering by spontaneous ventilatory effort, but weaning is inappropriate at this point, and applied PEEP may increase peak airway pressures. Increasing minute ventilation will worsen risk for barotrauma, and a lower PCO_2 is not necessary at this point. Paralysis sometimes is necessary to facilitate mechanical ventilation. However, the combination of systemic corticosteroid treatment with a neuromuscular blocking agent has been associated with prolonged neuromuscular weakness and should be avoided whenever possible. (*See textbook page* 601.)

3. **E.**   Pregnancy does not alter management of uncomplicated status asthmaticus. Maintenance of oxygenation is crucial. National Institutes of Health guidelines recommend 120 to 180 mg of methylprednisolone daily as standard therapy. Although intravenous magnesium sulfate is unconventional therapy for status asthmaticus, it has been used for years for the prevention of seizures in severe preeclampsia. Inhaled albuterol is a mainstay of therapy. The appropriate management of mechanical ventilation is essential for the maintenance of maternal and fetal tissue oxygenation. (*See textbook page* 599.)

Chapter 56

1. **B.**   Cefuroxime covers the most likely pathogens for this patient, including *Streptococcus pneumoniae, Haemophilus influenzae* and *Moraxella catarrhalis.* β-Lactamase production is common in hospital isolates of *H. influenzae* (up to 40%) and in *M. catarrhalis* infection (80% to 90%). This Gram stain is most suggestive of *M. catarrhalis.* Ampicillin is not an effective agent against β-lactamase-producing strains, and penicillin and erythromycin do not adequately cover the gram-negative possibilities. Other appropriate antibiotics for patients at high risk include second-generation macrolides such as azithromycin or clarithromycin, quinolones, second- and third-generation cephalosporins, and ampicillin-clavulanate. (*See textbook page* 610.)

2. **D.**   The length of stay for acute exacerbations of COPD has not been shown to be reduced by the use of supplemental oxygen. Use of supplemental oxygen leads to (a) a decrease in anaerobic metabolism and lactic acid production; (b) improvement in brain function; (c) a decrease in risk for cardiac arrhythmia and ischemia; (d) a decrease in risk for pulmonary hypertension; (e) improvement in right-sided heart function with improvement in right-heart failure; (f) a decrease in the release of antidiuretic hormone and an increase in the ability of the kidney to clear free water; (g) a decrease in the formation of pulmonary edema; (h) improvement in survival rate; (i) a decrease in red blood cell mass and hematocrit. (*See textbook page* 611.)

Chapter 57

1. **C.**   Pseudocholinesterase deficiency prolongs the action of succinylcholine, the only commonly used depolarizing neuromuscular blocker. Pancuronium is a non-

depolarizing neuromuscular blocker and is not degraded by pseudocholinesterase. Approximately 1 of 3,000 persons is homozygous for pseudocholinesterase deficiency. Pancuronium and its metabolites are primarily excreted through the kidneys, and prolonged neuromuscular blockade has been associated with concomitant renal failure. Myopathy has been associated with use of pancuronium. This has been described most commonly in association with corticosteroid use. Prolonged administration of a neuromuscular blocker also might be responsible; most reports describe patients who were not closely monitored with peripheral nerve stimulation and who received the medication for more than 2 days. (*See textbook page* 621.)

2. **A.**   Plasma exchange in patients with Guillain-Barré syndrome accelerates recovery and decreases time on mechanical ventilation if done early in the disease course. Intravenous immunoglobulin G may be just as effective. Corticosteroids and azathioprine have not been shown to be effective in Guillain-Barré syndrome. Pyridostigmine is an anticholinesterase useful in the management of myasthenia gravis, which also responds acutely to plasmapheresis when patients have an exacerbation. Pyridostigmine has no role in the management of Guillain-Barré syndrome. (*See textbook page* 619.)

Chapter 58

1. **B.**   The patient has likely had an amniotic fluid embolism, which may occur before or during labor or in the early postnatal period. The cause of hypoxemia often is noncardiogenic edema. Clinical evidence of disseminated intravascular coagulation also is common and occurs among as many as 50% of patients. It has been suggested that multiparous patients and those undergoing cesarean section are at increased risk. Although thrombotic pulmonary embolism is possible, the associated findings suggestive of disseminated intravascular coagulation make this less likely. The patient has no history of vomiting or aspiration, and this sudden change in status is unlikely to be caused by aspiration without a more obvious or witnessed event. Clinically significant air embolism is possible during normal labor and delivery but is highly uncommon. (*See textbook pages* 634, 635.)

2. **D.**   The $\dot{V}/\dot{Q}$ scan shows a high probability for pulmonary embolism, and the duplex ultrasound scan depicts a nonocclusive thrombus. One could argue about the necessity for the $\dot{V}/\dot{Q}$ scan under these circumstances, but the radiation exposure is low. Warfarin crosses the placenta and is associated with increased risk for fetal hemorrhage and birth defects. It is contraindicated throughout pregnancy. Heparin is the drug of choice and should be given intravenously initially for 10 to 14 days followed by adjusted-dosed subcutaneous heparin to maintain the partial thromboplastin time at 1.5 to 2.5 times control. Placement of an inferior vena caval filter is not indicated unless anticoagulation fails. Thrombolytic drugs are not indicated if the patient is in hemodynamically stable condition and has a nonocclusive thrombus. (*See textbook pages* 642, 645, 666.)

Chapter 59

1. **True.**   A $\dot{V}/\dot{Q}$ lung scan would be indeterminate given the chest radiographic findings, so a pulmonary arteriogram would almost certainly be necessary to document pulmonary embolism. However, a noninvasive lower extremity study indi-

cating the presence of proximal lower extremity deep venous thrombosis leads to the same treatment as does one that indicates pulmonary embolism—systemic anticoagulation. Thus, this would be the most appropriate first step. If the duplex scan has normal findings, pulmonary arteriography is indicated. Findings at non-invasive lower extremity testing might be normal in the presence of pulmonary embolism if all proximal lower extremity clots have already embolized or if the source of the clot was in the pelvis. (*See textbook page* 655.)

2. **False.** A chest radiograph in acute pulmonary embolus usually is abnormal, but the findings are nonspecific for most patients and rarely provide enough information to confirm a diagnosis. (*See textbook page* 653.)

3. **True.** Most patients with acute pulmonary embolism are hypoxemic with a widened $PAaO_2 - PaO_2$, but occasionally patients have a normal PaO_2 or $PAaO_2 - PaO_2$. (*See textbook page* 653.)

4. **False.** Although most patients with a high-probability lung scan have a pulmonary embolus, most patients with pulmonary embolus do not have a high-probability scan. Low- and intermediate-probability scans are more common and cannot be dismissed. (*See textbook page* 654.)

5. **True.** Warfarin is the most commonly prescribed long-term therapy for venous thromboembolism, and the dosage should be titrated to an INR of 2 to 3 for maximal efficacy and safety. (*See textbook page* 660.)

6. **False.** Thrombolytic therapy hastens clot resolution immediately in most patients and may be indicated in the treatment of those with hemodynamic instability. Hypoxemia, unless severe or refractory, is not necessarily an indication for thrombolysis unless associated with hemodynamic instability. (*See textbook page* 661.)

Chapter 60

1. **C.** The massive hemoptysis is most likely caused by bronchiectasis, and the source of the bleeding is probably the bronchial arterial supply. Even though bronchoscopy did not provide enough information for diagnosis, bronchial arteriography can likely localize the bleeding site if this bleeding continues. Embolization of a bleeding vessel stops the bleeding more than 90% of the time. Even if a definitive bleeding site is not identified, empiric embolization of a large bronchial vessel may be successful. Because the bleeding is likely bronchial, pulmonary angiography would not be helpful. Thoracotomy and right upper lobectomy would not be appropriate for this patient, who does not have preoperative localization, and it is unlikely that computed tomography would be helpful. Selective intubation may be necessary in exsanguinating bleeding when localization is more definite, but it is not appropriate here. (*See textbook pages* 675, 680, 681.)

Chapter 61

1. **A.** Anaerobic bacteria and *Streptococcus pneumoniae* are the common causes of aspiration pneumonia in the community setting. Enteric Gram-negative bacilli are common causes in the hospital setting. Acute respiratory distress syndrome has been reported to recur as a result of aspiration of gastric material with a pH of 5.9. Cough is a secondary defense mechanism that is important when aerodynamic filtration and mucociliary clearance are overwhelmed. There is no definitive proof that rates of aspiration differ depending on the location of the tip of a nasally placed feeding tube. (*See textbook pages* 686–689.)

Chapter 62

1. **E.**   Thirty-seven to 47% of drownings are associated with ethanol use. The importance of illegal drugs is uncertain, and therapeutic drugs appear to be involved in less than 10% of cases. Inadequate adult supervision and child abuse are involved in a substantial number of pediatric cases but do not occur in adult cases. Ethanol use by an adult also may be a predisposing factor in both child abuse and inadequate supervision of children. Diving, surfing, and water skiing may cause a large number of orthopedic and central nervous system injuries that may predispose to near-drowning, but the estimated numbers of these do not approach those involving ethanol. (*See textbook pages* 692, 693.)

2. **A.**   In experiments, freshwater aspiration inactivates surfactant, and atelectasis, shunt, and hypoxemia follow. Fresh water also damages type II pneumocytes, and surfactant production decreases. Hypertonic sea water does not appear to directly inactivate or denature surfactant. Hemoconcentration and severe electrolyte disorders are uncommon in human seawater near-drowning because of the limited volume of fluid aspirated. (*See textbook pages* 694, 695.)

Chapter 63

1. **A.**   In left heart failure, pulmonary arterial occlusion pressure and pulmonary arterial diastolic pressure both are elevated. If there is no severe pulmonary vascular disease, the gradient between the two pressures should be minimal. All the other diseases listed imply that pulmonary arterial diastolic pressure is much higher than pulmonary arterial occlusion pressure. In pulmonary venoocclusive disease, pulmonary arterial occlusion pressure may be high, low, or normal, because the wedged catheter tip measures downstream pressures in larger veins, which are connected to vascular beds of obstructed vessels but may not be affected themselves because of the patchy nature of the disease. However, pulmonary venoocclusive disease usually causes reactive pulmonary hypertension, and pulmonary arterial end-diastolic pressure still is much higher than pulmonary arterial occlusion pressure. (*See textbook page* 707.)

Chapter 64

1. **B.**   Spontaneous esophageal rupture dictates immediate operative intervention. Less aggressive or delayed approaches are associated with increased mortality. Endoscopy is relatively contraindicated given the diagnostic radiographic study, and this procedure may further enlarge the esophageal defect, making surgical repair more difficult. (*See textbook page* 718.)

2. **B.**   This patient has manifestations of ventilator-induced lung injury and is at high risk for pneumothorax. It is important to attempt to decrease airway pressure by whatever means are possible and safe. Decreasing peak inspiratory pressure and PEEP decrease airway pressures but may also decrease minute ventilation and arterial oxygen saturation. The patient's acid-base status can tolerate mild to moderate respiratory acidosis, however, and oxygenation can be supported by means of increasing F_{IO_2}. These conditions are preferable to the current situation. Increasing $I:E$ ratio increases mean airway pressure and causes air trapping. There is no indication for increasing rate at the current time, and doing so might cause air trapping. (*See textbook page* 721.)

3. **D.** Oxygenation and acid-base status are stable, and the lung appears to be expanded. There is no urgent need for surgical intervention. Medication-induced pleurodesis rarely is effective in closing a bronchopleural fistula during mechanical ventilation. Increasing chest tube suction is not indicated and may make the fistula worse. Examples of successful bronchoscopy-directed occlusion of a bronchus leading to a bronchopleural fistula have been reported, but the overall efficacy is uncertain, and the procedure is not appropriate at this time. If this patient's lung function improves and he can be successfully weaned from positive-pressure ventilation, the fistula may close spontaneously. (*See textbook pages* 722–724.)

Chapter 65

1. **A.** Pressure-support is a pressure-preset breath triggered by patient effort. Airway pressure is set, and flow, volume, and rate are dependent variables. Inspiratory flow in pressure-support ventilation is turned off when it decreases to a predetermined level below the initial value. (*See textbook page* 731.)
2. **A.** PEEP decreases intrapulmonary shunt by recruiting previously atelectatic alveoli, and this process increases functional residual capacity and improves ventilation-perfusion matching. Peak and mean airway pressures rise when PEEP is used to treat patients with acute respiratory distress syndrome. Extravascular lung water is redistributed in the lung by PEEP but is not reduced. (*See textbook page* 735.)
3. **D.** Patients with severe intrinsic PEEP and subsequent dynamic hyperinflation and airway compression at end expiration, must generate negative airway pressure sufficient to overcome this positive recoil pressure to trigger an inspiratory cycle during weaning. This can be extremely difficult for some patients and can dramatically increase the work of breathing. The application of extrinsic PEEP at 50% to 75% of measured intrinsic PEEP, counterbalances the positive recoil pressure present at end expiration without greatly affecting expiratory flow-volume events. It also decreases the magnitude of negative pressure necessary to initiate inspiratory flow for patients making spontaneous efforts. This level of applied pressure does not necessarily alter alveolar distention or lung compliance. Peak airway pressure may not change, but it will not fall. If airway pressure does rise considerably, the applied PEEP is probably in excess of the intrinsic PEEP and should be reduced. (*See textbook pages* 734, 736.)

Chapter 66

1. **C.** Respiratory muscle fatigue is the likely cause of inability to discontinue mechanical ventilation after a prolonged period. Nutritional, metabolic, and electrolyte disturbances may affect respiratory muscle function. Excessive work, superimposed illness affecting oxygen delivery or consumption by respiratory muscles, and associated cardiovascular disease also affect muscle function. Careful attention to mechanical ventilatory support while addressing factors that either decrease the strength or increase the work needed of the respiratory muscles is essential in weaning these patients. (*See textbook page* 742.)
2. **A.** This patient satisfies several of the most accurate criteria for success of complete liberation from mechanical ventilation. The respiratory rate to tidal volume ratio (f/V_T) spontaneous tidal volume, respiratory rate, and negative inspiratory

force, all suggest that the patient probably can discontinue mechanical ventilation and have the endotracheal tube removed. (*See textbook pages* 743–746.)

Chapter 67

1. B. This diver might have lung volume expansion, which often is caused by breath holding during ascent. From 40 feet (12 m) to the surface, lung volume doubles if gas is not vented by means of exhalation during ascent. Symptoms of lung damage occur immediately at the surface. Gas can enter the pulmonary veins and cause systemic gas embolism. Other forms of pulmonary barotrauma may occur. Immediate recompression may be life-saving. (*See textbook page* 756.)

Chapter 68

1. C. Although it currently is believed to have a role in the management of acute asthma, ipratropium bromide is recommended for use in addition to β_2 sympathomimetic drugs, not instead of those drugs. Albuterol administered through a nebulizer in standard doses and through an MDI with a spacer at appropriate doses (4 puffs) are thought to have equivalent efficacy. However, albuterol administered through an MDI is believed to be more cost effective. Two puffs of albuterol through an MDI is likely to be an inadequate dose to generate the desired clinical response. (*See textbook page* 764.)

2. A. Helium is less dense than nitrogen. Therefore in airways where flow is density dependent (large airways exhibiting turbulent flow), a mixture of helium and oxygen often improves flow and ventilation. Racemic epinephrine has been shown to be effective in reducing laryngeal edema, but that usually is not an issue for patients with paradoxic vocal cord movement. Speech therapy is essential for the long-term management of this condition but is unlikely to be effective in the setting described. Albuterol is most effective for small airway smooth-muscle relaxation. (*See textbook pages* 764, 771.)

Chapter 69

1. B. It is essential to know the position of the head and neck to evaluate properly the position of an endotracheal tube. Contrary to what intuition would suggest, when the neck moves from a neutral position to an extended position, the tip of the tube may ascend as much as 2 cm. Similarly, when the neck moves from a neutral position to a flexed position, the tip of the tube may descend as much as 2 cm. Therefore the following guidelines have been established to determine proper tip position: (a) When the neck is extended (inferior border of the mandible at level of C4), the tip of the endotracheal tube should be 7 ± 2 cm above the carina. (b) When the neck is in a neutral position (inferior border of the mandible at level of C5-6), the tip of the endotracheal tube should be 5 ± 2 cm above the carina. (c) When the neck is flexed (inferior border of the mandible at level of T1 or below), the tip of the endotracheal tube should be 3 ± 2 cm above the carina. (*See textbook page* 776.)

2. C. Chest radiographs are normal in 87.5% of cases of fat embolism diagnosed on the basis of the presence of lipiduria. In instances in which there are findings on a chest radiograph, widespread or patchy areas of alveolar filling are found. Oligemia may occur with thromboembolism not fat embolism. Bilateral pleural effusions are not common. (*See textbook page* 789.)

Chapter 70

1. A. The formation of carboxyhemoglobin results in increased affinity of the remaining sites for oxygen, shifting the oxyhemoglobin curve to the left. Total oxygen-carrying capacity is decreased, however, because of the higher affinity of carbon monoxide for the hemoglobin. Oxidative metabolism is decreased, partly because of the binding of carbon monoxide to cytochromes; this process interrupts the electron transport chain. (*See textbook page* 817.)

2. B. Noncardiogenic edema may develop several hours after extensive exposure to NO_2. Because of the poor water solubility of NO_2 there are few signs of upper airway or laryngeal edema or inflammation. Eosinophilia is not characteristic. The disease is caused by direct toxicity and not by hypersensitivity. (*See textbook page* 818.)

3. D. Most deaths due to smoke inhalation are related to severe carbon monoxide poisoning, sometimes associated with cyanide toxicity. Pulmonary edema may occur late, depending on the particular vapor exposure. Direct heat injury usually is confined to the upper airway and may occasionally cause problems with laryngeal edema and obstruction. (*See textbook page* 823.)

Chapter 71

1. True

2. False

3. True

4. True. The shivering phase of hypothermia usually occurs in the 35°C to 30°C range. Physiologic changes include marked increases in heat production, oxygen consumption, and metabolic rate. Cardiac output changes very little, however. Increased oxygen consumption without concomitant increased cardiac output leads to reduced mixed venous oxygen saturation and the development of lactic acidosis. (*See textbook page* 831.)

5. True

6. False

7. False

8. False. Compliance, airway resistance, lung volume, and $PaO_2 - PaO_2$ change little with hypothermia. Minute ventilation increases because of increased oxygen demand during shivering. (*See textbook pages* 831, 832.)

9. D. Despite decreased blood pressure and glomerular filtration rate, urine output is maintained in hypothermia (cold diuresis) because tubular defects in reabsorption result in diluted urine. Additional stimuli for this effect may be the triggering of volume receptors as central volume is increased in response to peripheral vasoconstriction and possibly insensitivity to antidiuretic hormone. The white blood cell count may be slightly elevated in mild hypothermia but is characteristically low at temperatures less than 28°C, and absolute neutropenia may result. Mild hyperglycemia is a common finding because of decreased insulin release, peripheral insulin resistance, increased glycogenolysis, and increased levels of counterregulatory hormones. Subclinical pancreatitis is common, perhaps partly because of alcohol ingestion by some patients. (*See textbook pages* 832, 833.)

Chapter 72

1. **C**
2. **A**
3. **D**
4. **C**
5. **C**
6. **B**
7. **B**
8. **B.** Malignant hyperthermia and neuroleptic malignant syndrome are characterized by excessive thermogenesis due to uncontrolled muscle contraction. Rhabdomyolysis is common in both disorders. Malignant hyperthermia is caused by a calcium transport defect in skeletal muscle that usually is triggered by exposure to general anesthetics or succinylcholine. This defect is inherited as an autosomal dominant trait with variable penetrance. Neuroleptic malignant syndrome is caused by hypersensitivity of dopaminergic receptors in the hypothalamus as a result of administration of agents designed to block dopamine receptors or withdrawal of drugs with dopaminergic effects. Extrapyramidal reactions are common in neuroleptic malignant syndrome. Dantrolene is a direct muscle relaxant and is effective in both conditions. Bromocriptine increases central dopaminergic tone, which decreases central drive, muscle rigidity, and thermogenesis. Pancuronium relaxes muscle in neuroleptic malignant syndrome but not in malignant hyperthermia because of the postsynaptic causation of the muscle rigidity in the latter syndrome. (*See textbook pages* 848, 849, 854.)

Chapter 73

1. **D.** *H. influenzae* infection is the most common identifiable infectious cause of acute epiglottitis among adults. (*See textbook page* 859.)
2. **A.** This patient has a submandibular space infection as a complication of an odontogenic infection. He needs additional imaging studies such as computed tomography of the neck to demonstrate the extent of infection and to search for any drainable abscess. These infections are usually polymicrobial, reflecting the common mouth flora of streptococcal and oral anaerobes. Some oral anaerobes show increasing resistance to penicillin, and a common oral gram-negative anaerobe, *Eikenella corrodens,* is resistant to clindamycin. Penicillin G is the best drug to cover the aerobic streptococci, and metronidazole is the best agent for anaerobes. This particular patient is at low risk for enteric gram-negative rod or *S. aureus* infection. Thus an initial antibiotic selection aimed at this spectrum is unnecessary. However, coverage of *S. aureus* is indicated for patients with penetrating trauma, vertebral disease, or a history of intravenous drug use. (*See textbook pages* 866, 867, 869.)

Chapter 74

1. **B.** Sucralfate use has not been associated with nosocomial pneumonia, although some studies have shown an increased pneumonia rate in association with use of H2 antagonists. The other factors listed have been associated with nosocomial pneumonia in most studies. Other cited conditions include recent thoracic or abdominal operation, head injury, shock, systemic antibiotic use, and prolonged mechanical ventilation. (*See textbook page* 882.)

2. **A.**   Concomitant use of antibiotics by a patient with suspected pneumonia may alter the result for any invasive diagnostic procedure. Bronchoalveolar lavage can be used to diagnose nonbacterial infectious diseases, most notably *Pneumocystis carinii* pneumonia and cytomegalovirus infection. There is poor discrimination between infection and colonization by culture. No studies have shown an effect of bronchoscopy on outcome among patients with suspected nosocomial pneumonia. (*See textbook pages* 890, 891.)

3. **D.**   The nasogastric tube itself may cause some incompetence of the lower esophageal sphincter, and neutralization of gastric acid by feedings may increase colonization by gram-negative rods. The effect of nutritional interventions on the outcome of pneumonia has not been proved. Maintenance of proper positioning in the semierect posture and close monitoring of gastric volume probably are important factors. Problems with gastric atony among critically ill patients and those recovering from an operative procedure make small-intestinal feeding more efficient for many patients. Small-intestinal feeding also provides more consistent results in attaining nutritional goals. (*See textbook page* 891.)

4. **A.**   Most studies have shown a decreased rate of pneumonia among some patients treated with selective decontamination of the digestive tract. Despite this, convincing evidence of decreased length of stay in the ICU or decreased overall mortality is lacking. Studies have documented increased numbers of resistant bacterial strains and a trend toward increased pneumonia from these organisms. There should be heightened concern over potential changes in resistance of hospital flora if routine use of selective decontamination of the digestive tract is initiated among a large number of patients in an ICU. Despite some positive trends in the overall incidence of pneumonia, more information is needed before this technique can be recommended. (*See textbook pages* 894, 895.)

5. **B.**   This patient has severe community-acquired pneumonia evidenced by multilobar infiltrates and hypoxemia. The clinical history and laboratory findings are nonspecific. There are no obvious risk factors for enteric gram-negative or anaerobic infection. Because of the severity illness, treatment should include a second-generation cephalosporin to cover *Haemophilus influenzae* and *Streptococcus pneumoniae* and erythromycin for the possibility of the presence of *Legionella* organisms. Sputum cultures are likely not to provide enough information to confirm a diagnosis based on the description of the inflammatory component. (*See textbook page* 892.)

Chapter 75

1. **B.**   Positive pressure ventilation is a relative contraindication but not an absolute contraindication. Transbronchial biopsies have been safely performed in this situation. (*See textbook page* 899.)

V. Renal Problems in the Intensive Care Unit

76. Physiologic Concepts in the Management of Renal, Fluid, and Electrolyte Disorders in the Intensive Care Unit

True or False

1. Angiotensin II has different effects on renal blood flow, depending on the local and systemic concentrations.
2. Digoxin, dopamine, and glucocorticoids act as diuretic agents.

Select the best answer

3. Regarding renal autoregulation:

   A. The term *autoregulation* encompasses the maintenance of renal blood flow, glomerular filtration, and solute excretion.
   B. Between mean arterial pressures of 60 mm Hg and 180 mm Hg, renal blood flow and glomerular filtration rate (GFR) are relatively constant.
   C. Separate exogenous mechanisms regulate the autoregulation of blood flow and filtration in the kidney.
   D. Diminished arterial pressure causes relaxation of the afferent arteriole and maintains glomerular blood flow.

4. Which of the following statements regarding atrial natriuretic peptide (ANP) is *true*?

   A. ANP enhances distal nephron reabsorption of sodium.
   B. Chronic congestive heart failure and hepatic cirrhosis are characterized by an increased responsiveness to ANP.
   C. When given intravenously into the renal artery, ANP promotes increased GFR and a substantial increase in urinary sodium secretion.
   D. ANP is not measurable in circulation.

5. Which of the following statements regarding diuretics is *true*?

   A. Mannitol is a polysaccharide freely filterable by the glomerulus and like glucose reabsorbable.
   B. Acetazolamide activates the enzyme carbonic anhydrase and causes a loss of tubular hydrogen ion secretion.

C. Loop diuretics inhibit the action of sodium-potassium adenosine triphosphatase and enhance sodium and chloride secretion.

D. Loop diuretics initially act to manage pulmonary congestion through brisk diuresis and subsequently through effects on venous capacitance and cardiac preload.

77. *Metabolic Acidosis and Metabolic Alkalosis*

True or False

1. The administration of sodium chloride is an effective treatment for chloride-resistant metabolic alkalosis after adequate repletion with potassium.

78. *Disorders of Plasma Sodium and Plasma Potassium*

True or False

1. The syndrome of inappropriate antidiuretic hormone (ADH) secretion is characterized by plasma hypoosmolality with urinary osmolality greater than 100 to 150 mOsm/kg, normal adrenal, renal, and thyroid function, hyperkalemia, and normal acid-base balance.

2. Hyperkalemia occurs among as many as one half of patients treated with amphotericin B.

Select the best answer

3. Which of the following statements regarding diabetes insipidus is *true*?

A. Glucose-induced osmotic diuresis is one form of diabetes insipidus.

B. Primary polydipsia, central diabetes insipidus, and nephrogenic diabetes insipidus cannot be differentiated on biochemical grounds.

C. Severe hypernatremia is common in diabetes insipidus and is a diagnostic criterion.

D. In central diabetes insipidus, both ADH release and thirst mechanisms may be impaired, leading to sodium concentrations that can exceed 160 mEq/L.

79. *Acute Renal Failure in the Intensive Care Unit*

True or False

1. In radiocontrast-induced nephropathy, serum creatinine level peaks 7 to 10 days after the procedure.

2. Myoglobin has direct toxic effects on the tubular epithelium.

80. *Drug Dosing in the Intensive Care Unit: The Patient with Renal Failure*

True or False

1. Aminophylline and theophylline may be given in their usual dosages in end-stage renal disease.
2. The half-life of amphotericin B is unaffected in end-stage renal disease.
3. The volume of distribution of a drug may be increased by ascites or edema.

81. *Dialysis Therapy in the Intensive Care Unit*

Select the best answer

1. Which of the following statements regarding hemodialysis is *true*?

   A. Observations suggest an important interaction between initiation of dialysis and the maintenance of residual renal function.
   B. Preserving residual renal function is of modest benefit only in the treatment of patients with advanced renal insufficiency.
   C. Residual renal function is of crucial importance only for clearance of larger solutes of greater than 500 daltons.
   D. It is less important to preserve residual renal function for patients undergoing peritoneal dialysis than it is for patients undergoing hemodialysis.

Answers
Chapter 76

1. **True.** Angiotensin II appears to selectively operate at the efferent sphincter or arteriole when locally produced. At higher circulating levels, sufficient to raise systemic blood pressure, angiotensin II also causes afferent vasoconstriction. (*See textbook page* 912.)
2. **False.** Diuretics promote the excretion of water by acting along distinct nephron sites. Agents such as digoxin, dopamine, and glucocorticoids enhance glomerular filtration and increase urine flow but are pharmacologically distinct from diuretics. (*See textbook page* 917.)
3. **D.** The term *autoregulation* encompasses the maintenance of renal blood flow and GFR over a wide range of arterial pressures, between 80 mm Hg and 200 mm Hg. Separate mechanisms regulate blood flow and GFR, but both appear to be intrinsic to the kidney. Diminished arterial pressure causes relaxation of the afferent arteriole and maintenance of glomerular blood flow in this manner. (*See textbook page* 911.)
4. **C.** When given intravenously into the renal artery, ANP promotes increased GFR and a substantial increase in urinary sodium secretion. This hormone is measurable with radioimmunoassay. Chronic congestive heart failure, nephrotic syndrome, and hepatic cirrhosis are characterized by a blunted response to ANP. Distal nephron reabsorption of sodium is inhibited by ANP. (*See textbook pages* 916, 917.)

5. **C.**   In the thick portion of the ascending limb of the loop of Henle, sodium and potassium cross the luminal cell membrane with two chlorides. The loop diuretics inhibit this cotransport system thereby enhancing sodium and chloride secretion. Mannitol is a polysaccharide, freely filterable by the glomerulus, but unlike glucose, it is not reabsorbable. Its osmotic activity thus constrains fluid absorption by the proximal nephron. Acetazolamide is secreted into the proximal nephron from the peritubular capillaries by a potent organic acid transport pathway. It inactivates the enzyme carbonic anhydrase, which catalyzes the conversion of carbon dioxide and water into bicarbonate. The loop diuretics stimulate renal prostaglandin synthesis thereby increasing renal blood flow. The loop diuretics increase systemic venous capacitance, reduce cardiac preload, and lower left ventricular end-diastolic pressure within 5 minutes of intravenous administration. This effect precedes the diuretic effect and can occur in anephric patients. This suggests that the vasodilator effects of the loop diuretics may be responsible for the acute amelioration of pulmonary congestion. (*See textbook pages* 917, 918.)

Chapter 77

1. **False.**   Patients with a urinary chloride concentration greater than 15 mEq/L are unlikely to respond to chloride-containing solutions such as physiologic saline solution. Because the effective perfusion volume is already normal or chloride reabsorption is impaired, the administered chloride is rapidly excreted in the urine. Management of these disorders depends on the cause. Only the chloride resorptive defect associated with severe hypokalemia is corrected with potassium chloride supplementation. Potassium repletion in that case will convert chloride-resistant alkalosis to a form of alkalosis that is responsive to sodium chloride. (*See textbook pages* 937–939.)

Chapter 78

1. **False.**   The syndrome of inappropriate ADH secretion is characterized by plasma hypoosmolality, urinary sodium concentration greater than 20 mEq/L, normal adrenal, renal, and thyroid function, and normal potassium and acid-base balance.
2. **False.**   Amphotericin B administration leads to an increase in membrane permeability that can promote potassium secretion from intracellular stores across the luminal membrane and into the tubular lumen. This has been shown to be caused by interaction between amphotericin and membrane sterols. (*See textbook page* 957.)
3. **D.**   Diabetes insipidus is a cause of hypernatremia that must be differentiated from other polyuric states. In the absence of glucose-induced osmotic diuresis in uncontrolled diabetes, the primary sources of true polyuria (>3 L/day) include primary polydipsia, central diabetes insipidus, and nephrogenic diabetes insipidus. Primary polydipsia is characterized by a primary increase in water intake. Thus, a low plasma sodium concentration with a history of polyuria is usually indicative of primary polydipsia. A high-normal plasma sodium concentration suggests diabetes insipidus. Marked hypernatremia is uncommon with diabetes insipidus because the initial water loss stimulates the thirst mechanism. An exception to this rule occurs among patients with trauma or a central nervous system lesion that impairs both ADH release and thirst. Among such patients,

plasma-sodium concentration can exceed 160 mEq/L. Nephrogenic diabetes insipidus is characterized by normal ADH secretion but varying degrees of renal resistance to ADH. (*See textbook page 951.*)

Chapter 79

1. **False.** The administration of intravascular radiocontrast agents leads to a syndrome of rapidly developing acute renal failure. The typical patient has a brief episode of oliguric acute renal failure. Serum creatinine level peaks approximately 4 days after the procedure. Most patients do not need dialysis. (*See textbook page 977.*)
2. **True.** On entering the distal nephron, myoglobin participates in the formation of proteinaceous casts that obstruct nephronal flow. In addition to this effect, myoglobin exerts direct cytotoxic effects on the tubular epithelium. This is thought to be caused by generation of reactive oxygen species. (*See textbook page 976.*)

Chapter 80

1. **True.** (*See textbook page 1019 and chapters 55 and 152.*)
2. **True.** Half-life is 24 hours in normal situations and with end-stage renal disease. (*See textbook page 1000.*)
3. **True.** Highly water soluble drugs may experience an increase in volume of distribution because of the increased fluid volume in edema states. Renal failure also may cause a change by decreasing plasma proteins available for drug binding; this alteration increases volume of distribution. An alternative explanation is that dehydration or muscle wasting states may lead to a decrease in volume of distribution and a subsequent increase in plasma or serum drug concentration. (*See textbook page 993.*)

Chapter 81

1. **A.** The influence of dialysis on residual renal function is critical. Observations have suggested an important and potentially deleterious interaction between dialysis and residual renal function. Investigators have observed that patients with posttraumatic acute renal failure treated by hemodialysis have pathologically demonstrable fresh focal areas of tubular necrosis 3 to 4 weeks after the original hemodynamic insult. Hemodialysis often is associated with an acute decline in urine output. Preservation of residual renal function is of great benefit in the care of patients with advanced renal insufficiency. Even a modest preservation of urine output simplifies management of volume status. For patients undergoing hemodialysis, effective residual renal function is even more important for the clearance of middle-molecular-weight solutes. For patients treated with peritoneal dialysis, which is less efficient than hemodialysis, preservation of renal function is an even more important aid in management of volume status. (*See textbook page 1029.*)

VI. Infectious Disease Problems in the Intensive Care Unit

82. Approach to Fever in the Intensive Care Patient

Select the best answer

1. Which of the following conditions is unlikely to produce fever of a noninfectious nature?

    A. Acute vasculitis
    B. Subarachnoid hemorrhage
    C. Acute alcohol withdrawal
    D. Myocardial infarction
    E. Atelectasis

83. Use of Antimicrobials in the Treatment of Infection in the Critically Ill

Select the best answer

1. Which of the following bacteria are covered by first-generation cephalosporins?

    A. Enterococci
    B. *Listeria monocytogenes*
    C. Community-acquired *Escherichia coli* infections
    D. Methicillin-resistant *Staphylococcus aureus*
    E. *Staphylococcus epidermidis*

2. Which of the following statements concerning cefoxitin is *false*?

    A. It is less potent than first-generation cephalosporins against *S. aureus*
    B. It is active against most strains of *Proteus* and *E. coli*
    C. It is usually effective against anaerobes
    D. It is a good single-agent choice for enterococcal infections
    E. It is actually a cephamycin

84. Prevention and Control of Nosocomial Infection in the Intensive Care Unit

Select the best answer

1. Which of the following organisms is not commonly observed to be etiologic in nosocomial infections?

   A. *Escherichia coli*
   B. Human immunodeficiency virus
   C. *Serratia marcescens*
   D. Methicillin-resistant *Staphylococcus aureus*
   E. *Candida albicans*

2. The patient factor that correlates most with the development of nosocomial infection includes:

   A. Shock on admission
   B. The presence of invasive monitoring devices
   C. Immunosuppression
   D. Renal insufficiency
   E. All of the above

3. Which of the following decreases the rate of bacterial transmission in nosocomial infections?

   A. Intensive care unit design
   B. Handwashing
   C. Prophylactic antibiotics
   D. Laminar flow environments
   E. Negative-pressure patient rooms

4. Which of the following measures is most effective at preventing the spread of *Clostridium difficile*?

   A. Vinyl gloves
   B. Handwashing
   C. Prophylactic vancomycin
   D. Prophylactic metronidazole
   E. Avoiding clindamycin use

85. Central Nervous System Infections

Select the best answer

1. The most common organism responsible for bacterial meningitis among older children and young adults is:

   A. *Haemophilus influenzae*
   B. *Neisseria meningitidis*
   C. *Streptococcus pneumoniae*
   D. *Listeria monocytogenes*
   E. *Staphylococcus aureus*

2. Which of the following statements concerning bacterial meningitis is true?

   A. A normal cerebrospinal glucose level eliminates the possibility of bacterial meningitis.
   B. Aztreonam is a reasonable choice for initial empiric therapy for bacterial meningitis.
   C. Dexamethasone therapy is contraindicated in meningitis.
   D. Patients with cerebrospinal fluid (CSF) shunts or intracranial pressure monitoring devices who contract meningitis should always have the devices removed to optimize the chances for cure.
   E. Respiratory isolation is recommended for patients with meningococcal or *H. influenzae* meningitis.

3. The most reliable and definitive way to prove the presence of herpes simplex encephalitis (HSE) is:

   A. The detection of antibodies to herpes simplex virus in blood
   B. The detection of antibodies to herpes simplex virus in CSF
   C. Electroencephalography
   D. The demonstration of viral antigen or recovery of virus in brain tissue obtained at biopsy
   E. Computed tomography

86. Infective Endocarditis

Select the best answer

1. A 46-year-old male user of intravenous drugs comes to medical attention with obtundation and fever. Physical examination reveals evidence of emaciation, the presence of splinter hemorrhages and petechiae on the plantar surface of the toes and the buccal mucosa, and a mitral regurgitant murmur. Laboratory data include hemoglobin 9.6 g/dL and serum creatinine 2.3 mg/dL. Findings at computed tomography of the brain are consistent with an acute infarction in the distribution of the middle cerebral artery. Blood cultures are repeatedly positive for *Streptococcus bovis*. Which of the following conditions should be considered in the care of this patient?

   A. Bacterial endocarditis
   B. Malignant gastrointestinal tumor
   C. Both
   D. Neither

2. Which of the following organisms is most likely to infect a previously normal heart valve?

   A. *Eikenella corrodens*
   B. *Staphylococcus aureus*
   C. *Candida albicans*
   D. *Haemophilus* species
   E. *Streptococcus pneumoniae*

3. Bacterial endocarditis of which valve has the worst prognosis?

   A. Tricuspid
   B. Pulmonary

C. Mitral

D. Aortic

4. A patient with known bacterial endocarditis is found to have a painful, tender, purplish nodule on the pad of his right great toe. This finding is known as:

   A. A Janeway lesion
   B. A Roth spot
   C. An Osler's node
   D. A splinter hemorrhage

5. Most cases of bacterial endocarditis require how many blood cultures for detection?

   A. One
   B. Two
   C. Three
   D. Four or more

87. Infections Associated with Vascular Catheters

Select the best answer

1. Which of the following agents has been shown to be most effective at preventing intravascular catheter-associated infections?

   A. Skin disinfection with 70% alcohol
   B. Prophylactic administration of intravenous clindamycin
   C. Skin disinfection with 2% aqueous chlorhexidine
   D. Prophylactic administration of intravenous penicillin
   E. Skin disinfection with 10% povidone-iodine solution

2. Which of the following conditions provides the greatest risk for the development sepsis related to central venous catheters?

   A. Using gauze dressings instead of transparent dressings
   B. Failing to use an antiseptic ointment over the insertion site
   C. Changing the infusion set every 72 hours instead of every 24 hours
   D. Leaving the catheter in place for longer than 72 hours
   E. None of the above

3. Which of the following statements concerning catheter-related infections is *true*?

   A. Arterial catheters should be suspected of being infected only if they show signs of local inflammation.
   B. Coagulase-negative staphylococci are the organisms most commonly associated with catheter-related infections.
   C. *Candida* and *Malassezia* species are uncommonly associated with infections of total parenteral nutrition catheters.
   D. Excision of the vein should never be performed if a patient has suppurative thrombophlebitis.
   E. All patients with catheter-related sepsis should be treated with a 2-week course of the appropriate antibiotic for the organisms isolated.

88. *Urinary Tract Infections*

Select the best answer

1. Which of the following statements concerning catheter-associated urinary tract infection (UTI) is *false*?

    A. Removal of the catheter results in eradication of the infection for only 15% of patients.

    B. Low bacterial colony counts among patients with urinary catheters progress to high-grade bacteriuria in most instances if the patient does not receive suppressive antimicrobial therapy.

    C. Polymicrobial bacteriuria occurs among more than 15% of patients with catheter-related UTI.

    D. Bacterial colony counts in the urine of less than 10^5 colony-forming units (CFU) per milliliter does not allow the urinary tract to be safely disregarded as a potential source of active infection in a patient who has a urinary catheter.

    E. None of the above.

2. UTI associated with the use of indwelling urinary catheters in the care of critically ill patients can best be prevented by:

    A. Effective care of the meatus with the application of antimicrobial povidone-iodine solution or topical polyantimicrobial ointments

    B. Avoidance of catheterization when possible

    C. Use of silicone rather than latex urinary catheters

    D. Systemic antimicrobial prophylaxis

    E. None of the above

3. Which of the following statements concerning *Candida* UTI is *true*?

    A. The isolation of *Candida* species from a sample of urine confirms the presence of invasive candidiasis, and the patient should be treated aggressively.

    B. The finding of urinary casts made up of *Candida* elements indicates invasive upper-tract candidiasis.

    C. Systemic amphotericin B should be avoided in the treatment of patients found to have fungus balls within the urinary collecting system.

    D. Fluconazole has been shown to be ineffective therapy for *Candida* cystitis.

89. *Life-Threatening Community-Acquired Infections*

Select the best answer

1. The differential diagnosis of toxic shock syndrome should include all but which of the following conditions?

    A. Rocky Mountain spotted fever

    B. Meningococcemia

    C. Acute pelvic inflammatory disease

    D. Streptococcal scarlet fever

    E. Rubeola

2. Which of the following is specific therapy for Rocky Mountain spotted fever?

   A. Penicillin
   B. Aztreonam
   C. Doxycycline
   D. Imipenem
   E. Ceftazidime

3. The main host defense against invasive meningococcal infection is represented by:

   A. Basophil activity
   B. CD4 lymphocytes
   C. Eosinophils
   D. The complement system
   E. Antibody production

4. Which of the following statements regarding malaria is *false*?

   A. Fever is present among 54% to 73% of patients when they arrive for medical care.
   B. Diagnosis is established by review of the peripheral blood smear.
   C. Clarithromycin has emerged as a first-line therapy for chloroquine-resistant falciparum malaria.
   D. The Middle East and Central America are endemic areas that do not show high rates of chloroquine resistance.
   E. As many as 50% of children with cerebral malaria have sequelae such as hemiparesis, seizure disorder, blindness, or spasticity.

90. Acute Infection in the Immunocompromised Host

Select the best answer

1. Infection with which of the following organisms is associated with defects in cell-mediated immunity?

   A. *Pneumocystis carinii*
   B. *Streptococcus pneumoniae*
   C. *Haemophilus influenzae*
   D. *Pseudomonas aeruginosa*
   E. *Neisseria meningitidis*

2. In an immunocompromised patient, bacteremia without an obvious source is most likely arising from which of the following sources?

   A. Intravenous catheter
   B. Foley catheter
   C. Gastrointestinal tract
   D. Lungs
   E. Surgical wound

3. Which of the following is *not* an acceptable broad-spectrum antibiotic regimen for treatment of a patient with neutropenia and a fever of unknown origin?

A. Ceftazidime and tobramycin

B. Imipenem

C. Aztreonam, tobramycin, and vancomycin

D. Clindamycin and vancomycin

E. Piperacillin and amikacin

91. Intensive Care of Patients with HIV Infection

Select the best answer

1. Which of the following statements regarding *Pneumocystis carinii* pneumonia (PCP) is *true*?

   A. The percentage of human immunodeficiency virus (HIV)–related deaths attributable to PCP increased from 13.8% to 32.5% during the period from 1987 to 1992.

   B. Prednisone 40 mg twice a day should be initiated in the care of patients with moderate or severe PCP.

   C. The yield of sputum induction for the diagnosis of PCP is generally thought to be less than 50%.

   D. Serum lactate dehydrogenase levels are elevated in 55% to 60% of instances.

2. Which of the following is the most common infection among patients with HIV infection who are admitted to the hospital with respiratory illness?

   A. Bacterial pneumonia

   B. Pulmonary tuberculosis

   C. PCP

   D. Cryptococcal pulmonary disease

   E. *Mycobacterium avium-intracellulare* lung disease

92. Infectious Complications of Drug Abuse

Select the best answer

1. Endocarditis developing as a consequence of intravenous drug abuse typically involves which heart valve?

   A. Tricuspid

   B. Pulmonic

   C. Mitral

   D. Aortic

   E. All are affected in equal proportion

2. Which of the following is the most common reason for hospital admission?

   A. Hepatitis A

   B. Hepatitis C

   C. Hepatitis B

   D. Hepatitis D (delta agent)

3. Which of the following is not a common pulmonary complication among abusers of intravenous drugs?

A. Acute pulmonary edema
B. Unilateral bacterial pneumonia
C. Septic pulmonary emboli
D. Tuberculosis
E. Pulmonary infection related to acquired immunodeficiency syndrome (AIDS)

93. Tuberculosis

Select the best answer

1. Which of the following statements concerning the current status of tuberculosis in the United States is *true*?

A. The incidence of active cases of tuberculosis is rising.
B. The incidence of active cases of tuberculosis is declining.
C. The incidence of tuberculosis has been unaffected by the human immunodeficiency virus (HIV) epidemic.
D. The incidence of active cases of tuberculosis is stable.
E. The incidence of multidrug-resistant tuberculosis is stable.

2. Which of the following statements regarding tuberculosis of the central nervous system is *true*?

A. The finding of an elevated spinal fluid glucose concentration excludes the possibility of tuberculosis of the central nervous system.
B. Tuberculoma of the central nervous system is readily detected with computed tomography.
C. Tuberculoma of the central nervous system is rarely detected with magnetic resonance imaging.
D. The number of spinal taps does not increase the likelihood of obtaining a specimen positive for acid-fast bacilli.
E. None of the above.

3. Antibiotic agents that have activity against *Mycobacterium tuberculosis* include:

A. Ciprofloxacin
B. Gentamicin
C. Rifampin
D. Isoniazid
E. All of the above

94. Botulism

Select the best answer

1. Which of the following conditions is necessary for the germination of *Clostridium botulinum* spores?

A. Low humidity
B. High temperature (>39°C)
C. Anaerobic conditions
D. A pH less than 4.0
E. Oxygen

2. Which of the following is the site of action of the *C. botulinum* toxin?

   A. Cortical motor strip
   B. Medulla oblongata
   C. Spinal cord
   D. Autonomic ganglia
   E. Neuromuscular junction

3. In the care of a patient who has signs of botulism, the most sensitive indicator of the need for mechanical ventilation is:

   A. PaO_2
   B. Vital capacity
   C. Respiratory rate
   D. Dead space-to-tidal volume ratio
   E. Intrapulmonary shunt fraction

95. *Tetanus*

Select the best answer

1. Which of the following are the major complications of tetanus?

   A. Respiratory paralysis
   B. Seizures
   C. Cardiac arrhythmias
   D. Facial pain
   E. All of the above

2. Which of the following drugs is not often useful in the treatment of a patient with generalized tetanus?

   A. Diazepam
   B. Meperidine
   C. Propranolol
   D. Baclofen
   E. Penicillin G

3. Which of the following treatments is necessary in all cases of tetanus?

   A. Clindamycin
   B. Human tetanus immune globulin
   C. Metronidazole
   D. Penicillin

Answers

Chapter 82

1. **E.** Many noninfectious conditions can cause fever among patients in an intensive care unit, although acute bacterial infections are certainly the most common and serious causes of fever among critically ill patients. Many cardiovascular conditions can be associated with a noninfectious fever, such as acute vasculitis, dissection of an aortic aneurysm, mesenteric ischemia, deep venous thrombophlebitis, pulmonary embolism, or myocardial infarction. Also, hemorrhage into certain areas, such as the central nervous system, retroperitoneum, joint spaces, or lung, can cause temperature elevations. Certain metabolic conditions such as heat stroke, malignant hyperthermia, hyperthyroidism, adrenal insufficiency, and alcohol withdrawal can produce fevers. Conspicuously absent from the list presented in the text in Table 82-1 is atelectasis. Although this process has been widely regarded to cause fever among patients recovering from an operation, there is no clear evidence that this is true. Animal models of fever also do not support the hypothesis that atelectasis alone causes fever. (*See textbook pages 1053–1055.*)

Chapter 83

1. **C.** First-generation cephalosporins usually are very effective against a number of gram-positive aerobic bacteria, with some notable exceptions. Methicillin-resistant strains of *Staphylococcus,* such as methicillin-resistant *S. aureus,* usually also are resistant to first-generation cephalosporins. *S. epidermidis* also is frequently (approximately 50% of strains) resistant to methicillin and shares this resistance with first-generation cephalosporins. *Enterococcus* organisms, despite being gram-positive aerobes (once having been considered streptococci), is resistant to first-generation cephalosporins. *L. monocytogenes* usually is resistant to first-generation cephalosporins. Many community-acquired gram-negative organisms in the Enterobacteriaceae family are sensitive to first-generation cephalosporins, including *E. coli, Proteus mirabilis,* and even *Klebsiella pneumoniae,* although many hospital-acquired infective isolates of Enterobacteriaceae organisms are resistant to these agents. (*See textbook page* 1061.)
2. **D.** Cefoxitin is a popular cephamycin, although it usually is classified as a second-generation cephalosporin. It has broader activity against gram-negative aerobes than do the first-generation cephalosporins. Many of the gram-negative organisms in the Enterobacteriaceae family such as *E. coli* and *Proteus, Providencia,* and *Klebsiella* species are covered by cefoxitin. This drug usually is highly effective against anaerobes such as *Bacteroides fragilis.* As with virtually all the cephalosporin and cephalosporin-like antibiotics, cefoxitin has no independent activity against *Enterococcus* species. (*See textbook page* 1061.)

Chapter 84

1. **B.** Although the microbiologic features of nosocomial infections can vary greatly from institution to institution, a pattern of the organisms commonly involved has emerged. Gram-negative organisms tend to predominate in most clinical series of nosocomial infections, the most common of these being *E. coli,*

Klebsiella species, *Enterobacter* species, and *Serratia* species. *Pseudomonas* species also are found, although less frequently. Gram-positive organisms are responsible for roughly one fifth of nosocomial infections, led by *S. aureus*. Methicillin-resistant strains are commonly found in critically ill patients. *Candida* species are the most common fungal infections and appear to be increasing in importance over recent years. Although many critically ill patients may be infected with HIV, these infections rarely are nosocomial in nature. Universal precautions help to minimize risk for transmission, although only if health care workers change gloves between patient contacts. The antibody screening that is now routine in blood banks minimizes the risk for infecting hospitalized patients with this HIV. (*See textbook pages* 1074, 1075, 1158.)

2. **E.**   A large multivariate analysis performed by Craven et al. of 1,300 patients admitted to adult intensive care units at Boston City Hospital revealed the presence of invasive monitoring devices (e.g., urinary catheters, intracranial pressure monitors, arterial catheters, Swan-Ganz catheters) and patient factors (shock at admission, immunosuppression, and renal insufficiency) to be strongly correlated with the ultimate development of a nosocomial infection. The length of stay in the intensive care unit was another entity associated with nosocomial infection, independent of use of devices. (*See textbook page* 1075.)

3. **B.**   Various aspects of intensive care unit design have been attempted in an effort to reduce the bacterial transmission rate in nosocomial infections, including air filters, positive- and negative-pressure rooms, laminar flow environments, and individual room temperature and humidity controls. However, all of these have had an inconsistent effect on nosocomial infection rates. On the other hand, handwashing by health care workers has clearly been shown to be effective at reducing transmission of bacteria. (*See textbook pages* 1075, 1076.)

4. **A.**   *C. difficile* causes pseudomembranous colitis, which can be a severe problem and is associated with increased morbidity and costs. The colitis is produced by exotoxins elaborated by the organism. Although this condition commonly is associated with clindamycin use, nearly all antibiotics have been found to be capable of altering the colonic flora sufficiently to allow *C. difficile* to emerge. Oral vancomycin or oral metronidazole is effective treatment, although prophylactic use of these agents does not prevent infection. Handwashing is not effective at removing the organism from the hands of health care workers who care for patients with pseudomembranous colitis; most such personnel have positive hand cultures. Only the use of vinyl gloves by health care personnel has been shown to be effective at limiting the spread of the organism from patient to patient. (*See textbook page* 1079.)

Chapter 85

1. **B.**   The most common bacterial cause of meningitis among older children and young adults is *N. meningitidis* infection. This organism is a relatively uncommon cause of meningitis among those older than 45 years. *H. influenzae* had been the most common cause of bacterial meningitis among children between the ages of 3 months and 6 years until the introduction of new vaccines reduced the incidence among that age group. Among adults *Strep. pneumoniae* is the most common cause. *L. monocytogenes* is more common among neonates and immunologically compromised persons. *S. aureus* meningitis is less common, occurring primarily among patients undergoing neurosurgical procedures or sustaining head trauma. (*See textbook pages* 1081, 1082.)

2. **E.**   Although extremely low, CSF glucose levels (e.g., >20 mg/dL) provide strong evidence of bacterial infection, a normal level does not exclude the possibility—13% to 40% of patients with bacterial meningitis have normal CSF glucose levels. Aztreonam can achieve bactericidal concentrations in the presence of inflamed meninges; however, clinical experience with it in the management of meningitis is limited. It provides no coverage against *Strep. pneumoniae,* a frequent causative agent of bacterial meningitis. Therefore, aztreonam should not be used as an initial empiric agent for the management of meningitis. Dexamethasone may be useful in the treatment of adult patients with very severe forms of bacterial meningitis and potentially for all children with meningitis. Among children, the use of dexamethasone has been shown to improve cerebral perfusion pressure and reduce the incidence of subsequent neurologic abnormalities. In general, patients who contract meningitis with CSF shunts or intracranial pressure monitoring devices in place should have such devices removed. On occasion, however, removal of these devices would severely adversely affect the patient's outcome, and treatment without removal, effective among nearly 30% of patients, can be attempted. Respiratory isolation until 24 hours after the initiation of antibiotic therapy is recommended for patients with bacterial meningitis due to *N. meningitidis* or *H. influenzae* because the disease is highly contagious. (*See textbook pages* 1083, 1085.)

3. **D.**   Confirming the diagnosis of HSE can be difficult because the evidence often is indirect or difficult to demonstrate consistently. The most reliable and definitive method of establishing the diagnosis is through demonstration of viral antigen or recovery of virus during biopsy of the brain. The detection of antibodies to herpes simplex in blood is unreliable for the diagnosis of HSE because a positive serologic result at the onset of the disease is 70% in both biopsy-positive and biopsy-negative cases. Even CSF antibody determination is imperfect, because this technique may be insensitive during the first week of the illness. Anatomic techniques such as electroencephalography, computed tomography, and magnetic resonance imaging have been attempted to demonstrate the focus of the disease, although these are imperfectly sensitive and specific tests. (*See textbook page* 1087.)

Chapter 86

1. **C.**   The patient has classic signs of acute bacterial endocarditis. Because he is a man and a user of intravenous drug, the patient is in a high-risk category for the condition. The physical findings of a regurgitant murmur and evidence of embolization (petechiae, splinter hemorrhages, cerebral infarction, and impaired renal function) should provoke an evaluation of the heart valves as the source of the emboli. The distribution of the petechiae in bacterial endocarditis tends to be different from that seen in thrombocytopenia, with a greater predilection for the plantar surfaces of the toes and fingers and the buccal and conjunctival mucosa. The presence of fever and positive blood cultures make the diagnosis of bacterial endocarditis highly likely. The finding that *Strep. bovis* is the organism responsible, should alert the physician to the possibility of a malignant gastrointestinal tumor because of the high association rate of this organism with benign and malignant gastrointestinal growths. The malignant growth actually may be identified months to years after the episode of bacteremia.(*See textbook page* 1093.)

2. **B.**   Bacterial endocarditis can be produced by any organism. However, most cases require a preexisting congenital or acquired heart valve abnormality to establish a nidus for the infectious process. Still, *S. aureus* is particularly virulent and appears to be able to infect even previously normal heart valves. *S. aureus* can account for up to one-half the cases of bacterial endocarditis in some series.

Gram-negative bacilli, especially those in the HACEK (*Haemophilus* species, *Actinobacillus actinomycetem comitans, Cardiobacterium hominis, Eikenella corrodens, Kingella kingae*) are an increasingly recognized cause of infective endocarditis. However, these organisms rarely cause endocarditis among patients without pre-existing valve disease or in the absence of predisposing factors. Pneumococci are relatively uncommon as causative agents of bacterial endocarditis. Endocarditis due to *Candida* species can be particularly difficult to diagnose, because blood cultures frequently may be negative despite the presence of the disease. (*See textbook pages* 1092–1094.)

3. **D.** Although bacterial endocarditis of any valve is a serious problem, aortic valve infections have the worst prognosis. Aortic insufficiency is more poorly tolerated by the heart than insufficiencies of the other valves. With erosion of a sinus of Valsalva aneurysm into the pericardium or right atrium, pericardial tamponade or a large left-to-right shunt may develop. Invasion by the aortic abscess into the conducting system can produce heart block. Vegetations on the aortic valve also can be easily dislodged into the coronary arteries, easily producing an infarction for the overstressed left ventricle. (*See textbook page* 1094.)

4. **C.** Patients with bacterial endocarditis can have a variety of clinical findings related to embolization of valvular vegetation material. The lesion described is an Osler's node. Janeway lesions are similar, although they are painless and commonly involve the palms and soles. Roth spots are a pale area within a retinal hemorrhage. Splinter hemorrhages are linear hemorrhages under the nail bed. (*See textbook pages* 1095, 1096.)

5. **B.** Studies have demonstrated that 99.3% of all septic episodes are detected with the first two blood cultures. Some rare cases can appear to be culture-negative and should provoke involvement by a clinical microbiologist for special growth conditions. Fungal forms often can be culture-negative on multiple repeated samples; cultures are positive among only 50% of patients with *Candida* endocarditis. (*See textbook page* 1096.)

Chapter 87

1. **C.** Several techniques have been used in an effort to reduce the ultimate incidence of infections caused by intravascular catheter insertion. In one study, chlorhexidine was shown to be more effective than alcohol or povidone-iodine at reducing the incidence of catheter-associated infection and bacteremia. This effectiveness may be the result of greater persistence of the antiseptic effect known to exist with chlorhexidine. Prophylactic administration of intravenous antibiotics has not been definitively shown to be effective at preventing infections caused by use of intravascular catheters. (*See textbook page* 1111.)

2. **E.** Proper maintenance of an indwelling intravascular catheter is an area in which knowledge is still incomplete. Several factors have been evaluated as to their potential role in preventing or promoting catheter-related sepsis. Many institutions have used transparent, semipermeable polyurethane dressings rather than traditional gauze dressings. Although they can allow for better monitoring of the appearance of the insertion site, these transparent dressings may trap moisture and actually may be associated with higher infection rates than for gauze dressings. Several antiseptic ointments have been evaluated with respect to ability to minimize catheter infection rates, and use of these agents often is considered standard practice. However, evidence of a statistically significant rate of effectiveness of these ointments at reducing the rate of catheter-associated infection is not overwhelming. Although initial recommendations were to change every 24 hours,

infusion sets associated with long-term use of indwelling catheters, subsequent studies showed that in many circumstances, such sets can be left in place for as long as 72 hours with no discernible effect on the rate of catheter-associated infection. Use of central catheters carries a risk from new insertion as well as from infection. The relative risks of catheter placement versus those of catheter infection are not known with certainty. One large study did not detect a difference in rates of infection between catheters changed to a new site every 7 days, those changed over a guide wire every 7 days, and those not changed on a scheduled basis. Therefore, no firm recommendations for routine rotation of central catheters currently exist. (*See textbook pages* 1111, 1112.)

3. **B.**   In most series, coagulase-negative staphylococci are the organisms most commonly associated with catheter-related infections, although other organisms certainly can be isolated. In particular, *Candida* and *Malassezia* species are the organisms most commonly associated with infections of total parenteral nutrition catheters. Many arterial catheters can be infected even though they have an innocuous clinical appearance. Excision of the vein has been advocated in the care of patients with suppurative thrombophlebitis in which gross purulence is present or sepsis persists despite adequate antibiotic treatment. Removal of the offending catheter is almost always necessary to eliminate the infection, although there is substantial controversy regarding the nature and duration of any accompanying antibiotic regimen. (*See textbook pages* 1110, 1112, 1113.)

Chapter 88

1. **A.**   The main risk factor for UTI is the presence of an indwelling urinary catheter. Therefore, removal of the catheter can by itself eliminate the presence of a UTI among as many as 70% of patients treated. Because of the persistent source of barrier violation provided by the catheter, initially low bacterial colony counts progress to high-grade bacteriuria in most patients unless suppressive antimicrobial therapy is provided. The presence of high-grade bacteriuria does not confirm the presence of bacterial infection, however. Although more than than 10^5 CFU/mL of urine indicates that the urinary bladder is colonized with a large number of bacteria and that active UTI is likely, a smaller number does not exclude the possibility in a patient who has a catheter. Polymicrobial bacteriuria occurs among a large number of patients with catheter-related UTI. (*See textbook pages* 1121, 1123, 1124.)

2. **B.**   Because the urinary catheter represents the main risk factor toward the development of a catheter-related UTI, avoidance of catheterization whenever possible is the best means of preventing such infections. The use of condom catheters may be beneficial to many patients, although problems with use of these devices (kinking, leakage, or penile maceration) may lead to other problems, and use of condom catheters may not appreciably reduce risk for UTI among many patients. Topical antimicrobial agents applied to the urethral meatus have not been shown to provide effective prophylaxis of catheter-associated UTI. Alternative catheter design or manufacture, as with siliconized materials rather than latex, has not yet been shown to be effective at significantly reducing the incidence of catheter-related UTI. Although systemic antimicrobial prophylaxis may reduce the incidence of symptomatic bacteriuria, especially among patients who have a catheter in place for only a short time, the subsequent development of widespread antibiotic resistance limits the utility of this preventive measure. (*See textbook pages* 1122, 1124.)

3. **B.**   *Candida* species are normal inhabitants of the vaginal tract and therefore may merely be contaminants of a urine specimen. Moreover, *Candida* species frequently colonize the urinary tract without causing invasive infection. Therefore,

the finding of *Candida* in a urine sample is not an indication of invasive candidiasis. However, the presence of urinary casts made up of *Candida* organisms does indicate invasive upper-tract candidiasis. Fungus ball formation from *Candida* species is associated with ascending candidal infection and warrants systemic amphotericin B therapy. Fluconazole often is effective therapy for *Candida* cystitis. Bladder irrigation for 2 days with 50 mg amphotericin B in 1,000 mL of sterile water also is safe, effective, and nontoxic in eradicating *Candida* infection of the bladder. (*See textbook pages* 1124, 1125.)

Chapter 89

1. **C.** Toxic shock syndrome presents a dramatic and distinct syndrome similar to only a few other diseases. The primary clinical hallmarks of fever, rash, orthostatic hypotension, and systemic signs of toxicity are mimicked by a few conditions. These include Rocky Mountain spotted fever, meningococcemia, streptococcal and staphylococcal scarlet fever, leptospirosis, rubeola, and rash-associated viral infections. Conditions such as acute pelvic inflammatory disease can produce severe illness, fever, and toxicity, although a rash is not a common finding, and evidence of pelvic inflammation should be detectable at physical examination. Therefore pelvic inflammatory disease should not be included in the typical differential diagnosis of toxic shock syndrome. (*See textbook page* 1128.)

2. **C.** The etiologic organism of Rocky Mountain spotted fever is *Rickettsia rickettsii,* an obligate intracellular bacterium. Lacking a typical bacterial cell wall, it is not affected by β-lactam agents, such as penicillin, aztreonam, ceftazidime, or imipenem. Rather, specific treatment is the use of tetracycline or doxycycline. Chloramphenicol is an alternative drug for those unable to take tetracyclines. (*See textbook page* 1131.)

3. **D.** Although all parts of the immune system are important barriers to infection, the complement system provides the most important defense against meningococcal infection. Patients with deficiencies of a single late complement component are at 7,000 to 10,000 fold greater risk for meningococcal infection than those with an intact complement system. (*See textbook page* 1131.)

4. **C.** Accepted therapies for chloroquine-resistant *Plasmodium falciparum* malaria are quinine sulfate, quinidine sulfate, mefloquine, and halofantrine. Recommended second agents in these cases include pyrimethamine-sulfadoxine, tetracycline, doxycycline, and clindamycin. Use of tetracycline derivatives is contraindicated during pregnancy and in the treatment of children younger than 8 years. Fever and chills are the classic presenting symptoms; fever is present among 54% to 73% of patients when they come to medical attention. The diagnosis is established by means of review of the peripheral blood smear, including both thick and thin smears. The Middle East and Central America are the only endemic areas that do not show high rates of chloroquine resistance. The most fearsome complication of malaria is the development of cerebral malaria. This condition produces hemiparesis, seizure disorder, blindness, or spasticity among 6% to 50% of children who contract it. (*See textbook pages* 1135, 1136.)

Chapter 90

1. **A.** *P. carinii* infection is associated with defects in cell-mediated immunity. Defects in cell-mediated immunity include abnormalities in T cells, such as cytotoxic killer T cells, and macrophages. Such defects usually are associated with infections with viruses, protozoa, fungi, helminths, mycobacteria, and intra-

cellular bacteria. *P. carinii* is a protozoan that commonly produces infections in patients with cell-mediated immunity, such as those infected with human immunodeficiency virus 1. Infection due to extracellular bacteria such as *Strep. pneumoniae, H. influenzae, N. meningitidis,* and *Ps. aeruginosa* may occur among patients with altered humoral immunity (deficient B-cell lymphocyte function and antibody production). (*See textbook page* 1143.)

2. **C.**   Although bacteremia can have a number of different sources, in many cases an obvious infection can be established. For example, the presence of white cells and bacteria in the urine or endotracheal secretions can establish the urinary tract or the lungs as a source of bacteremia. However, among immunocompromised patients, bacteremia without an obvious source usually originates in the gastrointestinal tract. Chemotherapy and neutropenia appear capable of producing a breakdown in the normal intestinal mucosal barrier to bacterial invasion. Most of the breaches in the barrier may be clinically undetectable. Some that may be clinically apparent, however, include typhlitis, anorectal cellulitis or abscess formation, pseudomembranous colitis, and necrotizing colitis. (*See textbook page* 1144.)

3. **D.**   Because a patient with neutropenia has little in the way of endogenous antibacterial defenses, antibiotic coverage must be sufficiently broad to cover all possible offending organisms when their precise identity and sensitivity are unknown. Of the combinations listed, only clindamycin and vancomycin stand out as being deficient because that combination lacks effective gram-negative coverage. All the other combinations and imipenem alone represent a sufficient breadth of coverage for empiric antibiotic treatment of a patient with a fever and neutropenia. (*See textbook page* 1145.)

Chapter 91

1. **B.**   Therapy with 40 mg prednisone twice a day should be initiated in the care of patients with moderate or severe PCP. The percentage of HIV-related deaths attributable to PCP decreased from 32.5% to 13.8% during the period from 1987 to 1992. The yield of sputum induction for the diagnosis of PCP generally is thought to be 50% to 80%, although reports vary widely. Serum lactate dehydrogenase levels are elevated in more than 90% of cases. (*See textbook pages* 1151–1153.)

2. **A.**   In two retrospective analyses of patients with HIV infection admitted to the hospital with respiratory illnesses, bacterial pneumonia was the most common diagnosis, and most of the patients were users of injected drugs. Although HIV targets the cell-mediated immune system, qualitative and functional defects in helper T cells also impair humoral immunity and predispose the patient to infection with encapsulated organisms such as *Streptococcus pneumoniae* and *Haemophilus influenzae*. The incidence of bacterial pneumonia may be reduced among patients who take trimethoprim-sulfamethoxazole prophylaxis of PCP. (*See textbook page* 1154.)

Chapter 92

1. **A.**   Endocarditis in a patient who abuses parenteral drugs is different from endocarditis in a person who is not a drug abuser in that the underlying valve does not have to be diseased. Another likely consequence of the frequent peripheral venous accesses made by drug users is that the tricuspid valve is more commonly involved; left-sided valves are more commonly involved in persons who are not abusers of drugs. Because of the right-sided nature of tricuspid endocarditis, the

typical stigmata of other forms of endocarditis, such as Osler's nodes, Janeway lesions, and Roth spots, are rarely observed. Rather, multiple patchy infiltrates can be seen on a chest radiograph, suggesting multiple pulmonary emboli more consistent with tricuspid disease. Left-sided endocarditis can occur among persons addicted to drugs and may accompany tricuspid endocarditis. Such patients often have a history of underlying heart disease. (*See textbook page* 1166.)

2. C. Hepatitis B remains a principal pathogen responsible for hospital admissions among drug users in the United States. Estimates consider 60% to 80% of users of parenteral drugs to be infected with hepatitis B and 10% to be chronic carriers. Hepatitis C also is highly prevalent among drug users; some surveys have found as many as 83% of drug users to be infected. Hepatitis B, however, tends to cause fulminant acute disease more often, whereas hepatitis C is more likely to lead to chronic liver disease. Hepatitis A has also been documented as a cause of acute hepatitis among users who inject their drugs. (*See textbook page* 1168.)

3. E. Several pulmonary complications occur frequently among abusers of intravenous drugs. Acute pulmonary edema is commonly seen as a result of drug injection, but it is not usually infectious in nature and clears within 24 to 48 hours. Unilateral bacterial pneumonia can develop as a result of exposure to pathogens in the community. Septic pulmonary emboli may arise as a result of bacterial endocarditis of the tricuspid valve, although they may occasionally develop as a result of mycotic aneurysms in the peripheral circulation. In a study involving abusers of intravenous drugs, approximately 10% were found to have tuberculosis. A strange finding, however, was that pulmonary infections related to AIDS were not common in that study. (*See textbook page* 1169.)

Chapter 93

1. B. Until recently, tuberculosis appeared to be becoming so infrequent that the practice of routine screening for tuberculosis among health care workers was being increasingly questioned. However, the decline in the incidence of tuberculosis that had been apparent in previous decades ended in 1984. From 1985 through 1992 the number of new cases of tuberculosis increased each year. The main influences on this transition appear to be increased immigration into the United States, the HIV epidemic, and a deterioration in the health care delivery infrastructure marked by a reduction in the funding of tuberculosis control programs. The incidence of multidrug-resistant tuberculosis also has increased. Fortunately, annual decreases in tuberculosis morbidity resumed in 1993. (*See textbook page* 1172.)

2. B. The central nervous system manifestations of tuberculosis include tuberculous meningitis and tuberculoma. Typical spinal fluid analysis reveals lymphocytic pleocytosis, low glucose concentration, and elevated protein level. However, none of these findings is absolute, because tuberculous meningitis can have a polymorphonuclear predominance, an elevated glucose concentration, or a low protein concentration. Acid-fast bacilli can be detected in cerebrospinal fluid, although it appears that the likelihood of detection is increased if multiple spinal taps are performed (e.g., up to 87% with four spinal taps). Tuberculoma of the central nervous system can be readily detected with either computed tomography or magnetic resonance imaging. (*See textbook pages* 1176, 1177.)

3. E. Drugs commonly used in the management of tuberculosis include isoniazid, streptomycin, ethambutol, rifampin, and pyrazinamide. However, it is important to realize that several commonly used antibiotics also possess activity against *M. tuberculosis.* In addition to streptomycin, other aminoglycosides, such as gentamicin and amikacin, can ameliorate a course of tuberculosis. Fluoroquinolones, such as ciprofloxacin and ofloxacin, also possess antituberculous activity. (*See textbook pages* 1178, 1179.)

Chapter 94

1. **C.**   The spores of *C. botulinum* are highly heat resistant, able to survive boiling for hours. Yet their germination conditions require a favorable environment. An anaerobic environment is essential, because oxygen inhibits growth. Other conditions include adequate water and nutrients, a high pH (>4.6), a reasonable temperature (although very cold, nonfreezing temperatures can be tolerated), and a lack of inhibitory substances for growth. (*See textbook page* 1184.)

2. **E.**   The site of action of the potent neurotoxin produced by *C. botulinum* is the neuromuscular junction. The neurotoxin appears to inhibit the release of acetylcholine by the nerve cell at the cholinergic synapses. The toxin does not act centrally, nor does it act on adrenergic nerves. The toxin is distributed by the lymphatic and circulatory systems to the neuromuscular junctions. It usually is absorbed from the small intestine, although it may arise from growth of *C. botulinum* within a wound. (*See textbook page* 1184.)

3. **B.**   Because botulism interferes with muscle activity, measurements of ventilatory muscle strength and activity are better suited to monitor the clinical progress of the disease. For this reason, vital capacity is the most sensitive of the indices listed. When vital capacity drops to 30% of the patient's predicted value, intubation and mechanical ventilation are prudent. The respiratory rate also may be sensitive for respiratory muscle fatigue, although it is less specific. Because the lung is not the primary site of action of the toxin, gas exchange may be relatively unimpaired initially, and therefore arterial blood gas analysis is not as sensitive an indicator as vital capacity. (*See textbook page* 1186.)

Chapter 95

1. **E.**   All of these complications occur. Headaches, muscle aches, muscular rigidity including trismus, and respiratory and urinary infections also may occur. (*See textbook page* 1187.)

2. **E.**   Effective ventilatory support is key to the management of generalized tetanus. Sedatives such as diazepam often are useful to produce adequate sedation and prevent seizures. Pain from excessive contractures should be relieved with narcotic agents such as meperidine. Drugs such as baclofen administered intrathecally may reduce muscle contractures. Excess sympathetic activity should be managed with a β-blocker, such as propranolol. The use of antibiotics such as penicillin to specifically target the causative organism usually is of little value. Most often, there is a wound site of probable entry of the organism, and this area should be surgically opened, débrided, and cleansed as primary treatment against the infection itself. In rare instances in which there is no obvious portal of entry of the organism, empiric penicillin administration may be attempted, although there is no evidence that such an approach is effective. (*See textbook page* 1188.)

3. **C.**   Patients with tetanus should receive 500 units of human tetanus immune globulin by means of intramuscular injection as soon as the diagnosis of tetanus is made. Larger doses or repeated doses are of no value. Immunization with tetanus toxoid should be simultaneously started intramuscularly at another site. The use of antibiotics is of little value, because the most beneficial antiinfective therapy is effective débridement of the wound that served as the portal of entry of the organism. (*See textbook page* 1188.)

VII. Gastrointestinal and Hepatobiliary Problems in the Intensive Care Unit

96. Gastrointestinal Bleeding: Principles of Diagnosis and Management

Select the best answer

1. Which of the following statements regarding gastric lavage for a patient with upper gastrointestinal bleeding is *true*?

    A. Gastrointestinal lavage through a nasogastric tube often is essential in stopping upper gastrointestinal hemorrhage.
    B. Gastric lavage with iced saline solution prolongs bleeding time.
    C. Gastric lavage is necessary for endoscopic visualization of the bleeding lesion.
    D. The gastric vasoconstriction produced by ice-water lavage helps to stop active bleeding.
    E. None of the above.

2. Which of the following statements regarding inhibition of gastric acid production during acute upper gastrointestinal hemorrhage is *true*?

    A. Use of H2-receptor antagonists can stop or prevent rebleeding.
    B. Use of omeprazole can reduce transfusion requirements.
    C. Ulcers that are found to be actively bleeding during endoscopy should be managed with omeprazole.
    D. Prescribing patterns suggest that H2-receptor antagonists are administered primarily to stop bleeding rather than to manage peptic ulcer disease.
    E. H2-receptor antagonism is effective during acute upper gastrointestinal bleeding episodes because blood clots poorly in an acid medium.

3. Which of the following endoscopic findings carries the greatest risk for continued bleeding or rebleeding from gastric or duodenal ulcers?

    A. Oozing
    B. Nonbleeding visible vessel
    C. Arterial bleeding
    D. Flat, pigmented spot
    E. Adherent clot

97. *Stress Ulcer Syndrome*

Select the best answer

1. Endoscopic features used to differentiate stress ulcers from chronic peptic ulcers include:

    A. Multiple lesions
    B. Little surrounding inflammation
    C. Proximal location in the stomach
    D. Infrequent duodenal location
    E. All of the above

2. Which of the following conditions is considered a potential complication of stress ulcer prophylaxis with H2-receptor antagonists?

    A. Urinary tract infection
    B. Acidosis
    C. Gram-negative nosocomial pneumonia
    D. Coagulopathy
    E. Alkalosis

3. Which of the following choices is the best regimen to use in attempting to prevent stress gastritis?

    A. Antacids
    B. H2-receptor antagonists
    C. Sucralfate
    D. All of the above in combination
    E. None of the above

98. *Variceal Bleeding*

Select the best answer

1. What percentage of patients with cirrhosis who have varices eventually have bleeding variceal bleeding?

    A. 10%
    B. 20%
    C. 50%
    D. 70%
    E. 90%

2. Which of the following is *not* an adverse effect of the use of vasopressin?

    A. Arterial hypotension
    B. Myocardial ischemia
    C. Electrolyte abnormalities
    D. Congestive heart failure

3. The best initial treatment of a patient with acutely bleeding esophageal varices is:

    A. Placement of a Sengstaken-Blakemore tube
    B. Insertion of a distal splenorenal shunt
    C. Endoscopic sclerotherapy or band ligation

D. Placement of a Linton-Nachlas tube
E. Performance of a Sugiura procedure

---

99. *Intestinal Pseudoobstruction (Ileus)*

Select the best answer

1. In a patient with possible intestinal pseudoobstruction, the most useful clue to the presence of hollow visceral disease is:

   A. Whether nausea is present
   B. Whether diarrhea is present
   C. The frequency of urination
   D. Whether constipation is a problem
   E. Whether frequent belching occurs

2. Which of the following intestinal segments returns motility most quickly after laparotomy?

   A. Stomach
   B. Cecum
   C. Rectum
   D. Small intestine
   E. Colon

3. Which of the following agents is most likely to improve intestinal motility in cases of paralytic ileus?

   A. Naloxone
   B. Erythromycin
   C. Simethicone
   D. Rectal suppositories
   E. Atropine

---

100. *Fulminant Colitis and Toxic Megacolon*

Select the best answer

1. Which of the following conditions is the greatest risk factor for mortality in toxic megacolon?

   A. Bleeding
   B. Ileus
   C. Diarrhea
   D. Fluid sequestration
   E. Perforation

2. Reasons that may justify the use of corticosteroids in the treatment of patients with toxic megacolon include the following:

   A. Parenteral corticosteroids are accepted therapies for Crohn's colitis and ulcerative colitis, and a many patients with toxic megacolon have one of these diseases.
   B. Most patients with toxic megacolon were receiving steroids before the condition developed, and augmented steroid dosing may be necessary for the additional stress.

    C. Use of steroids may reduce mortality and the need for surgical intervention.
    D. All of the above.
    E. None of the above.

3. Which of the following are indications for emergency surgical treatment of patients with toxic megacolon?

    A. Perforation
    B. Septic shock
    C. Colon diameter greater than 12 cm
    D. All of the above
    E. None of the above

101. Evaluation and Management of Liver Failure

Select the best answer

1. Which of the following statements regarding fulminant hepatic failure is *true*?

    A. Higher survival rates have been quoted for patients with fulminant hepatic failure caused by hepatitis C.
    B. The single most important predictor of outcome is the degree of encephalopathy.
    C. Sepsis is rarely a cause of mortality after liver transplantation for fulminant hepatic failure.
    D. Survival rates for patients with fulminant hepatic failure without transplantation are excellent.
    E. Identification of the cause of fulminant hepatic failure is rarely important for clinical management.

2. In fulminant hepatic failure, the most sensitive method for detecting the presence of elevated intracranial pressure is:

    A. The neurologic examination
    B. Computed tomography
    C. The grade of encephalopathy
    D. Routine clinical examination
    E. Intracranial pressure monitoring

3. Renal failure in fulminant hepatic failure:

    A. Is a marker of a poor prognosis
    B. Occurs among only 25% of patients with liver failure due to acetaminophen toxicity
    C. Occurs among 60% of patients with fulminant hepatic failure of other causes
    D. Cannot be managed with continuous forms of dialysis
    E. Is rarely caused by intravascular volume depletion

102. Diarrhea

Select the best answer

1. The most common nonhemorrhagic gastrointestinal complication in the intensive care unit is:

A. Acalculous cholecystitis
B. Diarrhea
C. Hepatitis
D. Constipation
E. Intolerance of enteral feedings

2. Which of the following drugs may promote the development of antibiotic-associated (pseudomembranous) colitis?

   A. Clindamycin
   B. Metronidazole
   C. Ampicillin
   D. Vancomycin
   E. All of the above

3. The most important early step in the treatment of patients with diarrhea of any type is:

   A. Prompt diagnostic sigmoidoscopy
   B. Empiric administration of oral vancomycin
   C. Empiric administration of oral metronidazole
   D. Discontinuation of enteral feedings
   E. Correction of fluid and electrolyte abnormalities

103. Severe and Complicated Biliary Tract Disease

Select the best answer

1. Which of the following studies are preferable in the initial evaluation of critically ill patients with suspected biliary tract disease?

   A. Endoscopic retrograde cholangiopancreatography
   B. Hepatobiliary scan
   C. Computed tomography
   D. Abdominal ultrasonography
   E. Percutaneous transhepatic cholangiography

2. A 52-year-old man has the findings of fever, chills, jaundice, and right upper quadrant abdominal pain. His serum bilirubin level is 6.3 mg/dL, 5.2 mg/dL being conjugated. A technetium Tc 99m iminodiacetic acid (HIDA) scan demonstrates a lack of drainage into the small intestine, although a trickle of flow was detected on delayed images. Initial treatment should consist of:

   A. Oral lactulose and neomycin
   B. Intravenous fluid resuscitation and broad-spectrum antibiotics
   C. Monoclonal antibodies to endotoxin
   D. Cholestyramine
   E. Intravenous heparin

3. After 6 hours of appropriate initial treatment, the patient described in question 2 remains febrile, with evidence of worsening renal and respiratory function. What should be done at this time?

A. A pulmonologist should be consulted to help manage the respiratory failure.
B. A nephrologist should be consulted regarding the possibility of impending acute renal failure.
C. Plans should be made for biliary lithotripsy.
D. The patient should undergo emergency biliary decompression.
E. A pulmonary arterial balloon flotation catheter should be inserted to more effectively manage the resuscitation effort.

104. Complications of Gastrointestinal Procedures

Select the best answer

1. Which of the following statements regarding conscious sedation is *true*?

   A. Midazolam is more likely to produce cardiopulmonary complications than is diazepam.
   B. Patients with chronic obstructive pulmonary disease are more likely to experience respiratory depression during endoscopy than are patients without such a condition.
   C. The presence of the endoscope in the hypopharynx is the most important factor contributing to hypoxemia during endoscopy.
   D. Anaphylaxis due to exposure to contrast material during endoscopic retrograde cholangiopancreatography is common.
   E. Allergy to sedative or narcotic premedication during endoscopy is not infrequent.

2. For patients who may have sustained an overdose of benzodiazepines during conscious sedation for a procedure, an agent that can reverse the oversedation is:

   A. Lorazepam
   B. Naloxone
   C. Dextrose
   D. Flumazenil
   E. Atropine

3. Which of the following findings during or after colonoscopic polypectomy mandate surgical management?

   A. Localized abdominal pain
   B. Tachycardia
   C. Guarding
   D. Visualization of the peritoneal cavity during colonoscopy
   E. Free intraperitoneal air

105. Hepatic Dysfunction

Select the best answer

1. The most striking abnormality observed that differentiates ischemic hepatitis from other forms of liver dysfunction that occur among the critically ill is:

A. A marked rise in serum bilirubin level

B. A marked rise in serum alkaline phosphatase level

C. A marked rise in serum aspartate aminotransferase (AST) and alanine aminotransferase (ALT) levels

D. An extended period of impaired synthetic function, marked by prolongation of prothrombin time, even after other markers have normalized

E. A marked rise in unconjugated bilirubin

2. Which of the following statements regarding hepatic function during total parenteral nutrition (TPN) is *true*?

A. Abnormalities in liver function tests occur among approximately one third of patients receiving TPN for 2 weeks or longer.

B. The most common abnormalities in liver function test results are coagulation abnormalities.

C. Liver biopsy demonstrates findings consistent with cirrhosis.

D. After 6 or more weeks of TPN, biliary sludge can form and cause acalculous cholecystitis or even cholelithiasis.

E. There is no benefit to enteral feeding if the patient is already receiving TPN.

3. Which of the following statements regarding sepsis-induced liver dysfunction is *not true*?

A. Between 15% and 20% of patients with bacteremia have abnormalities of liver function tests.

B. Hepatomegaly is absent in as many as one half of patients.

C. Serum bilirubin is typically elevated into the range of 5 to 10 mg/dL.

D. Clotting function often is preserved.

E. Chemical markers of liver function return to normal in 1 to 2 weeks.

Answers

Chapter 96

1. **B.** Although nasogastric lavage is frequently used, the absolute value of this procedure has never been substantiated. Among patients who do not have hematemesis or melena, a nasogastric tube may be helpful in confirming the presence of upper gastrointestinal hemorrhage. Although it may appear that nasogastric lavage would be helpful in clearing clots and thus facilitate visualization during endoscopy, many gastroenterologists do not consider it necessary. There also is the possibility that the tube might produce suction artifacts that produce confusion for the endoscopist. Contrary to common belief, iced saline lavage does not help slow upper gastrointestinal bleeding. Rather, iced saline lavage prolongs bleeding time, increases clotting time, and prolongs bleeding from ulcers. (*See textbook page* 1191.)

2. **D.** Although prescribing patterns for H2-receptor antagonists suggest that these drugs are administered in an effort to stop acute upper gastrointestinal bleeding, there is little clinical or scientific evidence to support this practice. Although it is true that blood clots poorly in an acid environment, it has not been shown that inhibition of acid production in a patient with an acutely bleeding ulcer slows the rate of bleeding, changes transfusion requirements, or affects the operative or mortality rates. This inability to see a beneficial effect from acid inhibition during an acute bleeding episode might occur because the neutralizing effect of blood itself may diminish any further beneficial effect produced by drugs or antacids. Therapy directed at reducing gastric acidity may be helpful in healing an ulcer,

but it is difficult to demonstrate that such therapy stops bleeding or prevents rebleeding. Omeprazole was found to be ineffective in the care of patients with ulcers that are actively bleeding or oozing. (*See textbook pages* 1191, 1192.)

3. C.   Several endoscopic findings can be associated with upper gastrointestinal bleeding from gastric or duodenal ulcers. Some, such as the presence of oozing, an adherent clot, a clean ulcer base, or a flat, pigmented spot are associated with relatively low (<25%) incidences of continued bleeding or rebleeding. However, a visible blood vessel in the ulcer crater is associated with rebleeding 40% to 50% of the time, even though it may not be actively bleeding at the time of endoscopy. The endoscopic finding of active arterial bleeding is most highly associated with persistent or recurrent rebleeding, which was present among 90% of patients with the finding. (*See textbook page* 1192.)

Chapter 97

1. E.   Stress ulceration can have a typical endoscopic appearance that is quite distinct from that associated with chronic peptic ulcers. Because stress ulcers usually occur in association with a more acutely stressful state, they do not have many of the stigmata of chronicity that occur with chronic peptic ulceration. Often more than 10 lesions are found at endoscopy. They tend to appear more in the proximal stomach, rather than in the distal antrum and duodenum, as is true of peptic ulcer disease. The histologic appearance of stress ulcers is minimal inflammatory cell infiltrate in contrast to the marked inflammation that occurs with chronic peptic disease. This histologic finding is consistent with the acutely ischemic nature of the stress gastritis process. (*See textbook pages* 1195, 1196.)

2. C.   Although the issue is quite controversial, there is a great deal of concern that stress ulcer prophylaxis with H2-receptor antagonists may predispose patients to gram-negative nosocomial pneumonia. This complication would presumably not be an issue if sucralfate were to be used. The presence of an acid stomach appears to inhibit all organisms from growing in large concentrations. However, when gastric pH is neutral, it appears that gram-negative organisms have some survival advantage over gram-positive organisms. These organisms are thought to have a causal role in the development of pneumonia. Studies have yielded conflicting results regarding the effect of stress ulcer prophylaxis on risk for pneumonia. Even metaanalyses have come to different conclusions on this topic. Therefore, the relation between pneumonia and stress ulcer prophylaxis with H2-receptor antagonists must be clarified before a firm recommendation can be made favoring one method of prophylaxis over another. (*See textbook pages* 1197, 1198.)

3. E.   At the current time, no one method for preventing stress gastritis appears to have any advantage over any other. Combinations of agents appear to provide no appreciable added benefit. The combination of sucralfate with agents that increase gastric pH is particularly unsound, in that sucralfate requires a pH less than 4.5 for effective activity. Thus no specific recommendations for the choice of a prophylactic agent can be made at this time. (*See textbook pages* 1198, 1199.)

Chapter 98

1. B.   Upper gastrointestinal bleeding develops in at least 20% of all patients with cirrhosis that leads to varices. (*See textbook page* 1200).

2. B.   Vasopressin is normally produced by the posterior pituitary gland in the regulation of the body's water balance (antidiuretic hormone). It also acts as a potent vasoconstrictor and can reduce portal venous blood flow. It may be useful in the management of acute gastroesophageal variceal bleeding due to portal hypertension, although there is a great deal of controversy over the absolute utility of this approach. Because the vasoconstriction that vasopressin produces is nonselective, it can constrict the vessels and impair tissue perfusion to other vital organs besides the gastrointestinal tract, such as the heart and brain. Therefore, its use is contraindicated in the treatment of patients with preexisting conditions that impair circulatory oxygen delivery, such as severe peripheral vascular disease and coronary artery disease. Use of vasopressin may cause hypertension, myocardial ischemia, electrolyte abnormalities, and congestive heart failure. (*See textbook page* 1202).

3. C. Most patients with variceal bleeding stop bleeding spontaneously, and only supportive care is necessary. In cases of severe or persistent bleeding, endoscopic visualization usually is necessary to determine the cause of the gastrointestinal hemorrhage. Not all patients with varices who have acute upper gastrointestinal bleeding are actually bleeding from the varices. If variceal bleeding is found, sclerotherapy is effective for many patients. Studies have found band ligation to be equal or superior to sclerotherapy. Placement of a Sengstaken-Blakemore (or Minnesota) tube for gastroesophageal variceal tamponade or a Linton-Nachlas tube for gastric varices alone may be useful when endoscopic sclerotherapy has failed, although the complication rates are higher. Insertion of a distal splenorenal shunt and the Sugiura procedure are operations reserved for patients for whom other nonoperative methods have failed to control the hemorrhage. (*See textbook pages* 1201–1203.)

Chapter 99

1. C. Patients with diseases of hollow viscera can have intestinal pseudoobstruction, but they also have problems with the motility of other hollow organs. The single most useful observation with which to identify this pattern from the patient's history is frequency of urination. Urination that occurs considerably more or less frequently than the normal five to six times per day (in the absence of acute cystitis) is a sign of abnormalities in smooth-muscle motility. Problems with ptosis or ophthalmoplegia occasionally can provide clues to the presence of hollow visceral disease. (*See textbook page* 1209.)

2. D. Surgical opening of the abdomen and handling of intestine appears to arrest intestinal contractile activity. However, most of this slowing appears to involve the colon and the stomach. The small intestine regains its function rapidly and may never really lose much activity after an uncomplicated surgical procedure. Because of this, enteral feedings can be used very early in the postoperative period, even in the recovery room. This is especially true of enterally delivered nutrients that bypass the stomach (e.g., in jejunal tubes) and contain little residue to be deposited in the atonic colon. (*See textbook page* 1207.)

3. B. Intravenously delivered erythromycin appears to stimulate motor activity in the stomach and small intestine and may be beneficial in cases of paralytic ileus. A macrolide antibiotic, erythromycin acts as a motilin agonist in the intestinal tract. Naloxone, a narcotic antagonist, may be marginally beneficial when excessive narcotic has led to intestinal slowing, although it would not be expected to work in other types of ileus. Simethicone can absorb excessive gas within the intestine and thus may provide some marginal benefit, although in serious cases of ileus it is not of great help. Use of rectal suppositories is strongly discouraged. Atropine would be contraindicated in cases of ileus because it acts as a cholinergic antagonist and would aggravate the intestinal atony. (*See textbook page* 1211.)

Chapter 100

1. **E.** Colonic perforation is the greatest risk factor for death in cases of toxic megacolon. The mortality rate is 50% among patients who have perforation before surgical intervention is undertaken. Other factors associated with increased mortality include age older than 40 years and a delay in surgical intervention. Early recognition and management of toxic megacolon have reduced the overall mortality of the condition to less than 15%. (*See textbook page* 1213.)

2. **D.** Corticosteroids are frequently used to manage toxic megacolon, although the issue of use of these agents is subject to some controversy. In many cases of toxic megacolon, it is prudent to administer augmented doses of steroids to patients who were taking steroids before the onset of the toxic condition. Parenteral administration of corticosteroids is accepted therapy for Crohn's colitis and ulcerative colitis, and many patients with toxic megacolon have one of these diseases. However, prospective randomized trials of use of corticosteroids as therapy for toxic megacolon are lacking, so the controversy is far from settled. (*See textbook pages* 1213–1215.)

3. **D.** Perforation is an absolute indication for surgical intervention in the care of patients with toxic megacolon. However, because the mortality rate is so high once perforation occurs, efforts at preventing this complication should be undertaken. The sign of impending perforation is enlargement of the colon diameter to more than 12 cm, which is an indication for emergency surgical intervention to prevent the disastrous consequences of perforation, such as peritonitis, extreme fluid and electrolyte imbalance, and hemodynamic instability. Septic shock should be an indication to desist from nonoperative therapy in an effort to eradicate the source of the septic complication. Some authors believe that conditions such as severe malnutrition or pregnancy also mandate emergency surgical treatment of patients with toxic megacolon. (*See textbook page* 1215.)

Chapter 101

1. **B.** Fulminant hepatic failure is a severe complication of liver disease that has devastating consequences. The single most important predictor of clinical outcome is the degree of encephalopathy. Higher survival rates are reported when fulminant hepatic failure is caused y hepatitis A, hepatitis B, and acetaminophen toxicity, but not failure caused by idiosyncratic drug reactions, acute Wilson's disease, halothane hepatitis, and non-A, non-B hepatitis. In addition to helping to assess the overall prognosis, etiologic identification is important for effective clinical management. Patients with fulminant hepatic failure caused by toxicity may benefit from potential antidotes. If a patient has failure caused by infectious agents, adequate public health measures may have to be taken. Liver transplantation is an important therapeutic tool; survival rates exceed 50% in most series but are less than 20% without transplantation. Mortality after liver transplantation for fulminant hepatic failure usually is caused by sepsis and neurologic complications. (*See textbook page* 1217.)

2. **E.** For patients with fulminant hepatic failure, the most sensitive method for detecting the presence and degree of intracranial pressure elevations is through the use of intracranial pressure monitoring. The grade of encephalopathy can sometimes be a guide to the need for intracranial pressure monitoring, although it is neither sensitive nor specific. In general, patients with grade 3 or 4 encephalopathy should be observed with an intracranial pressure monitor. Typical clinical manifestations of increased intracranial pressure, such as papilledema, bradycardia,

vomiting, and headache, frequently are not evident in fulminant hepatic failure. Findings at computed tomography of the brain of a patient with fulminant hepatic failure do not appear to correlate well with the presence of increased intracranial pressure. (*See textbook page* 1218.)

3. A. Acute renal failure in a patient with fulminant hepatic failure is an ominous sign. It occurs among as many as 75% of patients with fulminant hepatic failure due to acetaminophen toxicity, but only about 30% of patients with fulminant hepatic failure of other causes. The most common causes of renal failure are intravascular volume depletion, acute tubular necrosis, and hepatorenal syndrome; many cases have a multifactorial cause. The technique of continuous hemodiafiltration may offer advantages to patients with fulminant hepatic failure and renal failure who need dialysis. (*See textbook page* 1220.)

Chapter 102

1. B. Diarrhea is the most common nonhemorrhagic gastrointestinal complication among critically ill patients. It occurs among 40% to 50% of patients in an intensive care unit, although clinicians often overlook it as a problem. Definitions of what constitutes diarrhea seem to vary, confusing the establishment of this clinical entity as a problem necessitating clinical attention. Failure to properly identify and manage diarrhea for a critically ill patient usually leads to severe fluid, electrolyte, and nutritional abnormalities that further complicate the patient's course. (*See textbook page* 1225.)

2. E. Antibiotic-associated, or pseudomembranous colitis is most notoriously linked to the use of clindamycin with the subsequent emergence of *Clostridium difficile*. However, it appears to develop after the use of other antibiotics such as ampicillin. It even occurs after the use of agents that are commonly used to manage antibiotic-associated colitis—vancomycin and metronidazole. Broad-spectrum cephalosporins also have been implicated in the development of pseudomembranous colitis. It is important to realize that this disease can occur as late as 6 weeks after discontinuation of the responsible antibiotic. (*See textbook page* 1226.)

3. E. Although the treatment of critically ill patients with diarrhea can be complex, the most important early issues concern effective management of fluid and electrolyte disturbances. Replacement of water, sodium, potassium, phosphorus, magnesium, and bicarbonate may be necessary to varying degrees. In states of severe volume depletion, invasive hemodynamic monitoring may be necessary to accurately guide resuscitation measures. Diagnostic procedures such as sigmoidoscopy may be necessary to establish the cause of the diarrhea, but this is never the initial procedure. Agents such as vancomycin and metronidazole can be effective at controlling pseudomembranous colitis caused by the emergence of *C. difficile*. These agents themselves, however, have been implicated in the causation of some cases of pseudomembranous colitis. Although enteral feeding intolerance is frequently implicated in cases of diarrhea, enteral feedings should not be arbitrarily stopped until a clear relation is established between the rate of infusion and the onset of diarrhea. (*See textbook pages* 1226, 1229.)

Chapter 103

1. D. Ultrasonography of the abdomen can be very helpful in the evaluation of critically ill patients who may have a biliary disorder. It is highly sensitive and specific for ascertaining the presence of dilated bile ducts and of gallstones. Hepatobiliary scanning is useful for demonstrating patency of the cystic duct and the presence of normal function of the biliary tract. Both tests are noninvasive and can be performed at the bedside for a critically ill patient, providing a substantial advantage to this patient population. Although computed tomography also is non-invasive and can show highly specific findings, it is not a portable technique. Thus, ample justification should exist for performing it over portable studies in the care of a critically ill patient whose condition may deteriorate during transport. One reason to perform computed tomography would be to provide a better view of the head of the pancreas than can be achieved in many ultrasound examinations. Both endoscopic retrograde cholangiopancreatography and percutaneous transhepatic cholangiography are invasive tests that necessitate fluoroscopy. As such, they are not usually used as the initial diagnostic maneuver in the care of critically ill patients with suspected biliary tract disease. (*See textbook pages* 1233, 1234.)

2. **B.**   This patient has the classic signs of acute cholangitis (fever, right upper quadrant abdominal pain, and jaundice), also known as *Charcot's triad.* Under such circumstances, initial stabilization efforts should be concentrated on maintaining an effective circulating volume status with intravenous fluids. The systemic sepsis should be approached initially with broad-spectrum intravenous antibiotics after blood cultures are obtained. In many cases, a response occurs, and the antibiotic regimen can be tailored pending further identification of the offending organism. (*See textbook page* 1234.)

3. **D.**   When the initial approach of fluid and antibiotic administration fails to achieve a marked beneficial response or when a patient clearly has complete obstruction of an infected biliary tree, emergency decompression of the biliary tract should be performed. This can be accomplished by means of a variety of different approaches—endoscopic, percutaneous, or surgical depending on the patient's condition and the available local resources and expertise. Removal of the gallbladder is not necessary in the initial setting. Rather, efforts to decompress the biliary tract must be the focus of the intervention. The gallbladder can be removed at a later date if the patient survives. (*See textbook page* 1234.)

Chapter 104

1. **B.**   One of the greatest risks of performing procedures on critically ill patients is production of hypoxemia. Patients with chronic obstructive lung disease and elderly patients are more likely to have respiratory depression during endoscopy. Premedication is responsible for the greatest number of hypoxic events, although other factors can sometimes play a role, such as the presence of the endoscope in the hypopharynx or the use of topical anesthesia. Although it was initially thought to be more causative of respiratory depression, midazolam was shown in a large clinical study to be no more likely to be responsible for cardiopulmonary complications than was diazepam. Allergy to sedation or narcotic premedication is extremely rare. However, allergy to intravenous contrast agents is not unusual. Nevertheless, anaphylaxis during endoscopic retrograde cholangiopancreatography has not been reported.(*See textbook page* 1237.)

2. **D.**   Flumazenil is a benzodiazepine-receptor antagonist that can block the action of benzodiazepines at receptor sites. This makes it useful for complete or partial reversal of oversedation due to benzodiazepines. However, it may be ineffective at reversing any hypoventilation and accompanying hypoxemia due to benzodiazepines. Patients who have taken benzodiazepines for a long time may have seizures when given flumazenil. Naloxone is a narcotic antagonist and is not

expected to reverse the action of benzodiazepines, although it might be useful if excessive narcotics are used in addition to the benzodiazepines. (*See textbook page* 1238.)

3. D.   Visualization of the abdominal viscera or peritoneum during colonoscopy indicates free perforation into the peritoneal cavity and necessitates immediate surgical intervention to minimize the potential for overwhelming iatrogenic peritonitis. The finding of free intraperitoneal air after colonoscopic polypectomy indicates the presence of an intestinal perforation. Perforations found on radiographs after a procedure often are microperforations that may be successfully managed with conservative measures. The other symptoms listed may suggest the presence of a serious complication after colonoscopic polypectomy but may not mandate surgical exploration. These symptoms may be related to what has been called *postpolypectomy coagulation syndrome,* which can occur within a few hours of colonoscopy. Treatment with antibiotics, bowel rest, and close observation for 48 to 72 hours usually is sufficient. (*See textbook page* 1239.)

Chapter 105

1. C.   The diagnosis of ischemic hepatitis often can be made on clinical grounds, making liver biopsy unnecessary in many cases. The syndrome occurs in response to a period of reduced liver perfusion. The most striking finding is a pronounced rise in serum AST and ALT. These can rise to levels 40 or more times the normal level. In contrast, serum bilirubin and alkaline phosphatase levels are normal or modestly elevated. The elevations in transaminase levels are brief and self-limited, usually lasting only 1 to 2 weeks at most. Prolongation of prothrombin time occurs early but promptly corrects itself with recovery. (*See textbook page* 1242.)

2. D.   TPN can produce abnormalities in liver function tests among 68% to 93% of patients who receive it for more than 2 weeks. Elevations of ALT and to a lesser extent AST typically develop with variable changes in serum bilirubin and alkaline phosphatase levels. No specific effect of TPN on coagulation values has been determined. With prolonged administration, cholelithiasis or acalculous cholecystitis can develop, presumably because of gallbladder disuse and the development of biliary sludge. The pathophysiologic mechanisms underlying the effects of TPN on liver function are not known, although recent interest focuses on the effect of intestinal rest on hormone secretion and bacterial overgrowth. Liver biopsy shows either fatty infiltration or no significant abnormalities. Progression to cirrhosis has been reported only rarely. Enteral nutrition may help to prevent many of the abnormalities in liver function that occur with TPN, although this is not always possible. (*See textbook page* 1242.)

3. A.   As many as 54% of patients with bacteremia have abnormalities of liver function tests. Hepatomegaly is absent in as many as one half of patients. Serum bilirubin level typically is elevated into the range of 5 to 10 mg/dL, whereas ALT, AST, and alkaline phosphatase levels increase as much as threefold. Clotting function often is preserved, as are cytosolic and microsomal function. Chemical markers of liver function usually return to normal in 1 to 2 weeks if there is no underlying disease. (*See textbook page* 1243.)

VIII. Endocrine Problems in the Intensive Care Unit

106. Approach to the Acutely Ill Patient on Chronic Steroid Therapy

True or False

1. Patients receiving pharmacologic doses of glucocorticoids for only 10 days may have an abnormal cortisol response to corticotropin (ACTH) infusion.
2. Hypotension during surgical stress is uncommon among adrenal-suppressed patients who chronically receive physiologic replacement doses of steroid (20 mg hydrocortisone daily or equivalent).
3. A glucocorticoid dose-equivalent to 300 mg intravenous hydrocortisone every 8 hours is necessary for adequate stress coverage.
4. Alternate-day therapy with glucocorticoids reduces the possibility of adrenal suppression.

107. Management of Diabetes in the Critically Ill Patient

Select the best answer

1. Compensatory mechanisms to maintain normal blood concentrations of glucose during fasting and starvation include all of the following *except*:

    A. Mobilization of hepatic glycogen
    B. Release of amino acid precursors for gluconeogenesis
    C. Inhibition of lipolysis
    D. Central nervous system utilization of ketone bodies

2. An 88-year-old man with a history of asthma and non-insulin-dependent diabetes mellitus underwent laparotomy for perforated colonic diverticulum that resulted in partial colectomy and descending colostomy. Two days postoperatively, worsening bronchospasm developed despite frequent doses of nebulized albuterol; methylprednisolone treatment was begun. Three days postoperatively, enteral feeding was initiated. The following day, the morning blood sugar was 410 mg/dL. The most appropriate management is:

A. To discontinue methylprednisolone
B. Continuous intravenous infusion of insulin
C. To discontinue enteral feeding
D. Intermittent subcutaneous insulin

108. The Diabetic Comas

Select the best answer

1. Alcoholic ketoacidosis is characterized by all of the following *except*:

   A. Dehydration
   B. Hyperglycemia
   C. Lactic acidosis
   D. Increased free fatty acids

2. Insulin deficiency results in:

   A. Decreased lipolysis
   B. Accelerated gluconeogenesis
   C. Reduced glucagon secretion
   D. Metabolic alkalosis

3. A 29-year-old man arrives at the emergency department with weakness, nausea, anorexia, thirst, and weight loss that has been progressive over the last 2 weeks. He denies prior clinically significant medical problems and takes no medication. At examination, he appears to be in moderate respiratory distress. Blood pressure is 96/64 mm Hg supine. Pulse is 150 beats/min and regular, respirations are 38 breaths/min, and temperature is 36.6°C. The lungs are clear, the heart shows only regular tachycardia, and the abdomen is mildly and diffusely tender. Initial laboratory studies show serum sodium 142 mEq/L, potassium 6.2 mEq/L, carbon dioxide 5 mmol/Liter, chloride 105 mEq/L, blood urea nitrogen 62 mg/dL, creatinine 2.1 mg/dL, and glucose 820 mg/dL. Arterial blood gas analysis reveals PO_2 106 mm Hg; PCO_2 21 mm Hg; and pH 7.02. Urinalysis shows the presence of sugar and ketones. The most appropriate immediate management is:

   A. Intravenous calcium for severe hyperkalemia
   B. Intravenous bicarbonate for severe acidosis
   C. Intravenous isotonic saline solution for dehydration
   D. Intravenous insulin for severe hyperglycemia

109. Thyroid Storm

Select the best answer

1. A 67-year-old woman with a history of insulin-dependent diabetes mellitus comes to medical attention with a 2-week history of polydipsia and polyuria and a 1-week history of palpitations, fever, nervousness, and insomnia. Her temperature is 37.8°C. Pulse is 140 beats/min, and rhythm is irregular. An electrocar-

diogram shows atrial fibrillation. Serum thyroxine level is markedly elevated. A *true* statement concerning this patient's condition is:

A. Worsening diabetic control may occur in hyperthyroidism.
B. Tachycardia out of proportion to fever makes thyroid storm unlikely.
C. Atrial tachyarrhythmias during thyroid storm usually require less propranolol than is given to typical patients.
D. A patient should not be treated for the fever of thyroid storm.

2. True statements concerning management of thyroid storm include all of the following *except*:

A. Salicylates should not be used to manage the fever.
B. β-Blockade should not be used in the setting of congestive heart failure.
C. Iodide is useful to decrease thyroid hormone release.
D. Plasmapheresis, dialysis, or both, remove thyroid hormone from the circulation.

110. Myxedema Coma

Select the best answer

1. A patient with a history of hypothyroidism and bipolar disorder treated with lithium carbonate arrives in the emergency department with a 7-day history of lethargy progressive to obtundation. The patient had not been seen by a physician in more than 1 year. A history of fatigue and weight gain over the previous 6 months is elicited from a family member. At examination the patient is difficult to arouse. Blood pressure is 88/50 mm Hg, pulse is 55 beats/min, respirations 14 breaths/minute, and temperature 32.8°C. Laboratory values include blood sugar 50 mg/dL, mildly elevated lithium level, markedly elevated thyroid-stimulating hormone, and a low serum-free thyroxine index. True statements about this condition include all of the following *except*:

A. Lithium may be responsible.
B. Hypothermia is common and is associated with a decrease in basal metabolic rate, myocardial irritability, and blood pressure alterations.
C. Severe infections may precipitate this state.
D. Administration of concentrated dextrose solutions is contraindicated.

111. Hypoadrenal Crisis

Select the best answer

1. A principle in the treatment of patients with adrenal insufficiency is:

A. One must confirm the diagnosis before initiating treatment.
B. Methylprednisolone 300 to 400 mg per day is equivalent to maximum adrenal glucocorticoid release.
C. When the result of a corticotropin (ACTH) stimulation test reveals an increase in plasma cortisol levels from 8 μg/dL to 12 μg/dL, this test indicates adrenal insufficiency.
D. Secondary adrenal insufficiency from pituitary dysfunction often necessitates additional mineralocorticoid replacement.

112. Disorders of Mineral Metabolism

Select the best answer

1. Elevated serum calcium level:

   A. Is caused by primary hyperparathyroidism or a malignant tumor in nearly 90% of cases
   B. May be managed for extended periods of time (>1 month) with calcitonin
   C. Associated with spinal cord injury is most likely to occur at least 6 months after the initial injury
   D. Is managed the same way regardless of the underlying disease or mechanism

113. Lactic Acidosis

Select the best answer

1. Bicarbonate therapy for severe lactic acidosis:

   A. Improves cardiovascular hemodynamics
   B. May worsen metabolic acidosis
   C. Improves tissue hypoxia
   D. May cause hyponatremia

114. Hypoglycemia

Select the best answer

1. Identify the correct statement regarding hypoglycemia.

   A. Excessive production of endogenous insulin is usually caused by a malignant process.
   B. Providing intravenous or oral carbohydrates is adequate treatment of most patients with hypoglycemia.
   C. Infusion of intravenous pentamidine may cause hypoglycemia.
   D. The diagnosis of hypoglycemia is made by means of measurement of plasma glucose level.

115. Sick Euthyroid Syndrome in the Intensive Care Unit

Select the best answer

1. Changes in thyroid function test results among critically ill patients can include all of the following except:

   A. Decreased serum triiodothyronine (T_3) level
   B. Decreased serum thyroxine (T_4) level
   C. Increased thyrotropin (TSH) level
   D. Increased serum (T_4) level

Answers

Chapter 106

1. **True.**   Patients receiving therapeutic glucocorticoids for as few as 5 days have shown abnormal cortisol responses to ACTH infusion. As a rule, however, those who have taken glucocorticoids for at least 4 weeks are at greater risk. (*See textbook page* 1250.)

2. **True.**   It is rare for patients receiving only replacement doses of steroids to experience hypotension during surgical stress, but supraphysiologic perioperative dosing still is recommended. (*See textbook page* 1249.)

3. **False.**   The maximal adrenal stress equivalent is 300 to 400 mg hydrocortisone equivalent per day. (*See textbook page* 1250.)

4. **True.**   Alternate day dosing of glucocorticoids generally decreases adrenal and immune suppression. (*See textbook page* 1250.)

Chapter 107

1. **C.**   Lipolysis is accelerated, not inhibited, and peripheral tissues use free fatty acids for fuel. Glycogenolysis proceeds until hepatic glycogen stores are exhausted, and subsequent gluconeogenesis supplies glucose for obligate glucolytic tissues such as those of the central nervous system. If starvation lasts for more than 72 hours, the brain utilizes ketone bodies as alternative fuel. (*See textbook page* 1251.)

2. **B.**   The patient needs corticosteroids for asthma control and needs continued enteral feeding for intestinal mucosal integrity and nutrition. He needs insulin to decrease the blood sugar level to 150 to 250 mg/dL range to avoid metabolic, electrolyte, and possible infectious complications. Continuous intravenous insulin infusion is the preferred route to avoid large swings in control of glycemia. Fingerstick blood glucose concentration should be measured every 1 to 2 hours to ensure safety and efficacy. (*See textbook pages* 1254, 1255.)

Chapter 108

1. **B.**   Patients with alcoholic ketoacidosis often have hypoglycemia. Persons who are fasting and exhaust their glycogen stores depend on generation of glucose through gluconeogenesis, which is impaired in the presence of alcoholic ketoacidosis because nicotinamide adenine dinucleotide in the oxidized form (NAD+) is not available. NAD+ is reduced during the metabolism of ethanol. Insulin levels are low, and free fatty acid levels are high. Lactic acidosis contributes to the metabolic acidosis, perhaps because of poor tissue oxygenation from dehydration or impaired hepatic and renal lactate clearance. (*See textbook pages* 1258, 1259.)

2. **B.**   Insulin deficiency is the cause of diabetic ketoacidosis. When there is a lack of insulin, no glucose enters cells. Glucagon secretion is increased, and gluconeogenesis is accelerated. Blood sugar level rises and causes osmotic diuresis and water and electrolyte loss. To conserve muscle mass, free fatty acids are released and become the primary fuel source. Free fatty acids are metabolized in the liver to ketoacids, and metabolic acidosis occurs. (*See textbook page* 1259.)

3. **C.**   This patient has diabetic ketoacidosis and is severely dehydrated. Volume resuscitation with isotonic saline solution is the most important initial therapy. Hyperkalemia probably reflects systemic acidemia, but total body potassium is

severely depleted. The serum potassium value will fall rapidly with volume resuscitation, glucose control, and improving acidemia. Bicarbonate is not indicated for this level of acidemia. The metabolic acidosis will improve with volume and glycemic control. Insulin is essential in this patient's care, but volume resuscitation takes precedence in the initial emergency treatment. (*See textbook page* 1263.)

Chapter 109

1. **A.**   Diabetes mellitus and hyperthyroidism may occur in the same patient perhaps because of a common autoimmune cause. Glycemic control is more difficult if the patient has hyperthyroidism. Tachycardia out of proportion to fever is characteristic of thyroid storm. A high fever should be aggressively treated to control the component that drives oxygen utilization. Atrial tachyarrhythmias during thyroid storm may necessitate use of higher doses and higher plasma levels of propranolol for rate control than are used in the treatment of a patient with normal levels of thyroid hormones. (*See textbook pages* 1272, 1273.)

2. **B.**   β-Blockade stops the peripheral effects of excess thyroid hormone, the cause of the congestive heart failure. β-Blockers, sometimes combined with digoxin and diuretics, can be used. Large doses of salicylates displace thyroid hormones from serum-binding proteins, and an alternative antipyretic should be used. Iodide is important in the early management of severe hyperthyroidism and acts by blocking hormone release from the gland. Plasmapheresis and dialysis may be useful in the care of the rare patients who do not respond to conventional treatment. (*See textbook pages* 1273, 1274.)

Chapter 110

1. **D.**   This patient is in myxedema coma, and hypoglycemia is not uncommon. Supplemental concentrated dextrose or glucose should be administered if the serum value is low. Hypothyroidism is induced among 5% to 30% of patients undergoing long-term lithium therapy. Trauma, infection, and cold exposure may precipitate myxedema coma if a patient has hypothyroidism. Lithium may precipitate this syndrome, but the syndrome typically occurs only when the patient has preexisting thyroid disease. Hypothermia may be overlooked if careful attention is not given to the technique of temperature measurement. (*See textbook pages* 1276, 1277.)

Chapter 111

1. **C.**   Normal adrenal function shows cortisol levels rising by 7 µg/dL above baseline or reaching a level greater than 18 µg/dL in response to ACTH. Adrenal insufficiency is suspected on clinical grounds, and treatment including saline infusion, glucose supplementation, and glucocorticoid placement should be given quickly to seriously ill patients. Diagnostic tests such as checking the 1-hour cortisol response to synthetic ACTH infusion can be initiated, but treatment should proceed on clinical grounds before results are available. The most appropriate replacement steroid is intravenous hydrocortisone 300 to 400 mg/day in divided doses. This also supplies mineralocorticoid replacement if it is needed. The maximal dose of methylprednisolone needed for glucocorticoid replacement is 60 to 80 mg/day. Pituitary dysfunction resulting in adrenal failure rarely involves mineralocorticoid deficits, because ACTH is not critical to mineralocorticoid control. (*See textbook pages* 1280, 1281.)

Chapter 112

1. **A.** Elevated serum calcium level is caused by primary hyperparathyroidism or malignant parathyroid tumors in nearly 90% of cases. Other potential causes include sarcoidosis, vitamin D intoxication, thyrotoxicosis, Addison's disease, immobilization, and other less common causes. Management of hypercalcemia involves minimizing the central nervous system, renal, and cardiovascular affects. This includes increasing renal clearance by means of saline hydration and addition of loop diuretics when intravascular volume has been expanded. Calcitonin generally is effective for 4 to 7 days and then loses its effect because of down-regulation of calcitonin receptors. Hypercalcemia due to spinal cord injury usually occurs within 4 months of the injury. (*See textbook page* 1285.)

Chapter 113

1. **B.** Bicarbonate therapy for lactic acidosis is probably ineffective and may be harmful. A randomized trial showed no improvement in hemodynamic values among patients with lactic acidosis treated with bicarbonate. Bicarbonate may paradoxically worsen metabolic acidosis by increasing carbon dioxide at the tissue level (carbon dioxide crosses the cell membrane). Bicarbonate also may transiently shift the oxyhemoglobin curve to the left, resulting in less tissue oxygen availability. Administration of sodium bicarbonate can cause hypernatremia. (*See textbook page* 1294.)

Chapter 114

1. **C.** Infusion of intravenous pentamidine may damage pancreatic islet cells and release stored insulin, causing transient hypoglycemia. Excessive chronic production of insulin is usually caused by insulinoma, which is a small pancreatic islet cell tumor. Less than 10% of these are malignant. The biggest mistake in the management of hypoglycemia is failing to identify and address the cause of hypoglycemia, thus relapses occur. The diagnosis of hypoglycemia is made through observation of the triad of decreased plasma glucose levels, symptoms of hypoglycemia, and correction of symptoms with the administration of glucose. (*See textbook pages* 1297, 1299, 1301, 1304.)

Chapter 115

1. **C.** TSH levels usually are normal in early acute illness but often fall as the illness progresses. Dopamine and glucocorticoids have a direct inhibitory effect on TSH secretion. Thyrotropin-releasing hormone levels also may be depressed. Acute illness causes impairment of T_4 to T_3 conversion as the result of inhibition of the enzyme 5'-deiodinase. Therefore, T_3 levels fall soon after the onset of severe illness. Reverse T_3 (rT_3) levels increase because of unaffected conversion from T_4 and slow degradation. T_4 levels may be elevated in early acute illness because of increased thyroxine-binding globulin levels or the inhibition of 5'-deiodinase. Late in severe illness, however, T_4 level declines because of decreased binding to carrier proteins, decreased TSH level, and increased numbers of nondeiodinase metabolic pathways. (*See textbook pages* 1308, 1309.)

IX. Hematologic Problems in the Intensive Care Unit

116. Acquired Bleeding Disorders

True or False

Regarding hemostatic and fibrinolytic processes:

1. Thromboxane A_2 activates other platelets.
2. Fibrinogen is the bridge that mediates platelet aggregation.
3. All of the clotting factors are serine proteases.
4. Activated procoagulants do not inhibit their own further generation.
5. Antithrombin III appears to inhibit other clotting factors and not just inhibit activated thrombin.
6. Compartmentalization of reactions helps to limit the degree of coagulation.
7. Plasminogen formation of plasmin is an abnormal process that predisposes to clinical bleeding.

Select the best answer

8. Regarding acquired bleeding disorders:

   A. The most common cause of qualitative platelet disorders is autoimmune disease.
   B. Desmopressin (DDAVP) offers no benefit to patients with functional platelet disorders.
   C. Vitamin K deficiency is common among critically ill patients.
   D. The diagnosis of disseminated intravascular coagulation is easily made from the clinical appearance of the patient.
   E. Aprotinin is of little value in the control of postbypass bleeding.

117. The Congenital Coagulopathies

True or False

1. Female carriers of hemophilia can manifest some bleeding tendencies.
2. Spontaneous hemorrhage does not usually occur among persons with hemophilia unless the factor levels are less than 1% of normal activity.
3. Patients with factor levels at 5% of normal activity or more often do not bleed unless stressed by a surgical procedure or trauma.

4. Intracranial bleeding is the single most important cause of death from bleeding in hemophilia.
5. For the management of life-threatening bleeding in an intensive care unit, a factor VIII level of at least 80% should be achieved.

Select the best answer

6. Hemophilia A:

   A. Is an X-linked recessive disorder caused by decreased levels of properly functioning factor IX.
   B. Is an X-linked recessive disorder caused by decreased levels of properly functioning factor VIII.
   C. Is a Y-linked recessive disorder caused by decreased levels of properly functioning factor VIII.
   D. Is a Y-linked dominant disorder caused by decreased levels of properly functioning factor VIII.
   E. Is an X-linked dominant disorder caused by decreased levels of properly functioning factor VIII.

7. Which of the following statements is *true*?

   A. Hemophilia A is the most common congenital coagulopathy.
   B. Factor VIII inhibitor antibody tends to develop in patients older than 50 years who have received fewer than five treatments with factor concentrate.
   C. Approximately 70% of all persons in the United States who have hemophilia have positive serologic results for the human immunodeficiency virus.
   D. Patients with type I von Willebrand disease do not respond to desmopressin (DDAVP).
   E. Patients with type III von Willebrand disease do not respond to DDAVP.

118. Thrombocytopenia

True or False

1. Prophylactic platelet transfusions are contraindicated in the care of patients with heparin-induced thrombocytopenia.
2. Use of desmopressin (DDAVP) can lower bleeding time among patients with uremia.
3. Management of vancomycin-induced thrombocytopenia does not necessitate discontinuation of vancomycin.
4. If necessary, patients with heparin-induced thrombocytopenia incited by unfractionated heparin may be treated with the low-molecular-weight heparin enoxaparin.

Select the best answer

5. Which of the following is a *true* statement regarding thrombocytopenia?

   A. Thrombocytopenia is defined as a platelet count less than 250×10^9/L.
   B. Thrombocytopenia occurs only when excessive platelet destruction occurs in the circulatory periphery.

C. Thrombocytopenia should be initially evaluated with bone marrow biopsy.
D. Thrombocytopenia is rarely caused by increased platelet destruction in intensive care unit patients.
E. Thrombocytopenia is differentiated from pseudothrombocytopenia on the basis of a review of a blood film.

6. Thrombocytopenia:

A. Is most likely cured by means of splenectomy when idiopathic thrombocytopenic purpura is the underlying condition.
B. Is usually mild and brief in cases of posttransfusion purpura.
C. Due to thrombotic thrombocytopenic purpura typically occurs among male children.
D. Due to massive transfusion can be effectively prevented by means of prophylactic administration of platelets to patients who receive large volumes of fluid by means of intravenous infusion.
E. Due to hypersplenism can cause severe bleeding and should be aggressively managed by means of splenectomy.

119. Antithrombotic Therapy

True or False

1. Thrombolytic agents have been shown to reduce mortality from acute pulmonary embolism.
2. Large loading doses of streptokinase are necessary to overcome antistreptococcal antibodies.
3. Thrombolytic therapy does not usually require close monitoring of coagulation values.

For questions 4 through 8, match each antithrombotic agent with its primary target (s). Each item in the second column should be used only once.

4. Heparin   **A.** Cyclooxygenase
5. Warfarin   **B.** Factors IIa, IXa, Xa, XIa, and XIIa
6. Dextran   **C.** Factors II, VII, IX, and X
7. Aspirin   **D.** Plasminogen
8. Streptokinase **E.** Platelet adhesion and aggregation

Select the best answer

9. Heparin therapy:

A. Is best given in intermittent intravenous boluses.
B. Usually is started with an initial dose of 2,500 units/hour and titrated up or down as necessary.
C. Is most commonly monitored with activated partial thromboplastin time.
D. Is achieved when heparin concentration is 4 units/mL.
E. Should be given for at least 4 weeks to be effective.

120. Hypercoagulability and the Pathophysiology of Thrombosis in the Critically Ill Patient

True or False

1. Flow promotes dilution and reduces predisposition to thrombosis.
2. The activity of antithrombin III is inhibited by heparin.
3. Activated protein C neutralizes activated factors V and VIII.
4. Protein S inhibits the activity of protein C.
5. Natural inhibitors exist for both plasmin and its activators.

For questions 6 to 10, match the acquired thrombophilic disorder with its characteristic. Each item in the second column should be used only once.

6. Antiphospholipid syndrome   A. Budd-Chiari syndrome
7. Polycythemia vera   B. Megakaryocyte hyperproliferation
8. Paroxysmal nocturnal   C. Treated by means of phlebotomy
   hemoglobinuria   D. Presence of lupus anticoagulant
9. Trousseau's syndrome   E. Adenocarcinoma
10. Essential thrombocythemia

Select the best answer

11. Prophylaxis against venous thromboembolism:

    A. Is contraindicated in the care of patients undergoing neurosurgical procedures
    B. Requires the same dosage of anticoagulation needed for the management of thromboembolic disease
    C. Is of no benefit for patients recovering from myocardial infarction
    D. Has been shown to be beneficial to patients older than 40 years undergoing abdominal operations
    E. Is not warranted for patients with stroke in evolution

121. The Hemolytic Anemias

True or False

1. Intravascular hemolysis is characterized by increased plasma hemoglobin.
2. Extravascular hemolysis is characterized by elevated bilirubin.
3. In most cases of hemolysis, bone marrow examination is mandatory.
4. The direct Coombs' test is used to detect the presence of antibodies in the serum.

Select the best answer

5. Autoimmune hemolytic anemia:

    A. Is commonly associated with a negative result of a direct Coombs test
    B. Can be classified into six major categories
    C. Is characterized by the presence of IgA antibodies in the case of the cold-reactive form

D. Is characterized by the presence of IgM antibodies in the case of the warm-reactive form

E. Of the cold-reactive type is not effectively managed with steroids

Match each type of hemolytic anemia with its offending etiologic factor or associated clinical finding. Each item in the second column should be used only once.

6. Paroxysmal nocturnal hemoglobinuria

7. Osmotic erythrocyte injury

8. Erythroblastosis fetalis

9. Sickle cell anemia

A. Hemoglobin S
B. Sticky platelets
C. Rh incompatibility
D. Hypotonic intravenous infusions

122. Transfusion Therapy: Blood Components and Transfusion Complications

Select the best answer

1. The hemoglobin level at which transfusion is warranted in red cell transfusion therapy is:

A. 12 g/dL
B. 10 g/dL
C. 8 g/dL
D. 6 g/dL
E. Dependent on the patient's clinical situation

2. Which of the following statements regarding transfusion of red blood cells is *true*?

A. Delayed transfusion reaction usually occurs 24 to 48 hours after transfusion.
B. Graft versus host disease may occur after transfusion of peripheral blood.
C. Hepatitis C occurs among 1 per 1,000,000 transfusion recipients.
D. Transfusion from a donor infected with human immunodeficiency virus infects approximately 60% of recipients.
E. Clinically significant immunosuppression occurs among one in four recipients of more than 4 units of packed red blood cells.

123. Granulocytopenia

True or False

1. With most chemotherapeutic agents, the nadir of peripheral neutrophil counts occurs about 2 weeks after the beginning of therapy.
2. Neutrophil counts usually take longer to reach their nadir after treatment with *cis*-chloronitrosourea (CCNU) than with other chemotherapeutic agents.
3. The effect of chloramphenicol on leukocyte production is limited to the granulocyte line.
4. Penicillin in high doses can cause neutropenia.
5. H2-blockers have not been implicated in cases of neutropenia.

Select the best answer

6. Which of the following statements regarding cytokines is *false*?

    A. Granulocyte-macrophage colony-stimulating factor (GM-CSF) primarily affects the granulocyte pool.
    B. GM-CSF primarily affects the macrophage pool
    C. GM-CSF primarily affects the granulocyte pool.
    D. Macrophage colony-stimulating factor primarily affects the macrophage pool.
    E. The various colony-stimulating factors prevent apoptotic cell death.

7. A patient with oliguria and acute renal failure undergoes dialysis in which 2.5 L of fluid is removed. During dialysis, the patient became acutely short of breath. Arterial blood gas analysis reveals PaO_2 54 mm Hg with 60% oxygen by face mask and $PaCO_2$ 32 mm Hg. Assessment of vital signs reveals tachycardia of 110 beats/min, blood pressure 124/82 mm Hg, and a respiratory rate of 28 breaths/min. The patient has an indwelling pulmonary arterial catheter, which shows pulmonary capillary wedge pressure 7 mm Hg, cardiac index 4.9 L/min/m^2, and mixed venous oxygen saturation 74%. Which of the following tests is most likely to reveal the cause of the hypoxemia?

    A. Serum calcium measurement
    B. Hematocrit
    C. White blood cell count
    D. Colloid oncotic pressure measurement
    E. Serum albumin measurement

124. The Acute Leukemias

True or False

1. Patients with acute leukemia and hyperleukocytosis have a poor prognosis.
2. Patients can experience lethargy and obtundation caused by leukostasis within the cerebral circulation.
3. Patients can have disseminated intravascular coagulation (DIC) as a result of the release of a procoagulant from the primary azurophilic granules of leukemic promyeloblasts.

Select the best answer

4. Acute lymphoblastic leukemia (ALL):

    A. Primarily affects the elderly
    B. Has three distinct immunologic subtypes
    C. Is incurable among most patients
    D. Has a good prognosis when associated with a chromosomal marker of the Philadelphia type
    E. Is of the T-cell type in most instances

5. Acute myelogenous leukemia (AML):

    A. Primarily affects children
    B. Often is associated with DIC in its promyelocytic form

C. Has three subtypes in the French-American-British (FAB) classification system
D. Cannot be managed by means of bone marrow transplantation
E. Has an excellent response rate among the elderly

For questions 6 to 10, match the chemotherapeutic agent with its characteristic feature. Each item in the second column should be used only once.

6. Cytosine arabinoside   A. Toxicity managed with leucovorin
7. Daunorubicin   B. Toxic to bladder mucosa
8. Vincristine   C. Peripheral neuropathy
9. Methotrexate   D. Cardiotoxicity
10. Cyclophosphamide   E. Cerebellar toxicity

125. Oncologic Emergencies

Select the best answer

1. Which of the following statements regarding superior vena cava (SVC) syndrome is *false*?

   A. Most cases of SVC syndrome are caused by malignant tumors.
   B. The presence of a Swan-Ganz catheter can cause SVC syndrome.
   C. The presence of azygous occlusion increases the likelihood of problems.
   D. Thoracotomy is necessary to establish the cause.
   E. The mainstay of therapy is radiation.

2. Epidural metastatic tumor compression of the spinal cord:

   A. Usually is caused by metastatic prostate cancer
   B. Has autonomic dysfunction as the initial manifestation in most instances
   C. Is rarely detected on plain radiographs of the spine
   D. Mandates prompt lumbar puncture and myelography with neurosurgical backup
   E. Should be managed initially with radiation therapy in most instances

3. Which of the following statements regarding the hypercalcemia of malignant disease is *false*?

   A. Hypercalcemia usually occurs late in the course of the disease.
   B. Approximately 15% of patients with cancer and hypercalcemia do not have bone metastases.
   C. Hypercalcemia appears to be precipitated by hormonal therapy among approximately 25% of patients with breast cancer who have elevated calcium levels.
   D. Volume infusions and diuretic agents can help reduce calcium level.
   E. Approximately 80% of total serum calcium is bound to protein.

Answers
Chapter 116

1. **True.** Aspirin causes a mild platelet disorder by inhibiting synthesis of thromboxane A_2. (*See text page* 1319.)

2. **True.**   Platelet aggregation is defective when factors affect fibrinogen production or function. (*See text page* 1320.)
3. **False.**   The zymogens XII, XI, X, IX, II, prekallikrein, and factor VII are serine proteases (have serine at the active center of the enzyme). Factor XIII is a transglutaminase that introduces covalent bonds between lysine and glutamine residues. (*See text page* 1320.)
4. **False.**   Activated procoagulants do inhibit their own further generation. This serves as an important inhibitory mechanism that limits the process of fibrin deposition. (*See text page* 1321.)
5. **True.**   Antithrombin III is an important inhibitor of the activated serine proteases, including thrombin, Xa, Ixa, XIa, XIIa, and kallikrein, although its principal effect appears to be on factor Xa and thrombin. (*See text page* 1321.)
6. **True.**   Most coagulation reactions have specific requirements for optimal activity, such as phospholipid surfaces. Compartmentalization limits interaction of all necessary factors and can limit these reactions. (*See text page* 1321.)
7. **False.**   Plasmin activation from plasminogen is a normal part of the clotting process. It keeps fibrin formation from extending beyond areas where it is not being actively stimulated. (*See text page* 1322.)
8. **C.**   The most common cause of qualitative platelet disorders is drugs, aspirin and other nonsteroidal anti-inflammatory drugs being the main offenders. Desmopressin (DDAVP) is useful in the treatment of some patients with functional platelet disorders such as uremia. Vitamin K deficiency is common among critically ill patients because of the mechanisms that can produce this phenomenon, such as biliary disease, malnutrition, and antibiotic use. The diagnosis of disseminated intravascular coagulation is difficult and complicated by the fact that the clinical manifestations range from none at all to a severe hemorrhagic disorder. The definitive diagnosis is established in the laboratory. Aprotinin, a serine protease inhibitor that seriously affects plasmin, has been shown to decrease blood loss among patients recovering from cardiopulmonary bypass. (*See text pages* 1323–1325, 1327.)

Chapter 117

1. **True.**   Female carriers of hemophilia are not entirely immune from the condition. They may have bleeding tendencies after operations or trauma if their normal X chromosomes are more randomly expressed than normal. They may have factor levels less than 10%, similar to those of persons with mild hemophilia. (*See text page* 1330.)
2. **True.**   Spontaneous hemorrhage does not usually occur among persons with true hemophilia unless the factor levels are less than 1% of normal. (*See text page* 1330.)
3. **True.**   Persons with factor levels of 5% or more often do not bleed unless stressed by an operation or trauma. (*See text page* 1330.)
4. **True.**   Intracranial bleeding accounts for 25% of deaths of bleeding among persons with hemophilia. The mortality rate for central nervous system bleeding among persons with hemophiliacs is 34% of those who have such bleeding episodes; 47% of the survivors are left with severe neurologic sequelae. (*See text page* 1331.)
5. **True.**   Although most serious joint or muscle bleeding requires a factor VIII level of 50%, therapy for life-threatening bleeding in the intensive care unit requires a level of at least 80%. (*See text page* 1332.)

6. **B.** Hemophilia A is an X-linked recessive disorder caused by decreased levels of properly functioning factor VIII. This disorder accounts for approximately 80% of cases of bleeding hemophilia. Hemophilia B also is an X-linked recessive bleeding disorder; it is indistinguishable from hemophilia A in clinical manifestation. (*See text page* 1330.)

7. **E.** It is surprising for many to learn that the most common congenital coagulopathy is von Willebrand's disease and not hemophilia. Von Willebrand's disease occurs among approximately 1 in 200 persons in the general population, whereas hemophilia A occurs 10 to 15 times among every 100,000 boys and men. Repeated treatments in the management of hemophilia A can result in development of an inhibitor antibody to factor VIII. This typically occurs after 5 to 30 treatments with factor concentrates among patients younger than 5 years. About 20% of all persons with hemophilia in the United States have positive serologic results for human immunodeficiency virus. In the management of von Willebrand's disease, patients with the type I version respond well to DDAVP, whereas those with type III do not respond to DDAVP. (*See text pages* 1330, 1335–1337.)

Chapter 118

1. **True.** Although they may be necessary in many cases of thrombocytopenia, platelet transfusions are contraindicated in the care of patients with platelet-mediated thrombosis (heparin-induced thrombocytopenia, thrombotic thrombocytopenic purpura, hemolytic-uremic syndrome). This is because bleeding complications are relatively uncommon, and platelet transfusions may precipitate thrombosis. (*See text page* 1341.)

2. **True.** DDAVP may be useful in some instances of functional platelet disorders, such as uremia and cirrhosis. It can lower bleeding time as long as platelet count is not severely depressed ($>20 \times 10^9$/L). (*See text page* 1341.)

3. **False.** Vancomycin-induced thrombocytopenia appears to affect IgG Fab-binding to specific glycoprotein complexes (GPIIb/IIIa or GPIb/IX). Treatment includes discontinuation of vancomycin and replacement if necessary with a non-cross-reactive agent. (*See text page* 1343.)

4. **False.** Low-molecular-weight heparin should be considered contraindicated in the management of heparin-induced thrombocytopenia. *In vitro* cross-reactivity with antiplatelet IgG is 100% *in vivo*. There is a higher risk for persisting thrombocytopenia and progressing thrombosis with use of these agents. (*See text page* 1343.)

5. **E.** Thrombocytopenia can be defined in many ways. However, normal platelet counts range from 150×10^9/L to 400×10^9/L. Most clinicians agree that platelet counts less than 150×10^9/L are indicative of thrombocytopenia. This level is 2 standard deviations below the mean platelet count for a healthy population. Thrombocytopenia can develop through one of four mechanisms—inadequate platelet production, hemodilution, platelet sequestration, and increased platelet destruction. Most cases of thrombocytopenia can be diagnosed from the history, physical examination, complete blood cell count, and peripheral blood film. Bone marrow biopsy is warranted only when the mechanism of thrombocytopenia remains obscure or when a decrease in platelet production is suspected. Patients in intensive care units rarely need bone marrow biopsy because they most commonly have increased platelet destruction. Thrombocytopenia is differentiated

from pseudothrombocytopenia by means of review of the blood film. (*See text pages* 1338, 1339.)

6. **A.**   Idiopathic thrombocytopenic purpura is a relatively common autoimmune condition characterized by premature destruction of platelets. Although treatment usually is initiated with corticosteroids, splenectomy offers the best chance for lasting cure. Posttransfusion purpura produces severe, life-threatening thrombocytopenia that can last for days to weeks. Thrombotic thrombocytopenic purpura is a thrombotic microangiopathic disorder that occurs among middle-aged adults with a slight female predominance. Patients with thrombocytopenia due to dilution are treated when platelet counts become severely diminished in the presence of active bleeding, but prophylaxis is not warranted. Hypersplenism causes thrombocytopenia by means of sequestration of platelets. The platelet count usually is not severely depressed, and splenectomy is not often useful unless it somehow contributes to the management of other pathophysiologic conditions, such as portal hypertension. (*See text pages* 1344, 1346.)

Chapter 119

1. **False.**   Urokinase, tissue plasminogen activator, and streptokinase have been studied in the management of pulmonary embolism. Although they have shown some benefit, no data indicate improvement in mortality. (*See text page* 1356.)

2. **True.**   Large loading doses of streptokinase must be given to overcome antistreptococcal antibodies. Hydrocortisone should be given with streptokinase therapy to prevent side effects of the drug. (*See text page* 1356.)

3. **True.**   Thrombolytic therapy typically does not require close monitoring of coagulation values because a fixed dose usually is given. For long-duration therapy, monitoring either thrombin time or fibrinogen level may be beneficial in ensuring that a lytic effect has been achieved. (*See text page* 1356.)

4. **B**

5. **C**

6. **E**

7. **A**

8. **D.**   Several pharmacologic agents are used clinically in modulating the hemostatic process for therapeutic or prophylactic reasons. Heparin is administered intravenously and serves as the specific cofactor for antithrombin III in its activity against activated free forms of the serine proteases, specifically factors IIa, IXa, Xa, XIa, and XIIa. Thus heparin is useful in controlling uncontrolled activation of the clotting cascade and is useful only when adequate amounts of antithrombin III are present. Warfarin is the most commonly used oral anticoagulant. It interferes with production of the vitamin K–dependent clotting factors (inactivated factors II, VII, IX, and X) by the liver. Thus it is useful when oral administration is desired for long-term anticoagulation. Dextran is an intravenously administered polysaccharide that has mild effects on both platelet function and coagulation. Dextran appears to inhibit platelet adhesion and adenosine diphosphate–induced aggregation. Thus it is used after vascular surgical procedures when acute, mild impairment of hemostasis is consistent with safe postoperative patient care and inhibition of platelet adhesion as a primary effect is important. Aspirin irreversibly acetylates cyclooxygenase, the key enzyme in the initial stages of the prostaglandin synthesis pathway. Because this renders the platelet essentially nonfunctional for its lifetime (about 10 days), aspirin is more useful when chronic impairment of platelet adhesion and aggregation is desired. Streptokinase binds to plasminogen, pro-

moting formation of plasmin, the primary fibrinolytic agent in the circulation. Thus streptokinase and other plasminogen activators (urokinase and tissue plasminogen activator) are best used in the acute thromboembolic setting, in which clot lodgment threatens tissue or whole-body viability. (*See text pages* 1349–1352.)

9. **C.** Heparin was given in intermittent intravenous boluses until several clinical studies indicated that safer and more consistent management could be achieved with continuous intravenous infusion. A patient typically is given a bolus loading dose of heparin ranging from 50 to 125 units/kg and then is given a maintenance infusion of 1,000 to 1,200 units/hour. The dose is adjusted as necessary and usually is monitored by the patient's activated partial thromboplastin time (aPTT); an attempt is made to keep the aPTT 1.5 to 2.5 times control value. Therapeutic heparin concentrations usually range from 0.2 to 0.7 units/mL. Heparin usually is given for 5 to 14 days to ensure that the period during which the clot is nonadherent is fully covered with adequate anticoagulation. (*See text page* 1352.)

Chapter 120

1. **True.** Virchow's triad describes abnormalities that accelerate or promote *in vivo* clot formation, namely abnormalities of flow, abnormalities of the vessel wall, and abnormalities of the blood itself. The presence of flow tends to inhibit coagulation through local dilution of clotting factors. (*See text page* 1359.)

2. **False.** Antithrombin III is enhanced 1,000- to 10,000-fold by the presence of heparin. Heparin does not work without the presence of adequate amounts of antithrombin III. (*See text page* 1359.)

3. **True.** Activated protein C neutralizes activated factors V and VIII. (*See text page* 1359.)

4. **False.** Protein S is a cofactor for protein C. (*See text page* 1359.)

5. **True.** Plasminogen activation is inhibited by plasminogen activator inhibitor-1, whereas plasmin itself is inhibited by α_2 antiplasmin. (*See text page* 1359.)

6. **D**

7. **C**

8. **A**

9. **E**

10. **B.** A number of acquired thrombophilic disorders have been described, each having certain characteristics. The antiphospholipid syndrome defines a broad spectrum of abnormalities involving the presence of the lupus anticoagulant, thrombocytopenia, hemolytic anemia, leg ulcers, and a tendency for arterial and venous thrombosis. Polycythemia vera belongs to a group of myeloproliferative syndromes associated with recurrent thromboses; it often is managed by means of aggressive phlebotomy. Another myeloproliferative disorder, essential thrombocythemia, represents hyperproliferation of megakaryocytes and resultant thrombocytosis. Paroxysmal nocturnal hemoglobinuria tends to promote thrombosis of splanchnic vessels, particularly the hepatic veins, and produce Budd-Chiari syndrome. Trousseau's syndrome represents the hypercoagulability associated with adenocarcinoma. (*See text page* 1361.)

11. **D.** Because of the substantial morbidity and mortality that accompany venous thromboembolism, the potential to prevent these consequences has attracted a great deal of scientific interest. In general, a group of patients at risk for venous thromboembolic disease can have the risk markedly reduced through appropriate prophylactic measures. These measures consist of the use of anticoagulant

agents, although some patients, such as those undergoing neurosurgical procedures in which the risk for bleeding militates against use of anticoagulants, effective prophylaxis often can be achieved with intermittent pneumatic compression devices. It has been shown that the doses of anticoagulants necessary for prophylaxis are much lower than those usually needed for the management of thrombotic disease. The patients most thoroughly evaluated have been those undergoing elective abdominal operations, among whom prophylactic anticoagulation has been shown to be beneficial for patients older than 40 years. Patients with recent myocardial infarction and those with stroke in evolution also appear to be aided by the use of prophylactic anticoagulation. (*See text pages* 1363, 1364.)

Chapter 121

1. **True.** Hemolytic anemia can be characterized by whether the hemolysis occurs within or outside of blood vessels. Intravascular hemolysis is characterized by acute anemia associated with increased plasma hemoglobin levels, hemoglobinuria, and reduced plasma haptoglobin levels. (*See text page* 1366.)

2. **True.** Extravascular hemolysis develops more slowly than intravascular hemolysis, it is characterized by an elevated serum bilirubin level with a minimal increase, if any, in plasma hemoglobin level. (*See text page* 1366.)

3. **False.** In ascertaining whether anemia is caused by increased destruction or decreased production, reticulocyte count usually is a good index of bone marrow activity. A bone marrow examination is not needed. (*See text page* 1366.)

4. **False.** A direct Coombs' test is performed on red blood cells, whereas an indirect Coombs' test is used to detect the presence of antibodies in serum. (*See text page* 1366.)

5. **E.** Autoimmune hemolytic anemia can be broken down into two major categories: cold-reactive and warm-reactive. This classification is based on the best temperature range at which the offending antibodies react and agglutinate. In most cases of autoimmune hemolytic anemia, a positive direct Coombs' test result indicates the presence of antibodies to the patient's own red blood cells. Cold-reactive autoimmune hemolytic anemia is characterized by the presence of IgM antibodies that react best at low temperatures. Warm-reactive autoimmune hemolytic anemia usually is associated with the presence of IgG antibodies that react best at body temperature. Corticosteroids usually are of no benefit in the management of cold-reactive autoimmune hemolytic anemia. (*See text page* 1367.)

6. **B.** Hemolysis of red blood cells can occur through a variety of mechanisms, both congenital and acquired. Paroxysmal nocturnal hemoglobinuria is an acquired stem cell disorder manifested by severe intravascular hemolysis, thrombocytopenia, and thrombotic events. A peculiar characteristic, abnormally sticky platelets, may be responsible for many of the thrombotic consequences of this disease. (*See text page* 1368.)

7. **D.** Osmotic erythrocyte injury is a transient episode of intravascular hemolysis that occurs after intravenous infusion of hypotonic solutions. (*See text page* 1368.)

8. **C.** Erythroblastosis fetalis, or hemolytic disease of the newborn, occurs when an Rh-negative mother is sensitized to the presence of the Rh antigen in an Rh-positive fetus, affecting subsequent pregnancies. (*See text pages* 1368, 1369.)

9. **A.** Sickle cell anemia is caused by the homozygous presence of the abnormal hemoglobin, hemoglobin S. (*See text page* 1369.)

Chapter 122

1. **E.** A National Institutes of Health Consensus Development Conference reviewed the available information regarding perioperative red blood cell transfusion and came to the conclusion that the arbitrary hemoglobin level of 10 g/dL that clinicians have traditionally used is insupportable. The fundamental function of red blood cells is the transport of oxygen by hemoglobin to oxygen-dependent tissue beds, and transfusion should be performed only when oxygen delivery is seriously inadequate. Many otherwise healthy patients often can tolerate hemoglobin levels of 7 to 8 g/dL without adverse sequelae, and administering transfusions to such patients is wasteful. On the other hand, critically ill patients with circulatory insufficiency or impending organ failure may not have the reserve to tolerate even moderate degrees of anemia, and transfusion may be beneficial even if hemoglobin level already exceeds 10 g/dL. A rational approach to red blood cell transfusion therapy ignores an arbitrary hemoglobin level and concentrates instead on signs of inadequate oxygen delivery. (*See text page* 1373.)

2. **B.** Graft versus host disease may occur after transfusion of peripheral blood. This complication has been described as following bone marrow transplantation for quite awhile but is increasingly occurring among recipients of peripheral blood transfusions. Delayed transfusion reaction usually occurs 1 to 3 weeks after transfusion. Hepatitis C occurs among 1 per 100,000 transfusion recipients. Human immunodeficiency virus is transmitted efficiently by blood transfusion and infects approximately 90% of recipients. Clinically significant immunosuppression is suspected on the basis of retrospective studies of infection and results of *in vitro* experiments, but the clinical consequences have not been well proved. (*See text pages* 1375, 1376.)

Chapter 123

1. **True.** Granulocytopenia resulting from drug administration occurs through decreased production or increased destruction. Chemotherapeutic agents used in therapy for cancer are notorious for their ability to produce granulocytopenia, affecting as they do the more rapidly dividing cells. With most of these agents, the nadir of the white blood cell count occurs 10 to 14 days after the beginning of administration of chemotherapy, roughly paralleling the life span of neutrophils. (*See text page* 1381.)

2. **True.** Chemotherapeutic agents that affect stem cells, such as CCNU, carmustine (BCNU), melphalan, and busulfan, produce a nadir 30 to 36 days after the beginning of treatment. (*See text page* 1381.)

3. **False.** Chloramphenicol is traditionally thought to produce aplastic anemia, although cases of isolated neutropenia have been described. (*See text page* 1382.)

4. **True.** Antibiotics of many types can cause granulocytopenia. Even penicillin in high doses has been found to produce neutropenia through a drug-hapten mechanism. (*See text page* 1382.)

5. **False.** H2-blockers such as cimetidine and ranitidine appear to produce neutropenia through receptor blockade. (*See text page* 1383.)

6. **B.** It has been possible in recent years to isolate and purify several growth hormones that control white blood cell development. Several are now in clinical use, primarily for the treatment of patients with severe neutropenia. GM-CSF and granulocyte colony-stimulating factor primarily affect the granulocyte pool. Macrophage colony-stimulating factor appears to act primarily on the macrophage

population. These factors prevent apoptotic cell death in their respective cell lines. (*See text page* 1379.)

7. **C.**   On occasion, patients undergoing hemodialysis can have acute neutropenia associated with pulmonary sequestration of neutrophils. This appears to develop from complement activation through exposure of complement to the cellophane dialysis membranes. Hypoxemia and pulmonary infiltrates can be observed. The pulmonary edema that develops transiently is not likely to result from excessive hydrostatic forces. Because the patient's pulmonary capillary wedge pressure is 7 mm Hg, it is exceedingly unlikely that a low colloid oncotic pressure or low albumin is contributing to the pulmonary edema and hypoxemia. (*See text page* 1383.)

Chapter 124

1. **True.**   In general, patients with hyperleukocytosis have a worse prognosis than those without it. Leukemic infiltration in the pulmonary and cerebral circulations can produce symptoms referable to those organs, such as dyspnea and obtundation. (*See text page* 1392.)

2. **True.**   Impaired mental status may be caused by leukostasis in the cerebral circulation. This usually occurs with a blast count well in excess of 100,000/mm³. The other important, and more devastating, central nervous system complication is intracerebral hemorrhage. The incidence of this complication also is closely related to blast count. (*See text page* 1392.)

3. **True.**   The promyelocytic form of acute leukemia is associated with a high frequency of DIC because of the release of a procoagulant from the primary azurophilic granules of promyeloblasts. (*See text page* 1393.)

4. **B.**   ALL is primarily a disease of children, although it can affect adults on occasion. Sixty percent to 70% of children can now be cured of the disease. ALL can be characterized on the basis of immunologic characteristics into three different subtypes. The most common type, accounting for about 70% of cases, is caused by transport of CD10 antigen on the surface of pre-B cells. The next most common type (approximately 25% of cases) is T-cell ALL. The other types are B cell type ALL, which is likely a variant of Burkitt's lymphoma. The presence of a type of Philadelphia chromosome [t(9;22)] in the pre-B cell variety of ALL carries an especially poor prognosis. (*See text page* 1391.)

5. **B.**   AML primarily affects adults, although it occasionally occurs among children. The disease appears to be more resistant to chemotherapy among older patients. The FAB classification system identifies seven AML subtypes, differentiated primarily on the basis of the manifestations of the disease. The acute promyelocytic leukemia subtype often is associated with DIC. Bone marrow transplantation has been used as therapy for some cases of AML. The bone marrow used is obtained from an HLA-matched sibling or an unrelated donor. Another source is the patient's own remission bone marrow treated *in vitro* with chemotherapy or autologous monoclonal antibodies. (*See text page* 1392.)

6. **E**
7. **D**
8. **C**
9. **A**
10. **B.**   The chemotherapeutic agents used in the management of acute leukemia can all produce toxicities related to the general mechanisms of effectiveness. Cytosine arabinoside (ara-C, cytarabine) can cause severe intestinal mucositis, especially when used in a high-dose bolus regimen. In the worst cases, this therapy can produce severe ileus and gram-negative sepsis. Cytosine arabinoside also can produce

cerebellar toxicity. Daunorubicin and other anthracyclines and anthraquinones are prone to producing cardiotoxicity, especially as the cumulative dose increases. Vincristine, a vinca alkaloid, inhibits microtubular formation and can produce peripheral neuropathy. Methotrexate inhibits dihydrofolate reductase. Toxicity can include mucositis, hepatitis, and pulmonary fibrosis. Methotrexate-induced toxicity can be managed with leucovorin (folinic acid) to overcome the metabolic block produced by the chemotherapeutic agent. Cyclophosphamide can be toxic to bladder mucosa. (*See text pages* 1394, 1395.)

Chapter 125

1. **D.** SVC syndrome usually is an oncologic emergency because the most common cause is a malignant tumor of the upper thorax. Indwelling central catheters, such as Swan-Ganz catheters, have been implicated as causes of SVC syndrome. If patent, the azygous vein allows a collateral pathway for blood return, thereby minimizing symptoms. Thoracotomy is rarely necessary to establish the cause of SVC syndrome. The histologic diagnosis should be made with the simplest, least invasive method available. The mainstay of therapy for SVC syndrome is radiation, the dose and rate being determined by the histologic findings. (*See text pages* 1396–1399.)

2. **E.** Epidural compression of the spinal cord from metastatic tumors most commonly results from lymphoma, multiple myeloma, and among children, sarcoma and neuroblastoma. Pain is the initial symptom for more than 80% of patients. Weakness is a physical finding at presentation in most of these cases. Sensory deficits are rarely the presenting symptom, and autonomic dysfunction is a late and poor prognostic sign. Plain radiographs are beneficial in the evaluation of extradural compression, providing useful data in the cases of 80% of patients. Other diagnostic techniques useful for evaluation of this condition are bone scanning, computed tomography, magnetic resonance imaging, myelography, and cerebrospinal fluid analysis. Many experts believe that magnetic resonance imaging should be the primary radiologic procedure for ascertaining the location and extent of spinal cord compression. Although surgical decompression was initially the mainstay of therapy, radiation therapy is now considered the treatment of choice in most cases of epidural tumor compression of the spinal cord. (*See text pages* 1399–1401.)

3. **E.** Hypercalcemia is not an infrequent finding among patients with cancer, particularly those with bony metastases. The results of one study indicated that only 15% of patients with cancer who had hypercalcemia did not have evidence of bone metastasis. Elevated calcium levels typically occur late in the course of the malignant disease. About 98% of the patients already have had the cancer detected. Interpretation of the total calcium level requires judgment in that about 40% of the total calcium pool is bound to protein, mostly albumin; thus any reduction in albumin concentration reduces total calcium level, although the metabolically active ionized calcium may be normal or even elevated. Measurement of ionized calcium is physiologically more precise. Among as many as 25% of patients with breast cancer who have hypercalcemia, the condition appears to be precipitated by a course of hormonal therapy, as with androgens, estrogens, antiestrogens, progestins, or by an ablative surgical procedure. The combination of volume infusions and diuretic agents is given to patients with varying degrees of hypercalcemia. (*See text pages* 1401–1404.)

X. Pharmacology, Overdoses, and Poisonings

126. Applied Pharmacokinetics: Specific Application for the Intensive Care Unit

True or False

1. The bioavailability of prodrugs is usually less than 100% even though they have been administered intravenously.
2. With constant infusions of a drug, serum concentrations are assumed to have reached steady-state concentrations after three elimination half-lives of the drug.
3. Albumin concentrations have a negligible effect on free serum drug concentrations if the free fraction is less than 0.5.
4. Drugs that undergo substantial tubular secretion have renal clearance values that are greater than the glomerular filtration rate (GFR).

127. Using Physiologic Clearance and Pharmacokinetic Parameters to Individualize and Monitor Drug Therapy

True or False

1. The second phase of a two-compartment linear model is attributed to diffusion of the drug into the tissue compartment while it is being eliminated from the body.
2. Measurement of serum concentrations for drugs with low therapeutic indices is recommended for critically ill patients.
3. Acidic drugs bind to albumin.

Select the best answer

4. Which of the following drugs does not approximate a one-compartment model of elimination?

    A. Gentamicin
    B. Amikacin

C. Phenytoin
D. Penicillin
E. Tobramycin

Match each of the conditions in the first column with its influence on drug requirements in the second column.

5. Volume resuscitation
6. Hyperdynamic sepsis
7. Aggressive forced diuresis
8. Multiple organ failure
9. Major abdominal operation

A. Increases drug requirements
B. Decreases drug requirements
C. Can increase or decrease drug requirements
D. No effect

128. General Considerations in the Evaluation and Treatment of Poisoning

Select the best answer

1. The most effective gastrointestinal decontamination procedure for oral poisoning or overdosage is:

A. Activated charcoal
B. Saline gastric lavage
C. Syrup of ipecac
D. Lactulose

2. Which of the following is necessary to establish that a xenobiotic ingestion is nontoxic?

A. Absence of symptoms in both history and physical examination.
B. Amount and identity of all chemicals and time of exposure are known with a high degree of certainty.
C. Exposure dose is less than the smallest dose known or predicted to cause toxicity.
D. Time elapsed since exposure is greater than the longest known or predicted interval between exposure and peak toxicity.
E. All of the above.

129. Acetaminophen Poisoning

Select the best answer

1. Acetaminophen hepatotoxicity:

A. Correlates poorly with measured serum concentrations
B. Is associated with high hepatic levels of reduced glutathione
C. Uncommonly progresses to severe liver failure and death
D. Is characterized by an almost immediate increase in hepatic transaminases

2. *N*-Acetylcysteine (NAC) therapy for acute acetaminophen toxicity:

    A. Is associated with frequent anaphylactic or anaphylactoid reactions

    B. Is more effective when administered intravenously

    C. Should be administered even if more than 8 hours has elapsed since ingestion

    D. Is unnecessary if initial liver enzymes are normal and the patient has no symptoms

130. Alcohols and Glycols

Select the best answer

    1. An intoxicated patient with abnormal serum and urine ketone levels but no metabolic acidosis most likely has ingested:

        A. Isopropanol

        B. Methanol

        C. Ethylene glycol

        D. Ethanol

    2. Urgent hemodialysis is indicated for each of the following clinical scenarios *except:*

        A. Methanol ingestion with severe metabolic acidosis

        B. Ethylene glycol ingestion of approximately 175 mg/kg

        C. Visual acuity problems experienced by a patient with suspected methanol ingestion

        D. Ethanol ingestion with metabolic acidosis

131. Antiarrhythmic Poisoning

Select the best answer

    1. Polymorphic ventricular tachycardia (torsade de pointes) is associated with antiarrhythmic drug use and:

        A. Is most common with drugs that prolong repolarization

        B. Usually is associated with toxic antiarrhythmic drug levels

        C. Invariably is associated with baseline interval prolongation

        D. Rarely occurs in the first 4 weeks of antiarrhythmic therapy

    2. Lidocaine half-life is prolonged and risk for toxicity is increased in the setting of each of the following conditions *except*:

        A. Cirrhosis

        B. Congestive heart failure

        C. Old age

        D. Renal failure

132. Anticholinergic Poisoning

Select the best answer

1. The actions of physostigmine include which of the following?

    A. It reversibly blocks the action of acetylcholine at the motor end plate
    B. It decreases receptor sensitivity to acetylcholine
    C. It inhibits acetylcholine release from the presynaptic neuron
    D. It prevents enzymatic degradation of acetylcholine

133. Anticonvulsant Toxicity

Select the best answer

1. Soon into an intravenous loading dose of phenytoin, a patient has bradycardia and hypotension. The most likely cause is:

    A. Propylene glycol
    B. Metabolic acidosis
    C. Phenytoin metabolites
    D. Phenytoin anaphylaxis

2. A 32-year-old woman with a history of seizures arrives at the emergency department with a history of intentional carbamazepine overdose. She is comatose but in a hemodynamically stable condition. Carbamazepine level is 26 μg/mL. The patient's mental status gradually improves over the next 12 hours, but her condition worsens with increasing somnolence and hypotension. In addition to hemodynamic and airway support, the next most appropriate procedure is:

    A. Sodium bicarbonate administered intravenously
    B. More activated charcoal through the nasogastric tube
    C. Physostigmine administered intravenously
    D. Flumazenil administered intravenously

134. Antihypertensive Agents

True or False

1. Loop diuretics may potentiate the therapeutic effects of lithium.
2. Angiotensin-converting enzyme inhibitors may cause hyperkalemia.

Select the best answer

3. A 48-year-old male patient is admitted to the intensive care unit with severe hypertension with end-organ damage. He is treated with intravenous nitroprusside at 2 μg/kg per minute. Blood pressure is controlled, but the patient cannot be weaned from the nitroprusside. After 2 days of stability, the patient becomes agitated, disoriented, and tachypneic. Blood pressure control becomes increasingly difficult, and increasing doses of nitroprusside are necessary. The appropriate initial diagnostic step at this point is:

A. Renal angiography
B. Computed tomography of the abdomen
C. Measurement of serum potassium level
D. Measurement of thiocyanate level

135. *Antimicrobial Agents*

Select the best answer

1. Which of the following statements regarding vancomycin is *not true*?

   A. It has a distribution volume of 0.7 L/kg
   B. It can produce flushing and hypotension if infused rapidly
   C. It has to achieve peak serum levels of 5 to 10 mg/L for efficacy
   D. It is mostly eliminated by the kidneys
   E. It is not absorbed from the gastrointestinal tract

2. Which of the following statements regarding imipenem is true?

   A. It is structurally related to the aminoglycosides
   B. It may have to be given more frequently than usual to patients who are in a hyperdynamic state
   C. It has a clearly established therapeutic range
   D. It is well absorbed after oral administration
   E. It is primarily metabolized by the liver

136. β-*Blocker Poisoning*

Select the best answer

1. A 62-year-old man is brought to the emergency department after an intentional overdose of propranolol. At examination he is confused and has a blood pressure of 81/40 mm Hg and a pulse rate of 32 beats/min. An electrocardiogram shows sinus bradycardia with a PR interval of 0.28 second and an intraventricular conduction delay. Intravenous fluids are started, and 1.0 mg atropine is given intravenously with minimal results. The most appropriate drug to try to stabilize this patient's condition is:

   A. Isoproterenol
   B. Dopamine
   C. Glucagon
   D. Dobutamine

137. *Calcium Channel Blocker Poisoning*

Select the best answer

1. Acute cardiovascular toxicity from diltiazem may cause hypotension, bradycardia, and atrioventricular block. The most effective therapy for these complications is:

A. Glucagon
B. Calcium
C. Amrinone
D. Atropine

138. Cholinergic Agents

Select the best answer

1. A 65-year-old farmer is brought to the emergency department by his family 24 hours after spraying pesticide on several acres of crops. Three hours after he finished work, he experienced nausea, vomiting, and diarrhea. Since then he has reported blurred vision, shortness of breath, and mild weakness in his arms and legs. After the pesticide spraying, he removed his work clothes and bathed. Physical examination shows the patient to be diaphoretic and confused. His heart rate is 52 beats/min, blood pressure is 100/60 mm Hg, and respiratory rate of 30 breaths/min. Pupils are miotic, and there is excessive tearing. Scattered expiratory wheezes are present. Abdominal examination shows mild diffuse tenderness and hyperactive bowel sounds. There is diffuse symmetric extremity weakness. Results of routine blood studies are unremarkable, and a chest radiograph is normal. Serum and red blood cell cholinesterase levels are requested. The electrocardiogram shows sinus bradycardia. Initial treatment should include:

A. Pyridostigmine
B. A transvenous pacemaker
C. Succinylcholine and endotracheal intubation
D. Atropine

139. Cocaine Poisoning

Select the best answer

1. Chest pain after cocaine ingestion:

A. Is unlikely to represent myocardial ischemia among patients without a history of coronary artery disease
B. Should be managed presumptively with β-adrenergic blocking drugs
C. Usually occurs days after the acute ingestion
D. May represent coronary arterial spasm

140. Corrosive Poisoning

Select the best answer

1. A 24-year-old woman attempts suicide by ingesting acidic toilet bowl cleaner. Initial endoscopy shows diffuse, severe esophagitis and marked inflammation in the gastric antrum. The patient is treated with water dilution of the gastrointestinal tract, and total parenteral nutrition is begun. On the sixth postingestion day, the patient becomes more febrile and reports shortness of breath and substernal pain.

Crepitance is found on both sides of the neck. A chest radiograph shows pneumo-mediastinum and left pleural effusion. A contrast swallow study shows lower midesophageal perforation. The most appropriate management is:

A. Intravenous corticosteroids
B. Intravenous antibiotics and tube thoracostomy
C. Thoracotomy with drainage and an attempt at esophageal repair
D. Upper gastrointestinal endoscopy with stent placement

141. Cyclic Antidepressant Poisoning

Select the best answer

1. A 42-year-old man arrives at the emergency department after ingesting "a bottle" of imipramine tablets. He is somnolent but arousable. His blood pressure is 90/60 mm Hg, pulse is 130 beats/min, and respiratory rate is 18 breaths/min. Physical examination findings are unremarkable except for tachycardia. The electrocardiogram shows sinus tachycardia with a QRS interval of 0.14 second. Arterial blood gas analysis with 40% oxygen through a face mask shows pH 7.32, P_{CO_2} 42 mm Hg, and P_{O_2} 126 mm Hg. Intravenous access is established, and administration of normal saline solution is started. A nasogastric tube is placed and activated charcoal administered. A serum drug screen is requested. The most appropriate next procedure is:

   A. Intravenous administration of physostigmine
   B. Intravenous administration of sodium bicarbonate
   C. Intravenous administration of phenytoin
   D. To continue supportive therapy pending drug level

142. Cyclosporine

Select the best answer

1. Which of the following statements regarding cyclosporine is *incorrect*?

   A. Ingestion of cyclosporine with food decreases the amount of drug absorbed.
   B. Cyclosporine is primarily metabolized by the liver.
   C. Cyclosporine crosses the placental barrier and can be found in the amniotic fluid during pregnancy.
   D. Nephrotoxicity is the most common adverse effect.
   E. During the first 6 months after a solid organ transplant, serum concentrations of 200 to 400 ng/mL typically are maintained.

143. Digitalis Poisoning

Select the best answer

1. Cardiac glycoside-induced ventricular arrhythmias are most appropriately treated with:

   A. Phenytoin

   B. Procainamide
   C. Quinidine
   D. Bretylium

2. A 62-year-old man is hospitalized with an exacerbation of congestive heart failure. He has mild renal insufficiency with a serum creatinine level of 2.3 mg/dL. Several days later he experiences nausea, weakness, and dizziness on standing. His pulse rate is 42 beats/min and blood pressure 80/45 mm Hg. An electrocardiogram shows 2:1 atrioventricular block. Digoxin level is 6.4 mg/mL. Serum potassium level is 4.2 mEq/mL. Digoxin-specific Fab fragments are administered, and 1.0 mg atropine is given intravenously. Intravenous fluids are started, and the patient is moved to the intensive care unit. Within a few minutes, the patient is in sinus tachycardia with a normal PR and QRS interval, and his condition is clinically stable. A repeat digoxin level, however, is 14.8 mg/mL. The most appropriate treatment now is:

   A. Repeat digoxin-specific Fab fragment administration
   B. To continue current support
   C. Dilantin administration
   D. Hemodialysis

144. Envenomations

Select the best answer

1. A 27-year-old woman incurs a snakebite on the calf while hiking in the mountains near Denver, Colorado. She recognizes the snake as a rattlesnake and feels the bite is deep. Her hiking companions should:

   A. Capture the snake for identification, even if this takes some time.
   B. Place a tourniquet around the leg and use snow to immediately cool the limb.
   C. Immobilize and splint the extremity and make immediate arrangements for hospital transfer.
   D. Avoid incising and mechanically suctioning the bite, even if there is an anticipated delay in hospital transfer.

2. The patient in question 1 arrives in her companion's truck at an emergency department approximately 90 minutes after the snakebite. She is diaphoretic and confused. Her blood pressure is 82/52 mm Hg and pulse is 180 beats/min. A bloody discharge is coming from the bite wound. Large-bore intravenous lines are placed. A urinary catheter drains dark red urine. Blood studies show hematocrit 22%, prothrombin time 2.8 times control, and partial thromboplastin time 88 seconds. Proper management includes:

   A. Correcting coagulopathy first
   B. Intravenous volume expansion and administration of antivenin
   C. Immediate skin testing to antivenin to assess potential hypersensitivity
   D. Local administration of antivenin into the wound

145. Heavy Metal Poisoning

Select the best answer

1. Which of the following statements regarding arsenic ingestion is *incorrect*?

A. One of the primary cardiovascular manifestations is polymorphic ventricular tachycardia.
B. Activated charcoal is crucial to the decontamination effort.
C. The kidneys are the main route of excretion of arsenic compounds.
D. Neuromuscular respiratory failure may be delayed 1 to 2 months after ingestion.

---

146. Hydrofluoric Acid Poisoning

True or False

1. The toxicity of hydrofluoric acid exposure is roughly equal to that of similar magnitude exposure to hydrochloric acid.
2. The predominant route of exposure to hydrofluoric acid is inhalation.
3. Ingestion of milk may be helpful in decontaminating the gastrointestinal tract after hydrofluoric acid ingestion.

---

147. Hydrocarbons

Select the best answer

1. Which of the following tests is most likely to be useful in confirming the diagnosis of carbon tetrachloride ingestion 1 hour after the suspected event?

   A. Prothrombin time
   B. Serum aspartate aminotransferase
   C. Serum creatinine
   D. Supine plain radiography of the abdomen

---

148. Iron Poisoning

Select the best answer

1. Which of the following modalities is not recommended for use in the management of iron overdose by a pregnant patient?

   A. Desferoxamine
   B. Activated charcoal
   C. Whole-bowel irrigation
   D. Gastrotomy for tablet removal

---

149. Isoniazid Poisoning

Select the best answer

1. Which of the following is considered a specific antidote to the neurologic toxicity of isoniazid?

A. Vitamin B_1
B. Vitamin B_2
C. Vitamin B_6
D. Vitamin B_{12}

150. Lithium Poisoning

Select the best answer

1. A 28-year-old woman with a history of manic-depressive illness arrives at the emergency department 12 hours after intentional overdose of an unknown number of lithium tablets. She is confused and has slurred speech. Her vital signs are stable except for a pulse of 56 beats/min and a blood pressure of 100/60 mm Hg. Physical examination findings are unremarkable except for diffuse hyperreflexia. Laboratory studies show serum sodium 152 mEq/L, potassium 3.8 mEq/L, and creatinine 1.2 mg/dL. An electrocardiogram shows sinus bradycardia with an intraventricular conduction delay and a QT interval of 0.58 second. She is given intravenous fluids, nasogastric lavage, and activated charcoal down a nasogastric tube in the emergency department and is admitted to the intensive care unit. Serum lithium level is 3.9 mEq/L (therapeutic level 0.8 to 1.25 mEq/L). The most appropriate management is:

A. Emergency hemodialysis
B. Transvenous insertion of a temporary pacemaker
C. Subcutaneous administration of vasopressin
D. Administration of more activated charcoal

151. Local Anesthetics

Select the best answer

1. Which of the following is known to increase plasma lidocaine levels?

A. Famotidine
B. Ranitidine
C. Cimetidine
D. All of the above
E. None of the above

152. Methylxanthines

Select the best answer

1. A 52-year-old man with chronic obstructive pulmonary disease (COPD) arrives in the emergency department with shortness of breath, nausea, and tremors. He reports taking "extra" theophylline tablets for the previous 4 days because of worsening shortness of breath. At examination he has tachycardia and is tremulous but is awake and alert. Blood pressure is normal. A chest examination shows

decreased breath sounds, but the findings are otherwise clear. There is mild, diffuse abdominal tenderness. An electrocardiogram shows sinus tachycardia at 124 beats/min with occasional unifocal premature ventricular contractions. A chest radiograph shows changes typical of COPD and no infiltrates or edema. Theophylline level is 34.8 µg/mL. Serum potassium level is 3.6 mEq/mL. The most appropriate treatment is:

A. Administration of propranolol
B. Urgent hemodialysis
C. Administration of oral activated charcoal
D. Charcoal hemoperfusion

2. Which of the following is a *true* statement regarding theophylline-induced seizures?

A. They respond rapidly to intravenous diazepam
B. They occur only with theophylline levels greater than 35 µg/mL
C. They are an indication for charcoal hemoperfusion
D. They may respond to vecuronium

153. Monoamine Oxidase Inhibitor Toxicity

Select the best answer

1. Which of the following sympathomimetic drugs should be avoided by patients taking a monoamine oxidase inhibitor (MAOI) for depression?

A. Epinephrine
B. Dopamine
C. Norepinephrine
D. Isoproterenol

2. A severe drug reaction between meperidine and MAOIs that may lead to cardiovascular and neurologic crises has been described. Other agents that have been implicated in similar reactions include all of the following *except:*

A. Metoclopramide
B. Theophylline
C. Fluoxetine
D. Dextromethorphan

154. Neuroleptic Agents

Select the best answer

1. Ventricular arrhythmias among patients receiving neuroleptic agents may be managed with any of the following except:

A. Lidocaine
B. Electrical cardioversion
C. Magnesium
D. Isoproterenol
E. Metoprolol

155. Neuromuscular Blocking Agents

Select the best answer

1. Which of the following medications has been reported to antagonize the neuromuscular blockade of neuromuscular blocking agents?

    A. Diltiazem
    B. Doxycycline
    C. Ranitidine
    D. Quinidine
    E. Propranolol

156. Nonsteroidal Antiinflammatory Agents

Select the best answer

1. Metabolic acidosis caused by severe salicylate intoxication:

    A. Is not anion gap in character
    B. Occurs early after toxicity, when salicylate levels are high
    C. May be associated with hypoglycemia
    D. Is less common among children than among adults

157. Opioids

Select the best answer

1. Seizures associated with meperidine abuse or overdose are likely to be caused by:

    A. Idiosyncratic drug reaction
    B. Toxic metabolite accumulation
    C. Occult central nervous system lesion
    D. Drug adulterants

158. Pesticides

Select the best answer

1. Which of the following is not indicated for the initial management of organochlorine poisoning?

    A. Removal of clothing and wash with soap and water
    B. Cholestyramine
    C. Activated charcoal
    D. Milk of molasses
    E. Gastric lavage

159. Phencyclidine and Hallucinogens

Select the best answer

1. The use of activated charcoal is not recommended in the treatment of patients with minor patterns of phencyclidine (PCP) intoxication because:

   A. Activated charcoal does not adsorb PCP.
   B. The risk of aspiration of charcoal is too great.
   C. The patient is likely to have smoked PCP, and therefore gastric decontamination is unlikely to be beneficial.
   D. Activated charcoal will adsorb other medications being used as specific antidotes to this intoxication.

160. Sedative-Hypnotic Poisoning

Select the best answer

1. The properties of flumazenil include all of the following *except:*

   A. Half-life of 4 to 6 hours
   B. Reversal of benzodiazepine-associated sedation
   C. Potential for seizures among patients dependent on benzodiazepines
   D. Persistence of benzodiazepine-associated amnesia

161. Sympathomimetic Poisoning

Select the best answer

1. Which of the following medications should be avoided in the management of hypertension due to phenylpropanolamine overdose?

   A. Propranolol
   B. Labetalol
   C. Intravenous nitroprusside
   D. Phentolamine

162. Systemic Asphyxiants

Select the best answer

1. A chemist ingests 1 g potassium cyanide in a suicide attempt. A coworker calls an ambulance, and the patient arrives in the emergency department approximately 1 hour after the ingestion. He is anxious, tachycardic, and vomiting. A *true* statement about his poisoning is:

   A. One gram is not a fatal dose

B. Cyanosis should be present.

C. Hypoxemia should be present.

D. Metabolic acidosis should be present.

163. Withdrawal Syndromes

Select the best answer

1. Delirium tremens caused by alcohol withdrawal is commonly characterized by all of the following *except:*

   A. Hallucinations

   B. Seizures

   C. Autonomic instability

   D. Fever

2. The most appropriate agent for controlling the addiction associated with alcohol withdrawal and preventing progression to delirium tremens is:

   A. Chlorpromazine

   B. Haloperidol

   C. Lorazepam

   D. Ethanol

Answers
Chapter 126

1. **True.** The bioavailability of intravenously administered drugs is usually assumed to be 100%. Exceptions to this concept are drugs that are administered as pro-drugs, which need further processing before they are clinically active. An example of a prodrug is chloramphenicol succinate, which is inactive until it is cleaved by the liver to yield active chloramphenicol. Bioavailability of the drug depends on the ability of the kidney to eliminate the unchanged prodrug before it can be hydrolyzed to the active form. This agent, for example, is assumed to have a bioavailability of 60% to 90%. (*See textbook page* 1416.)

2. **False.** Intravenously administered drugs given as a continuous infusion are assumed to achieve a steady state with respect to the serum concentration values after five elimination half-lives of the drug have elapsed. The same time period is required for the achievement of a steady state when the drugs are given as intermittent infusions. Because the delay in achieving therapeutic concentrations may be disadvantageous with some drugs, a bolus often is administered at the initiation of therapy. Examples of such loading doses are the common methods of administering lidocaine and phenytoin. (*See textbook page* 1415.)

3. **False.** Most drugs bind to plasma proteins, and 95% of protein-bound drug is associated with one of two proteins, albumin or α-acid glycoprotein. The binding usually is reversible, a constant equilibrium existing between the proportion of free and bound drug. Only the free drug is active pharmacologically. The protein binding capacity usually is more than enough to remain unsaturated, although exceptions exist, such as with valproic acid and salicylates. If protein-binding saturation occurs, the total serum drug concentration can be in the normal range, but

the free fraction (the active component) is increased and potentially contributes to toxicity. If the free fraction is greater than 0.5, less than one-half of the drug is bound, and changes in albumin concentrations have little effect on free serum concentration. (*See textbook page* 1419.)

4. **True.**   The factors that influence the renal clearance of a drug are glomerular filtration, active tubular secretion, and passive reabsorption. Drugs that are filtered only by the glomerulus and neither secreted nor reabsorbed have a clearance equivalent to the GFR. Drugs that have considerable tubular secretion have renal clearance values higher than the GFR, whereas drugs that are reabsorbed have clearance values less than the GFR. (*See textbook page* 1420.)

Chapter 127

1. **False.**   A two-compartment model shows a biphasic relation between drug concentration and time. The first phase occurs as a result of the combination of drug diffusing into the tissue compartment while it is simultaneously being eliminated from the body. The second phase results from only drug elimination from the body. (*See textbook page* 1429.)

2. **True.**   Linear models commonly used to approximate the behavior of drug concentrations within the body are the one-compartment and two-compartment models. The one-compartment model is the simplest to apply and use. It assumes minimal to no tissue uptake and a linear relation between drug concentration and dosage. Because of the highly variable physiologic conditions common among critically ill patients, it is nearly impossible to apply the assumptions inherent in dosing nomograms for these patients. Therefore measurement of serum concentrations of drugs with low therapeutic indices is recommended for critically ill patients. (*See textbook pages* 1432, 1433.)

3. **True.**   Acidic drugs bind to albumin, the level of which is often decreased in critical illness. Basic drugs bind to α_1-acid glycoprotein, an acute phase reactant that is often increased in acute critical illness. (*See textbook page* 1433.)

4. **C.**   Most drugs used in the intensive care unit follow linear pharmacokinetic principles. This means that a change in serum concentration is directly proportional to a change in the patient's dosage regimen. Most antibiotics and analgesics used in the intensive care unit follow these linear principles. Phenytoin is nonlinear in epileptic patients. This indicates that there is some enzymatic metabolism of the agent that follows saturation kinetic principles (Michaelis-Menten concepts). However, among patients who are in a hyperdynamic state, it is possible that a nonlinear drug such as phenytoin can behave in a linear manner. (*See textbook page* 1428.)

5. **A**
6. **C**
7. **B**
8. **B**
9. **A.**   A patient's physiologic status can markedly affect the pharmacokinetic parameters that determine the serum concentration of any administered drugs. The disturbance can be so severe as to produce nontherapeutic drug concentrations, either subtherapeutic if the resulting concentration is too low to produce a pharmacologic effect or potentially toxic if the drug concentration is too high. Volume resuscitation tends to expand the apparent volume of distribution for drugs commonly used to treat patients in an intensive care unit, necessitating use of a larger drug dose if effective concentrations are to be ensured. Patients undergoing major abdominal operations usually have expanded volume requirements to maintain an adequate

circulation during the operation, and thus dosage requirements increase. Aggressive forced diuresis tends to contract a drug's apparent volume of distribution and reduce drug requirements. Patients with established multiple organ failure usually accumulate drug because of diminished clearance, and thus less drug may be necessary. If the synthetic capabilities of the liver are impaired, the reduction in albumin and other proteins can reduce the total pool requirements for the drug. Patients in a hyperdynamic septic state can have increased or decreased drug requirements, depending on the drug. Flow-limited agents usually have an expanded volume of distribution and a rapid elimination rate, and dosage requirements are increased. Capacity-limited drugs can have either increased or decreased clearance, depending on the effects of the hyperdynamic state on the enzyme system involved. (*See textbook pages* 1430–1433.)

Chapter 128

1. **A.**   Activated charcoal is probably the most effective single procedure for intestinal decontamination and prevention of chemical absorption. Gastric lavage may cause aspiration, especially among patients who are not awake and alert. There is no substantial evidence that gastric lavage improves outcome over that achieved with administration of activated charcoal alone. Use of syrup of ipecac likewise is associated with increased numbers of side effects and complications, but it continues to be useful for home management of some accidental ingestions. Cathartics may be helpful in enhancing intestinal motility of ingested toxins that have high anticholinergic activity, but they do not markedly affect intestinal chemical absorption. (*See textbook pages* 1450, 1451, 1455.)

2. **E.**   The overlapping components of the careful history, physical examination, and knowledge of the pharmacologic activity of the ingested substances provide the safeguards necessary to ensure patient safety when the patient is released from acute medical care. (*See textbook page* 1443.)

Chapter 129

1. **C.**   Although severe hepatitis is possible in acetaminophen toxicity, death is unusual. Reports of mortality among untreated patients have varied from 5.3% to 24%. Patients treated with *N*-acetylcysteine within 8 hours of drug ingestion have a mortality of less than 1%. The risk for liver injury correlates well with the measured blood levels of acetaminophen when the interval from ingestion is known. Reduced glutathione detoxifies reactive toxic acetaminophen metabolites oxidized by the cytochrome P-450 mixed-function oxidase system. Depletion of reduced glutathione is responsible for increased toxicity. Initial transaminase values often are normal after toxic acetaminophen overdose and may not increase until 24 to 36 hours after ingestion. (*See textbook pages* 1470, 1471, 1476.)

2. **C.**   Even if there is substantial delay from acetaminophen ingestion to initiation of NAC, antidote therapy decreases mortality and morbidity, presumably from effects other than those on acetaminophen metabolites and reduced glutathione stores. Serious side effects from NAC are rare. Although nausea and vomiting are common, the efficacy of oral NAC is the same as that of intravenous drug, and the intravenous form is not available in the United States. Initial liver enzyme levels may be normal even in the case of severe poisoning, and the need for therapy should be based on measured levels and nomogram interpretation. (*See textbook pages* 1471, 1473, 1475.)

Chapter 130

1. **A.** Isopropanol has twice the central nervous system depressant potency of ethanol. Acetone is the primary metabolite, and acetone cannot be further oxidized to an acid. Therefore ketone (acetone) levels are abnormal, but metabolic acidosis does not occur. Toxicity with methanol and ethylene glycol is associated with metabolic acidosis. These intoxicants are metabolized to acids, and methanol also interferes with the mitochondrial electron transport chain, producing lactic acidosis. Alcoholic ketoacidosis usually occurs when ethanol levels are low to absent and is attributable to liver glycogen depletion, impaired gluconeogenesis, free fatty acid mobilization, and subsequent ketoacid formation. (*See textbook pages* 1481, 1488, 1489.)

2. **D.** Ethanol is primarily metabolized and cleared by the liver. Therapy for alcohol ketoacidosis is supportive with intravascular volume and electrolyte replacement, glucose, and thiamine. Methanol and ethylene glycol are metabolized to acids that have the potential to produce severe end-organ damage and marked metabolic acidemia. Clearance is accelerated by hemodialysis, which should be performed early at any indication of substantial ingestion. (*See textbook page* 1481.)

Chapter 131

1. **A.** Polymorphic ventricular tachycardia occurs most commonly in association with class IA and class III antiarrhythmic drugs that prolong repolarization and increase the QT interval. The arrhythmia most often occurs with normal or therapeutic drug levels. One study found that less than half of patients with polymorphic ventricular tachycardia had baseline appreciable prolongation of the QT interval. Most episodes occur within the first 4 days of drug treatment, and almost all within the first month. (*See textbook page* 1497.)

2. **D.** Lidocaine is metabolized in the liver, and liver disease and congestive heart failure (decreased hepatic blood flow) prolong the drug half-life and lead to drug accumulation. The elderly also often metabolizes the drug more slowly. Renal failure does not affect levels or elimination of the active drug. (*See textbook page* 1502.)

Chapter 132

1. **D.** Physostigmine binds reversibly to acetylcholinesterase and prevents enzymatic degradation of acetylcholine. This results in persistent action of the enzyme. Physostigmine is used in selected cases of anticholinergic poisoning. The drug penetrates the blood-brain barrier more effectively than neostigmine or pyridostigmine. (*See textbook page* 1513.)

Chapter 133

1. **A.** Phenytoin is a weak acid and soluble only in alkaline media. Therefore, the parenteral form is delivered in propylene glycol. If the intravenous infusion is too rapid (>50 mg/min), hemodynamic and cardiac toxicity may be caused by the propylene glycol. Treatment is discontinuation of the infusion, at least temporarily, and routine hemodynamic support if necessary. (*See textbook page* 1515.)

2. **B.**   Carbamazepine may form concretions in the gastrointestinal tract that result in drug depots capable of persistent or intermittent release and absorption of drug over hours or days. A single dose of activated charcoal is inadequate to neutralize large amounts of ingested drug, and multiple doses are necessary. Because of the anticholinergic properties of carbamazepine, however, gastrointestinal decontamination procedures must be performed cautiously. Alkalinization does not affect carbamazepine clearance. Flumazenil and physostigmine are not recommended in the management of carbamazepine toxicity. (*See textbook page* 1522.)

Chapter 134

1. **True.**   Loop diuretics may increase the therapeutic and toxic effects of lithium. Toxic effects include gastrointestinal symptoms, polyuria, muscle weakness, lethargy, and tremor. Lithium levels should be monitored during concomitant therapy and dosages adjusted as needed. (*See textbook page* 1529.)
2. **True.**   Failure to monitor potassium levels adequately may cause hyperkalemia. This is especially likely if the patient is also receiving a potassium-sparing diuretic. (*See textbook page* 1536.)
3. **D.**   Regardless of the original reason for the patient's malignant hyperthermia, the combination of increasing dosage requirement for nitroprusside to maintain blood pressure with agitation, disorientation, and tachypnea indicates toxicity. Other findings include lethargy, disorientation, coma, and hypotension. (*See textbook pages* 1542, 1543.)

Chapter 135

1. **C.**   Vancomycin is a glycopeptide antibiotic effective in the management of infections due to several gram-positive organisms and some anaerobes. It has a relatively large volume of distribution, averaging about 0. 7 L/kg, or the amount represented by total body water. It has the peculiar property of producing the red man syndrome (rash, vasoflushing, nausea, facial edema, and hypotension) if infused too rapidly. In general, doses of 1 g or more should be infused over a period of 1 hour or more to avoid this syndrome. Peak serum levels for efficacy generally are considered to be between 30 and 40 mg/L. Vancomycin is mainly eliminated by the kidneys, and thus dosage adjustment often is made in the presence of renal failure. Oral administration of vancomycin is effective in the management of pseudomembranous colitis and staphylococcal enterocolitis. However, the drug is not absorbed from the gastrointestinal tract, making it ineffective through the oral route for other systemic infections. (*See textbook pages* 1552–1555.)
2. **B.**   Imipenem is the *N*-formimidoyl derivative of thienamycin, a carbapenem antibiotic that is a structural analogue of β-lactam antibiotics. There is no established therapeutic range for imipenem, although it is generally thought that the serum concentrations should remain above the minimal inhibitory concentration for the entire dosing interval. Imipenem is not well absorbed after oral administration and is therefore given by either the intravenous or the intramuscular route. It is predominantly eliminated by the kidneys. No studies have yet investigated the pharmacokinetics of imipenem in the treatment of patients in a hyperdynamic state. Because such patients may manifest flow-dependent glomerular filtration, more frequent dosing of imipenem may be necessary to maintain concentrations above the typical bacterial minimal inhibitory concentration. (*See textbook pages* 1556, 1557.)

Chapter 136

1. C. Glucagon exerts positive inotropic and chronotropic effects through activation of adenyl cyclase independent of β-adrenergic receptors. Therefore, glucagon increases cardiac contractility and heart rate even with complete β-adrenergic blockade. Other β-agonists may be helpful if given in large doses, but the effect is inconsistent. (*See textbook page* 1573.)

Chapter 137

1. B. Supplemental intravenous calcium improves negative inotropy and atrioventricular conduction disturbances in calcium channel blocker toxicity. The effect on heart rate is less predictable, and additional β-sympathomimetic treatment may be needed. Glucagon and amrinone may improve the hemodynamic complications of calcium channel blocker toxicity. Some patients with hypotension, may need sympathomimetic agents such as dopamine, norepinephrine, or epinephrine. (*See textbook pages* 1577, 1578.)

Chapter 138

1. D. Atropine is the primary therapy for cholinergic poisoning. Large doses sometimes are necessary, often in combination with pralidoxime, which reactivates acetylcholinesterase. Use of pyridostigmine, an anticholinesterase agent, clearly is contraindicated. Transvenous cardiac pacing may eventually be needed if the patient's condition is refractory to atropine and pralidoxime or more hemodynamic instability develops. Patients with severe bronchospasm or respiratory muscle weakness may need intubation and mechanical ventilation, but there is no definite indication in the care of this patient. Succinylcholine must be avoided because its effect may be very long lasting in the presence of cholinesterase inhibitors. (*See textbook pages* 1585, 1586.)

Chapter 139

1. D. Chest pain following cocaine use may represent myocardial ischemia regardless of the patient's age or cardiac history. The mechanisms of ischemia may be multifactorial and include coronary artery spasm, direct toxicity, or induced ischemia among patients with prior disease due to increased myocardial oxygen consumption. Patients most often report pain within 3 hours of ingestion, but in rare instances chest pain occurs days later. Use of β-blockers is controversial in the management of cocaine toxicity. Some authors have raised concerns about increased complications from unopposed α-adrenergic effects if β-blockade is imposed. (*See textbook page* 1591.)

Chapter 140

1. C. Caustic ingestion has resulted in esophageal perforation, a life-threatening complication. Immediate thoracotomy is indicated for an attempt at repair of the defect, isolation of the midesophagus, and possible colonic interposition. Intravenous corticosteroids may be useful in the management of some corrosive esophageal or gastric injuries, as to decrease stricture formation when started prophylactically. However, they have no place in this patient's treatment after perforation. Upper gastrointestinal endoscopy is unnecessary. The patient needs antibiotics and chest tube drainage, but thoracotomy and an attempt at repair are critical. (*See textbook page* 1599.)

Chapter 141

1. **B.** Cardiac arrhythmias and conduction abnormalities that occur with tricyclic antidepressant overdoses can be suppressed by means of increasing the arterial pH to alkalemic ranges. Increasing the pH also increases plasma protein binding of the drug and decreases the available amount of free drug. Increasing the extracellular sodium concentration has similar effects. Physostigmine antagonizes the sinus tachycardia and altered mental status, but the potential for cholinergic toxicity makes this agent rarely indicated. Phenytoin use is controversial and may actually increase the incidence of ventricular tachycardia. The central nervous system and cardiovascular manifestations show clearly that this patient has severe toxicity. Basing treatment decisions on a drug level is inappropriate at this time. (*See textbook page* 1609.)

Chapter 142

1. **A.** Ingestion of cyclosporine with food actually increases the amount of drug absorbed and leads to elevated serum levels. During the first 6 months following a solid organ transplant, serum concentrations of 200 to 400 ng/mL are typically maintained. After that time a range of 100 to 250 ng/mL usually is considered reasonable. Cyclosporine is metabolized by the liver with more than 90% of a dose excreted as metabolites into the bile and eliminated in feces. Cyclosporine crosses the placental barrier and can be found in the amniotic fluid during pregnancy, in the infant's blood 48 hours after birth, and in breast milk. Adverse reactions include renal dysfunction, tremor, hypotension, hepatotoxicity, and drug interaction. (*See textbook pages* 1615–1617.)

Chapter 143

1. **A.** Phenytoin increases the ventricular fibrillation threshold and speeds conduction through the atrioventricular node. Procainamide and quinidine decrease atrioventricular nodal conduction and are contraindicated. Lidocaine also has been used successfully to manage digoxin-induced ventricular arrhythmias and can be used safely in the presence of atrioventricular block. Bretylium also may be successful in some cases, but animal models of digoxin toxicity have shown some proarrhythmogenic effects of bretylium. (*See textbook page* 1621.)
2. **B.** Digoxin-specific Fab fragments rapidly bind free serum digoxin, and a concentration gradient results that moves tissue-based digoxin into the blood, where it is bound. Total bound and unbound digoxin is measured in the blood assay, and the level is markedly increased after Fab treatment. Further therapy should be based on the patient's clinical and electrocardiographic status, not the measured drug level. The Fab-digoxin complex is excreted by the kidneys, and the level

may be elevated for days. In severe renal failure, dissociation of the complex may occur over time, and increasing free digoxin levels can cause further toxicity. The digoxin-Fab complex is not cleared by dialysis. (*See textbook page* 1622.)

Chapter 144

1. **C.** The initial first aid for venomous snakebites includes placement of a wide constricting band on the extremity proximal to the bite with enough tension to occlude only superficial veins and lymphatic vessels. Use of an arterial tourniquet should be avoided. An involved extremity should be immobilized and splinted at heart level, and immediate transportation to an emergency department should be arranged. Cooling affected limbs is inappropriate. Some authors believe that cooling may actually drive venom deeper into tissues. Incision of the bite increases risk for infection and local necrosis. Mechanical suctioning for 30 to 60 minutes may be of benefit if a device with adequate suction is used and there is an anticipated delay in hospital transfer. Almost all venomous snakebites in the United States are inflicted by pit vipers. There should never be a delay in stabilization of the patient's condition or in hospital transfer while an attempt is made to capture the snake. (*See textbook pages* 1625, 1626.)

2. **B.** Systemic manifestations of envenomation include shock, hemolysis, consumptive coagulopathy, hemorrhage, and acute renal failure. Proper management includes volume expansion and administration of intravenous antivenin. Testing for potential hypersensitivity to antivenin is inappropriate in this clinical situation, because the patient needs the therapy. The patient must be monitored closely, and any reaction should be managed with epinephrine and slowing of the infusion rate. Administration of blood products to a patient who has experienced envenomation and has consumptive coagulopathy should follow treatment with antivenin. Local administration of antivenin is not helpful because binding of toxins occur rapidly and cannot be reversed. (*See textbook pages* 1627, 1628.)

Chapter 145

1. **B.** Results of animal and *in vitro* studies suggest that inorganic arsenicals are not well bound to activated charcoal. Therefore, gastric lavage seems to be the key element in gastrointestinal decontamination. Polymorphic ventricular tachycardia occurs and often necessitates overdrive pacing. A variety of antiarrhythmic agents have been used without clear success. Neurologic manifestations include confusion, delirium, convulsions, encephalopathy, coma, and neuropathy. The neuropathy tends to develop after the acute presentation and is the cause of the respiratory failure. (*See textbook pages* 1638–1640.)

Chapter 146

1. **False.** The corrosiveness of hydrofluoric acid is much greater than expected from its acidity alone. This is because although there is less hydrogen ion activity than with hydrochloric acid, the biologic activity of the fluoride ion is far greater, and much more toxic, than that of the other halides. Because it is less charged, hydrofluoric acid is more able to penetrate lipid barriers. Once inside tissue, it is able to attack many important molecules. (*See textbook page* 1653.)

2. **False.**   The predominant route of exposure to hydrofluoric acid is skin contact. The pulmonary toxicity of hydrofluoric acid occurs when the substance is heated, aerosolized, in the gaseous or anhydrous state, or present in concentrations greater than 60%. (*See textbook page* 1653.)
3. **True.**   Ingested hydrofluoric acid may be complexed and detoxified by calcium- or magnesium-containing substances, including milk. (*See textbook page* 1656.)

Chapter 147

1. Although the diagnosis of carbon tetrachloride ingestion usually is made from the history, an abdominal radiograph may be helpful because carbon tetrachloride is radiopaque. Liver function test results may begin to increase as early as the first day after ingestion, although clinical evidence of liver toxicity, including coagulopathy, usually occurs on days 2 to 4. Renal function can occur concomitantly with hepatic dysfunction. (*See textbook page* 1661.)

Chapter 148

1. **B.**   Treatment of a pregnant patient for iron overdose should be no different than the treatment of any other patient. Activated charcoal does not adsorb iron and therefore is of no use in iron ingestion. Whole-bowel irrigation is probably the most effective nonsurgical method of intestinal decontamination. If whole-bowel irrigation is ineffective, gastrotomy should be considered. Deferoxamine is generally considered the therapy of choice for serious ingestions. It acts as a chelating agent and removes a small amount of iron from the blood. However, its value has not been proved in any randomized prospective trial. (*See textbook pages* 1668–1671.)

Chapter 149

1. **C.**   Vitamin B_6 or pyridoxine can lessen the effect of isoniazid on τ-aminobutyric acid and therefore reverse the neurologic toxicities, including seizure, coma, and peripheral neuropathy. (*See textbook pages* 1674, 1676.)

Chapter 150

1. **A.**   Hemodialysis effectively removes lithium, and the patient has severe toxicity. Despite a lithium level less than 4.0 mEq/L, the neurologic and cardiovascular abnormalities may progress without prompt treatment. Lithium absorption may be delayed for up to 72 hours after ingestion, and the immediately determined level may not represent the peak potential for toxicity. Repeated dialysis sessions may be necessary, because lithium slowly leaves that tissue compartment for the circulation. A pacemaker may be necessary, but dialysis should be initiated first, because reduction of lithium levels may stabilize the cardiovascular toxicity. This patient might have drug-induced nephrogenic diabetes insipidus reflected by the elevated serum sodium concentration, but this does not respond to vasopressin.

Continued crystalloid volume replacement is the most effective therapy. Lithium is not bound effectively by activated charcoal, and additional treatment is necessary unless there is suspicion that additional drugs have been ingested. (*See textbook pages* 1680, 1681.)

Chapter 151

1. **C.** Cimetidine increases plasma lidocaine levels, the other H2-receptor antagonists have no effect. Cimetidine has no known effect on plasma bupivacaine levels. (*See textbook page* 1697.)

Chapter 152

1. **C.** Serial administration of oral-activated charcoal enhances elimination of theophylline by decreasing absorption and promoting the diffusion of theophylline out of the splanchnic circulation into the intestinal lumen. Theophylline clearance can be increased twofold with this treatment. Charcoal hemoperfusion is even more effective at drug removal, but the time and delay involved in initiating this procedure and the relatively mild nature of this patient's intoxication make hemoperfusion unnecessary. Hemodialysis accelerates clearance, but it is invasive. Propranolol may be useful in controlling toxic manifestations of theophylline, but it is not clearly indicated in the treatment of this patient at this time. (*See textbook page* 1704.)

2. **C.** Theophylline-induced seizures are a life-threatening complication, and hemoperfusion should be used to rapidly decrease theophylline level. Even with this intervention, seizures may be persistent and refractory. Failure to respond to usual doses of diazepam or phenytoin is typical. Anesthesia with a barbiturate such as pentobarbital may be the best anticonvulsant regimen. Theophylline-induced seizures have been described among patients with high-normal drug levels. Vecuronium is a nondepolarizing neuromuscular blocker, not an anticonvulsant. It may be useful for temporary control of refractory tonic-clonic activity, but it does not affect electric status epilepticus. (*See textbook pages* 1704, 1705.)

Chapter 153

1. **B.** Treatment with an MAOI results in decreased intraneuronal degradation of catecholamines. Administration of indirectly acting adrenergic agents such as dopamine causes release of stored catecholamines, which may precipitate a crisis. The other sympathomimetic drugs listed act directly on postsynaptic receptors. (*See textbook pages* 1708, 1709.)

2. **A.** All of the drugs listed except for metoclopramide have been associated with severe drug–MAOI reactions, although the data concerning morphine are inconsistent. The drug effect is believed to be an exacerbation of MAOI-induced increases in central nervous system serotonin level. In one experiment, metoclopramide decreased the symptoms of meperidine–MAOI interaction in an animal model. (*See textbook page* 1709.)

Chapter 154

1. E.   Use of type 1A (i.e. procainamide), type 1C (i.e. propafenone), and type II antiarrhythmic agents (i.e. metoprolol) should be avoided because of their ability to exacerbate prolongation of the QT interval. Isoproterenol may be used in cases of torsades de pointes to achieve chemical overdrive pacing. (*See textbook page* 1720.)

Chapter 155

1. C.   Ranitidine has been reported to antagonize neuromuscular blockade. All the other agents are considered to have the potential to potentiate the blockade. (*See textbook page* 1731.)

Chapter 156

1. C.   Anion gap metabolic acidosis characteristically occurs more than 24 hours after acute massive ingestion of salicylates. Hypoglycemia may be present. Because children tend to progress to severe intoxication more rapidly than adults, metabolic acidosis is more common and respiratory alkalosis less common among children. (*See textbook pages* 1737, 1738.)

Chapter 157

1. B.   Meperidine is metabolized to normeperidine, which has reduced analgesic and euphoric potency but twice the convulsant potential of the parent drug. Normeperidine also has a prolonged elimination half-life, so metabolite accumulates after repeated doses or a single large dose. The seizures usually are short-lived, but repeated events may necessitate anticonvulsant therapy. (*See textbook pages* 1749, 1751.)

Chapter 158

1. D.   Milk and oil-based cathartics should be avoided because their high lipid solubility can enhance intestinal absorption. Removal of clothing and washing the skin, hair, and nails are mandatory. Gastric lavage with a small nasogastric tube may be helpful, as may administration of activated charcoal. Cholestyramine may interrupt enteric circulation and limit absorption. (*See textbook pages* 1757, 1758.)

Chapter 159

1. C.   The patient is likely to have smoked PCP, to improve promptly after treatment for cerebral excitation, and therefore is unlikely to benefit from gastric decontamination. Activated charcoal does adsorb PCP and is indicated for the management of more severe intoxication due to oral ingestion. There is no specific antidote at this time. (*See textbook page* 1777.)

Chapter 160

1. **A.** Flumazenil is a competitive inhibitor at the benzodiazepine receptor and effectively reverses sedation. Amnesia, however, often is retained. Patients dependent on benzodiazepines are at risk for withdrawal seizures with flumazenil administration, and the drug should be avoided if dependence is suspected. The half-life is 1 to 2 hours, so rebound sedation may occur if the sedative being antagonized has a half-life longer than that. (*See textbook page* 1784.)

Chapter 161

1. **A.** Propranolol should be avoided because it blocks both the β_1 and β_2 receptors allowing unopposed ι-receptor activity. All the other agents listed are effective. (*See textbook page* 1295.)

Chapter 162

1. **D.** Cyanide binds to the ferric ion of mitochondrial cytochrome oxidase and blocks the terminal reaction of oxidative phosphorylation. Production of adenosine triphosphate is stopped, and anaerobic metabolism begins, leading to lactic acid production and metabolic acidosis in extreme poisoning. Tissue and mixed venous oxygen tensions may be slightly increased. The problem is not hypoxemia, which occurs in late poisoning complicated by respiratory arrest. Ingestion of as little as 200 mg of cyanide can be fatal to an adult. (*See textbook pages* 1797, 1798.)

Chapter 163

1. **B.** Delirium tremens usually begins 48 to 72 hours after the cessation or reduction in alcohol consumption. Seizures rarely occur during the delirium tremens phase. If they should appear, the concern is for a cause other than the alcohol withdrawal. The most common time for alcohol withdrawal seizures is 7 to 48 hours after cessation of drinking. The other signs and symptoms listed are characteristic findings. (*See textbook page* 180.)

2. **C.** Benzodiazepines are most effective at controlling agitation and potential self-harm, and they demonstrate cross-tolerance to ethanol, possibly preventing progression to delirium tremens. Phenothiazines and butyrophenones may lower the seizure threshold and do not prevent severe ethanol withdrawal. They should be avoided. Alcohol suppresses withdrawal reactions, but the duration of action is short and central nervous system side effects are common. Use of alcohol for therapy does not address the underlying abusive behavior. (*See textbook pages* 1809, 1810.)

XI. Surgical Problems in the Intensive Care Unit

164. Epistaxis

Select the best answer

1. Most posterior nosebleeds are due to rupture of the:

    A. Anterior ethmoidal artery
    B. Posterior ethmoidal artery
    C. Lateral branch of the sphenopalatine artery
    D. Septal branch of the sphenopalatine artery
    E. Greater palatine artery

2. Kisselbach's plexus is:

    A. A cluster of nerve fibers near the carotid body
    B. Considered an abnormality whenever it is encountered
    C. The area responsible for most nosebleeds
    D. Located on the superior-posterior portion of the nasal septum
    E. A site where ectopic pheochromocytoma is known to occur

3. Posterior epistaxis:

    A. Commonly results from branches of the superior labial artery
    B. Is usually controlled with balloon catheters
    C. Is best controlled with direct visualization and control of the bleeding vessel
    D. Is more easily controlled than is anterior epistaxis
    E. Is usually controlled with cotton strips soaked in cocaine or tetracaine-phenylephrine

165. Esophageal Perforation and Mediastinitis

Select the best answer

1. Which of the following is the most common mechanism of esophageal injury and esophageal perforation?

    A. Swallowing a foreign body

B. Perforation through intraluminal instrumentation
C. Perforation through penetrating trauma (extraluminal perforation)
D. Spontaneous rupture

166. Management of the Postoperative Cardiac Surgical Patient

Select the best answer

1. Which of the following does not reduce the endocardial viability ratio (EVR)?

   A. A decrease in aortic diastolic pressure
   B. An increase in heart rate
   C. An increase in aortic systolic pressure
   D. An increase in left ventricular diastolic pressure
   E. A decrease in heart rate

2. Prophylactic treatment with which of the following agents reduces the incidence of atrial fibrillation among patients recovering from cardiac operations?

   A. Lidocaine
   B. Procainamide
   C. Propranolol
   D. Digoxin
   E. Bretylium

3. Which of the following statements regarding postoperative bleeding among cardiac surgical patients is *false*?

   A. Heparin rebound is the most common cause of prolonged partial thromboplastin time and thrombin time.
   B. Platelets should be transfused when platelet dysfunction is suspected as a cause of bleeding diathesis.
   C. Patients who have undergone cardiac operations and undergo emergency exploration for bleeding in the intensive care unit have a poor survival rate, and this procedure should not be attempted.
   D. A normal reptilase time confirms the diagnosis of heparin rebound.
   E. Autotransfused blood has been extensively defibrinated.

167. Noncardiac Surgery in the Cardiac Patient

True or False

1. Transurethral resection of the prostate should be deferred for at least 6 months after myocardial infarction because of increased risk for perioperative death.
2. The presence of considerable valvular aortic stenosis appears to be the single preoperative factor of greatest importance in evaluating risk for cardiac complications of noncardiac surgical procedures.

Select the best answer

3. Which of the following has *not* been shown to be a predictor of increased risk for cardiac complications of surgical intervention?

   A. The presence of hyperlipidemia
   B. Age greater than 70 years
   C. Signs of chronic liver disease
   D. Intrathoracic operation
   E. Emergency surgical procedure

168. Diagnosis and Management of Intraabdominal Sepsis

Select the best answer

1. Which of the following statements regarding peritonitis is *false*?

   A. In cases of perforating diverticulitis, the complication rate from primary anastomosis is markedly higher than when resection with end colostomy is performed.
   B. Increased intraabdominal pressure can cause compression of mesenteric and renal veins.
   C. Planned relaparotomy has been shown to reduce the mortality of diffuse peritonitis.
   D. It is important to evacuate the peritoneal cavity of all purulent collections in the treatment of patients with diffuse peritonitis.
   E. Anastomotic leakage can increase mortality.

2. Which of the following statements regarding percutaneous drainage of intra-abdominal abscesses is true?

   A. Percutaneous drainage techniques are capable of removing infected necrotic tissue from the abdomen.
   B. Follow-up imaging rarely is necessary in percutaneous drainage of abdominal abscesses.
   C. It is not acceptable to cross the peritoneal space to drain an extraperitoneal abscess.
   D. Percutaneous drainage can be used as a temporizing measure before an operation for removal of infected tissue or management of the underlying cause of the peritonitis.
   E. Percutaneous drainage of lesser sac collections is not always possible.

3. Which of the following statements regarding the antibiotic management of intra-abdominal infections is *false*?

   A. The most common organisms isolated from intraabdominal infections are those of the Enterobacteriaceae family and *Bacteroides fragilis*.
   B. Aminoglycosides no longer represent the standard of therapy for intra-abdominal infections.
   C. Ceftazidime is recommended for general empiric therapy because of its broad spectrum of antimicrobial coverage.

D. Regimens for cell-wall-active agents in critically ill patients should have sufficiently short dosage intervals to ensure that serum levels remain above the minimum inhibitory concentration.

E. Most authorities believe that antienterococcal therapy should be given for intra-abdominal infection only when enterococci are the only organism isolated or when they are isolated from the blood.

169. Acute Pancreatitis

Select the best answer

1. Which of the following drugs is not currently thought to be capable of causing acute pancreatitis?

    A. Dideoxyinisine
    B. Pentamidine
    C. Azathioprine
    D. Furosemide
    E. H2-blockers

2. Which of the following techniques usually provides the best imaging of acute pancreatitis?

    A. Plain abdominal radiographs
    B. Abdominal ultrasonography
    C. Computed tomography
    D. Percutaneous transhepatic cholangiography
    E. Endoscopic retrograde cholangiopancreatography (ERCP)

3. Which of the following is not considered a grave prognostic sign in acute pancreatitis?

    A. Age older than 55 years
    B. Serum calcium level less than 8 mg/dL
    C. Pao_2 less than 60 mm Hg
    D. White blood cell count greater than 15,000/mm³
    E. Serum amylase level greater than 1,000 IU/dL

170. Mesenteric Ischemia

True or False

1. The mortality for nonocclusive mesenteric infarction necessitating surgical intervention approaches 70%.
2. Abdominal pain may be absent in 25% of cases of mesenteric ischemia.

Select the best answer

3. Which of the following is the diagnostic method of choice for patients with suspected colonic ischemia?

    A. Computed tomography of the abdomen and pelvis
    B. Arteriography

C. Colonoscopy

D. Exploratory laparotomy

E. None of the above

171. Compartment Syndrome of the Abdominal Cavity

Select the best answer

1. An increase in the thickness of the peritoneum of 0.5 cm due to edema or inflammation reflects retention of how much fluid is in that structure?

   A. 500 mL
   B. 1 L
   C. 5 L
   D. 9 L
   E. 18 L

172. Necrotizing Fasciitis and Other Soft Tissue Infections

True or False

1. The presence of gas in a soft-tissue infection is diagnostic of clostridial myonecrosis.
2. All clostridial infections occur in muscle.
3. A combination of streptococci and staphylococci can cause necrotizing fasciitis that is clinically identical to that produced by oral or enteric bacteria.
4. The mortality for nonclostridial myonecrosis appears higher than that of clostridial myonecrosis.

Select the best answer

5. The most effective means of establishing the diagnosis of necrotizing fasciitis is:

   A. Physical examination and needle aspiration
   B. Surgical exploration
   C. Plain radiographs of the area demonstrating gas
   D. Wound sonography
   E. Computed tomography

173. Arterial Diseases of the Extremities

True or False

1. Atrial fibrillation is associated with approximately 25% of instances of peripheral thromboembolism.

2. In the care of a patient with atrial fibrillation and no history of peripheral vascular disease, who experiences the acute onset of unilateral lower extremity arterial obstruction, arteriography provides useful information leading to appropriate treatment.
3. When lower extremity ischemia due to aortic dissection is suspected, aortography that includes the aortic arch is necessary.

174. Pressure Sores: Prevention and Treatment

Select the best answer

1. Which of the following statements regarding pressure sores is true?

   A. The elderly do not demonstrate increased risk for development of pressure sores.
   B. Skin necrosis is a sensitive indicator of tissue injury.
   C. A grade 3 ulcer indicates extension through the muscle down to the bone.
   D. Most ulcers that are treated surgically recur in the same location.
   E. All of the above.

175. Management of Pain in the Critically Ill

Select the best answer

1. A postoperative patient is to be treated with a continuous intravenous infusion of an opiate medication. The elimination half-life of the opiate is 4 hours. The patient needs 10 mg to initially obtain analgesia. What is the correct infusion rate?

   A. 1.25 mg/hour
   B. 2.50 mg/hour
   C. 4.25 mg/hour
   D. 6.25 mg/hour
   E. 7.25 mg/hour

176. Obstetric Problems in the Intensive Care Unit

Select the best answer

1. During pregnancy:

   A. Heart rate increases during the first and second trimesters.
   B. Systemic vascular resistance decreases during the first and second trimesters.
   C. Cardiac output increases during the first and second trimesters.
   D. Stroke volume increases during the first and second trimesters.
   E. All of the above are true.

2. Fetal blood oxygen content:

   A. Is highly dependent on the vascular tone of the maternal uterine vessels.
   B. Is lower than that of maternal blood because of the lower P_{O_2}.
   C. Is not dependent on maternal blood pressure.
   D. Is very close to that of maternal blood because of the greater oxygen affinity of fetal hemoglobin.
   E. Is lower than that of maternal blood despite a similar P_{O2}.

3. Which of the following drugs is *not* considered safe to administer to a pregnant patient?

   A. Diazepam
   B. Warfarin
   C. Penicillin
   D. Nitroglycerin
   E. Clindamycin

Answers

Chapter 164

1. D.   Five arteries supply the internal nose: the anterior ethmoidal and posterior ethmoidal arteries (both branches of the ophthalmic artery, which is a branch of the internal carotid artery), the sphenopalatine and greater palatine arteries (both branches of the internal maxillary artery, which is a branch of the external carotid artery), and the septal branch of the superior labial artery (coming from the facial artery, which is also a branch of the external carotid artery). The septal branch of the sphenopalatine artery supplies the posterior parts of the septum, the lateral nasal wall, and the sinuses. Thus, it is most commonly responsible for posterior nosebleeds. (*See textbook page* 1819.)

2. C.   Most nosebleeds occur in an area known as Kisselbach's plexus, or Little's area. It is located on the anterior-inferior portion of the nasal septum. It represents a plexus of the end branches of several different source vessels supplying the septum, such as the sphenopalatine, the anterior ethmoidal, the greater palatine, and the superior labial arteries. (*See textbook pages* 1820, 1821.)

3. B.   Posterior epistaxis is commonly responsible for bleeding that is more difficult to control than is anterior epistaxis. It usually is caused by rupture of the septal branch of the sphenopalatine artery. Although the same techniques used for anterior epistaxis should be initially attempted for posterior bleeding, they are often ineffective, and some form of posterior packing is used. The traditional technique of posterior packing involved pulling gauze packs into the posterior pharynx and securing them. These have been largely replaced with balloon catheters that can occlude both the posterior and anterior nasal passages. (*See textbook page* 1821.)

Chapter 165

1. B.   Esophageal perforation is a not uncommon consequence of esophageal instrumentation, such as upper gastrointestinal endoscopy and esophageal dilation. The potential for the existence of esophageal perforation should be considered when any patient who has undergone such a procedure suddenly has chest pain and dyspnea, although intraabdominal perforations can have signs of peritonitis and epigastric pain. (*See textbook page* 1824.)

Chapter 166

1. E. The EVR is defined as the ratio of diastolic pressure-time index to systolic pressure-time index. The pressure-time index is defined as the time-based integral of the area between the aortic pressure tracing and the left ventricular pressure tracing in either systole or diastole. The EVR represents the effect of hemodynamics on myocardial oxygen supply and demand. Myocardial perfusion depends on the integrated pressure difference between aortic diastolic pressure and left ventricular diastolic pressure. A longer diastole with a larger diastolic pressure gradient between the aorta and the left ventricle promotes improved myocardial blood flow and increases the EVR by increasing the numerator in the ratio. Conditions that reduce the EVR include a decrease in aortic diastolic pressure, an increase in left ventricular diastolic pressure, an increase in heart rate, an increase in aortic systolic pressure, and a decrease in left ventricular systolic pressure. A decrease in heart rate increases the EVR by providing a longer diastole for myocardial perfusion. (*See textbook page* 1831.)

2. C. Atrial fibrillation and other supraventricular tachycardias frequently occur in the initial days after a cardiac operation. Propranolol has been shown to reduce the incidence of atrial fibrillation among patients who have recently undergone a heart operation. This is an important consideration for patients taking β-blockers before an operation. Procainamide may be useful after the atrial fibrillation has occurred. Digoxin can slow the atrioventricular conduction of a rapid atrial fibrillation but is not effective as a preventive measure. Lidocaine and bretylium are used primarily to manage ventricular arrhythmias. (*See textbook page* 1838.)

3. C. Postoperative bleeding is a serious condition for a patient recovering from a cardiac operation. It can have multiple etiologic factors. Heparin rebound can occur postoperatively when a full reversal of heparin after the operation is overcome by release of heparin from body fat stores into the blood. This is the most common cause of a prolonged partial thromboplastin time and thrombin time. A normal reptilase time confirms that the prolonged thrombin time is caused by excessive heparin and not by fibrinolysis or consumption. Platelet dysfunction frequently occurs because of preoperative aspirin use or the effects of prolonged cardiopulmonary bypass. When this condition is suspected as a cause for excessive bleeding, platelets should be transfused. Autotransfusion is being used increasingly to transfuse autologous blood and reduce homologous blood use. Autotransfused blood appears to be extensively defibrinated, but it does not appear to contribute to coagulopathy when it is transfused. Rapid surgical bleeding that makes cardiac arrest imminent is best approached by means of immediate reopening of the sternotomy incision in the intensive care unit. Emergency therapy is finger control of the bleeding site and vigorous volume resuscitation to be followed by definitive control in the operating room. This practice appears to produce a survival rate of 60%. (*See textbook pages* 1840, 1841.)

Chapter 167

1. False. Thompson et al. showed that among a group of 192 men who underwent transurethral prostatic resection and who had a history of myocardial infarction, the mortality was no greater among patients who underwent an operation within 6 months of infarction than it was for the group as a whole. However, other factors may play a role in determining the timing of surgical intervention. (*See textbook page* 1848.)

2. **False.** In a classic study Goldman et al. created a point system for predicting cardiac risk. In that system, the presence of an S_3 gallop or jugular venous distention indicated impaired left ventricular function and is assigned 11 points and therefore carries the greatest weight in assessment of risk. The presence of substantial valvular aortic stenosis is assigned 3 points. (*See textbook page* 1848.)

3. **A.** In a follow-up report to their original article, Goldman et al. emphasized the lack of relation between the general cardiovascular risk factors, such as cigarette smoking and hyperlipidemia, and the risk of undergoing noncardiac operations. (*See textbook page* 1848.)

Chapter 168

1. **C.** Perforating diverticulitis usually produces severe contamination to the peritoneal cavity. It is important to resect the involved area and provide a diverting end colostomy to gain control over the septic state. The peritoneal cavity should be evacuated of all purulent collections to prevent persistent or recurrent infection. Attempts at primary anastomosis increase the complication rates, and high mortality is attributed to anastomotic leakage. Because of the intestinal and abdominal wall edema that occurs with diffuse peritonitis, it may be difficult to close many of these patients without exerting a severe amount of intraabdominal pressure. Such elevations in intraabdominal pressure can compress mesenteric and renal veins, potentially producing intestinal ischemia or renal failure. Because of this concern and because of the severe contamination that would be enclosed with primary fascial repair, many centers have attempted a technique of temporary fascial prosthetic closure with substances such as woven polypropylene (Marlex), polymeric silicone (Silastic), or polytetrafluoroethylene. Planned relaparotomy then can be easily performed to reduce the level of peritoneal contamination through irrigation and débridement, with removal of the prosthesis and definitive abdominal closure when the abdomen is less heavily contaminated and closure is mechanically feasible. Clinical studies have yet to demonstrate that this technique provides superior outcomes over more traditional methods of management. (*See textbook page* 1858.)

2. **D.** Percutaneous drainage of abdominal abscesses represents an important therapeutic improvement in the management of peritonitis. For some patients, the technique may allow avoidance of a laparotomy that would have been needed for drainage. For others, the presence of infected tissue prevents complete elimination of the infectious process by means of the percutaneous technique. A temporizing measure is a percutaneous method to relieve the pressure within the collection to reduce the infectious load. This measure might improve the patient's clinical condition before the required operation. Although it is generally not considered prudent to cross the pleural space with a percutaneous approach for fear of producing empyema, it is acceptable to cross the peritoneal space to drain an extraperitoneal collection. Lesser sac collections often can be approached by way of the transgastric or the transhepatic. (*See textbook pages* 1859, 1860.)

3. **C.** Intraabdominal infections represent serious clinical problems and often involve difficult decisions for clinicians, who are faced with a wide variety of antibiotic choices. The most common organisms isolated from these infections are members of the Enterobacteriaceae family and *B. fragilis*. Antimicrobial therapy should be aimed at these bacteria. Although aminoglycosides were the standard of management of gram-negative infections for 30 years, they no longer are the only or even the preferred therapy. Many other agents have been developed that effectively cover the spectrum with less toxicity. Third-generation cephalosporins such as cef-

tazidime offer a broad range of coverage; however, wide use of this agent is associated with diminishing susceptibility of *Pseudomonas aeruginosa* and emergence of enterococcal superinfections. Therefore, ceftazidime is not recommended for initial empiric therapy. β-Lactam agents should be given in adequate dosages and with sufficiently short dosing intervals to ensure that tissue levels remain consistently above the minimum inhibitory concentrations for the organisms being attacked. Although enterococci are frequently involved in intraabdominal infections, most authorities believe that these organisms should be covered only when they are the predominant organism on culture or they are isolated from the bloodstream. (*See textbook pages* 1867, 1868.)

Chapter 169

1. **E.**   Several drugs appear to be capable of causing acute pancreatitis. Diuretic agents such as furosemide and others once were considered the most likely drugs to produce acute pancreatitis. However, other drugs such as dideoxyinisine, pentamidine, and azathioprine have been found much more commonly to produce acute pancreatitis, although this may represent a shift in drug use patterns as the treatment of patients with acquired immunodeficiency syndrome and those undergoing transplantation has become more common. Once considered likely to cause pancreatitis, H2-blockers are no longer believed to be capable of doing so. (*See textbook page* 1872.)

2. **C.**   CT is the most useful imaging modality in early acute pancreatitis. The pancreas is depicted on CT scans without being obscured by overlying intestinal gas, as happens at ultrasound evaluation of acute abdominal pain. Plain abdominal radiographs are not helpful in evaluation of acute pancreatitis because they merely provide suggestions about etiologic factors, such as presence of a sentinel loop overlying the pancreas or retroperitoneal air if a gas-forming organism is involved. Percutaneous transhepatic cholangiography is unlikely to depict the pancreas or the pancreatic ducts. ERCP is more likely to depict the ducts, although this may not reveal the etiologic agent in cases of acute pancreatitis. ERCP also can exacerbate the inflammatory process in the pancreas. (*See textbook pages* 1875, 1877.)

3. **E.**   The clinical presentation of acute pancreatitis can vary widely. A worse outcome often can be predicted on the basis of indicators of a more severe disease state. Several grave prognostic indicators were identified by Ranson and by Imrie. These include findings such as age older than 55 years, white blood cell count greater than 15,000/mm^3, low arterial partial pressure of oxygen, low serum calcium level, and indicators of hypovolemia or fluid sequestration. It is interesting that the level of serum amylase does not appear to be a predictive factor, although it is commonly used to detect the presence and follows the course of acute pancreatitis. (*See textbook page* 1875.)

Chapter 170

1. **True.**   Ischemia can be caused by mechanical obstruction of a mesenteric vessel or more commonly by a derangement in regulation of the arteriolar tone of the mesenteric bed. Some of these obstructions progress to infarction of the mesentery, which necessitates surgical intervention and carries a mortality of 70%. (*See textbook page* 1883.)

2. **True.** If pain is absent, symptoms such as bloody diarrhea or abdominal distention and nonspecific signs such as changes in mental status, tachycardia, and fever may be the only clues to the diagnosis. (*See textbook page* 1884.)

3. **C.** Endoscopic evaluation of the colon has been used extensively in the diagnosis of ischemic colitis. This is the diagnostic method of choice for patients believed to have colonic rather than small-intestinal ischemia. These patients include those with left-sided abdominal pain and bloody diarrhea and those who have recently undergone an operation on the abdominal aorta. Colonoscopy can reveal a spectrum of mucosal changes indicative of the severity and duration of colonic ischemia. (*See textbook pages* 1884, 1885.)

Chapter 171

1. **D.** The peritoneum comprises a total area of approximately 1.8 m², an area approximately equal to that of the body surface. A 0.5 cm increase in the thickness of the peritoneum (almost entirely water) represents a 9000 mL increase in fluid. The calculation is as follows:

$$1.8 \text{ m}^2 = 18{,}000 \text{ cm}^2 \times 0.5 \text{ cm} = 9{,}000 \text{ cm}^3 = 9{,}000 \text{ mL} \ (\textit{See textbook page } 1891.)$$

Chapter 172

1. **False.** Although *gas gangrene* is an old and popular term for clostridial myonecrosis, clostridial soft-tissue infection can occur without the presence of obvious gas formation. Clostridial abscesses can occur without myonecrosis, and nonclostridial myonecrosis can produce gas in the wound. (*See textbook page* 1905.)

2. **False.** Not all clostridial infections occur in muscle; they also can occur in injured or ischemic subcutaneous tissue. In general, clostridia tend to thrive in poorly perfused tissue, because they are obligate anaerobes. (*See textbook page* 1906.)

3. **True.** The combination of streptococci and staphylococci can cause necrotizing fasciitis clinically identical to that produced by other organisms. Studies with animal models show that the fasciitis might be caused by synergistic effects of staphylococcal α-lysin and *Streptococcus pyogenes*. (*See textbook page* 1906.)

4. **True.** Nonclostridial myonecrosis can occur among patients with impaired host defenses, such as those with advanced age, diabetes, renal failure, obesity, or atherosclerosis. It is commonly caused by combination of mixed enteric bacteria. Probably because of the poor general health of the patients with the condition, nonclostridial myonecrosis appears to carry a mortality of approximately 76%; most of the survivors have extremity infections controlled by means of amputation. Clostridial myonecrosis has been reported to have a survival rate of 75% with aggressive treatment. (*See textbook pages* 1909, 1910.)

5. **B.** The physical examination findings of a patient with necrotizing fasciitis may be conclusive, especially if extensive superficial necrosis is evident, as with the scrotal skin infarction of Fournier syndrome. Needle aspiration of the inflamed area may recover fluid, but aspiration with normal results may have missed a deep area of necrosis. Gas and fluid may or may not be visible on plain radiographs, sonograms of the wound, or computed tomographic scans, but none of these conclusively eliminates the possibility of the presence of an infectious necrotic process. The most secure means of establishing or eliminating the diagnosis of necrotizing

fasciitis for patients who are at risk for the process is surgical exploration. (*See textbook page* 1908.)

Chapter 173

1. **False.**   Atrial fibrillation is associated with two-thirds to three-fourths of cases of peripheral thromboembolism. It is the single greatest risk factor for the development of arterial emboli. (*See textbook page* 1912.)
2. **False.**   This patient most likely has an embolic occlusion caused by embolism due to atrial fibrillation. The treatment is embolectomy under local anesthesia; arteriography is not necessary. When local thrombosis is highly suspected, arteriography is a necessary precursor to reconstructive surgical treatment under general anesthesia. (*See textbook page* 1915.)
3. **True.**   An aortogram obtained for the diagnosis of an aortic dissection should include the entire aortic arch and abdominal aorta to define the initial area of the intimal tear and associated arch and visceral and lower extremity arterial involvement. (*See textbook page* 1915.)

Chapter 174

1. **D.**   As many as 82% of surgically treated ulcers may recur at the same site. Elderly persons in nursing homes are prone to development of pressure ulcers, and the number of older adults in nursing homes is expected to increase as their population grows. A grade 3 ulcer indicates extension through the subcutaneous tissue to muscle. Extension through the muscle down to the bone qualifies as grade 4 ulcer. The skin may look normal despite extensive subcutaneous tissue injury. (*See textbook pages* 1923, 1924, 1927, 1928.)

Chapter 175

1. **A.**   The patient needs 10 mg to achieve analgesia. The elimination half-life is 4 hours. In 4 hours, or one elimination half-life, 5 mg of the drug is eliminated. Therefore an infusion of 5 mg/4 hours, or 1.25 mg, is needed. (*See textbook pages* 1939, 1940.)

Chapter 176

1. **E.**   Because of the increased demands for oxygen delivery that the placenta and developing fetus place on the maternal circulation, a number of hemodynamic commonly occur in a patient with an uncomplicated pregnancy. Both stroke volume and heart rate increase during the first and second trimesters. These changes combine to produce an increase in cardiac output that peaks during the second trimester to nearly 50% above normal values. In associated with these changes, calculated systemic vascular resistance decreases to a similar degree. In the later stages of pregnancy, cardiac output can be compromised whenever the patient assumes a supine position because of compression on the inferior vena cava produced by the gravid uterus. (*See textbook page* 1950.)

2. **D.**   Fetal oxygen delivery depends on arterial oxygen content, uterine arterial blood flow, placental transfer of oxygen, and the affinity of fetal hemoglobin for oxygen. Because uterine blood vessels are normally maximally dilated, uterine blood flow is directly related to maternal blood pressure. The greater oxygen affinity of fetal hemoglobin overcomes the relatively inefficient placental oxygen transfer and provides the fetus with a blood oxygen content very close to that of maternal blood. This occurs even though the P_{O_2} of fetal blood is substantially lower than that of the mother's blood. (*See textbook page* 1951.)

3. **B.**   Concerns are commonly expressed over drugs administered to pregnant women because of the potential for adverse effects on the developing fetus. In general, drug administration should be avoided for all patients unless the potential benefits outweigh the potential risks. For pregnant patients, however, the risks often are greater than for other patients because of the presence of the fetus. Several drugs have a long and established record of safety during pregnancy that makes their use acceptable. Among these are diazepam, penicillins and cephalosporins, clindamycin, and nitroglycerin. Warfarin is associated with a syndrome of developmental defects and should therefore be avoided in early pregnancy. (*See textbook page* 1952.)

XII. Shock and Trauma

177. Shock: An Overview

Select the best answer

1. Which of the following conditions would not be considered likely to produce a hypovolemic form of shock?

    A. Acute pancreatitis
    B. Bilateral femur fractures
    C. Intestinal obstruction
    D. Tension pneumothorax
    E. Second-degree burns covering 40% of body surface area

2. Which of the following statements concerning the compensatory stage of hypovolemic shock is *false*?

    A. Compensatory mechanisms preserve coronary and cerebral perfusion at the expense of perfusion to the skin, skeletal muscle, kidneys, and splanchnic viscera.
    B. Resuscitation efforts cannot usually be started until this stage is completed because it cannot be detected.
    C. Vasoconstriction and transcapillary refill can partially restore effective intravascular volume.
    D. A large blood volume may be shed in the absence of clinical signs.
    E. Myocardial contractility and heart rate usually increase in an effort to maintain cardiac output.

178. Hemorrhage and Resuscitation

Select the best answer

1. Which of the following statements regarding fluid resuscitation is *true*?

    A. Resuscitation of patients in hemorrhagic shock with isotonic crystalloid solutions increases the amount of pulmonary edema that develops over that which occurs among patients resuscitated with colloid solutions.
    B. Use of hypertonic saline solutions may provide effective resuscitation with relatively small fluid volumes.
    C. The mortality rate improves when trauma patients are resuscitated with colloid solutions.

D. The higher cost of colloid solutions is justified by the more rapid resuscitation achieved with them.

E. Colloid oncotic pressure is more important than capillary hydrostatic pressure in determining the amount of transvascular fluid movement in the pulmonary circulation.

2. Prophylactic administration of blood components is warranted in which of the following circumstances?

A. Platelet transfusion with every 6 units of red blood cell transfusion during an episode of massive transfusion.

B. Fresh-frozen plasma transfusion with every 6 units of red blood cell transfusion during an episode of massive transfusion.

C. Fresh frozen plasma transfusion with every 2 units of red blood cell transfusion during an episode of massive transfusion.

D. Cryoprecipitate transfusion with every 6 units of fresh frozen plasma transfusion during an episode of massive transfusion.

E. Platelet transfusion for any trauma patient with a platelet count less than 20,000/mm^3.

179. Trauma: An Overview

True or False

1. Immediate and early deaths are unlikely to be affected by the institution of a trauma care system.

2. Penetrating trauma distributes energy over a larger surface area than blunt trauma.

Select the best answer

3. The primary cause of immediate death among trauma patients is:

A. Major vascular injury
B. Cardiac injury
C. Brain injury
D. All of the above
E. None of the above

180. Critical Care of Patients with Traumatic Brain Injury

Select the best answer

1. The implementation of which of the following interventions is supported by class I evidence (randomized, prospective, controlled trials)?

A. Systemic corticosteroids
B. Prophylactic anticonvulsants
C. Keeping serum osmolality less than 320 mOsm
D. All of the above

2. Which of the following anatomic areas is least likely to depress into the cranial cavity when it is injured?

A. The cranial vault
B. The facial skeleton
C. The basilar skull
D. All of the above are equally likely to depress into the cranial cavity

181. Spinal Cord Trauma

Select the best answer

1. The skeletal and ligamentous elements that compose the middle column and provide spinal stability are the posterior longitudinal ligament, the posterior annulus fibrosis, and the:

    A. Anterior wall of the vertebral column
    B. Posterior wall of the vertebral column
    C. Anterior longitudinal ligament
    D. Ligamentum flavum
    E. Apophyseal joint capsules

2. Which of the following syndromes mimics peripheral nerve injury rather than spinal cord injury?

    A. Conus medullaris syndrome
    B. Brown-Sequard syndrome
    C. Anterior cord syndrome
    D. Central cord syndrome
    E. Cauda equina syndrome

3. Which of the following statements concerning corticosteroid use in spinal cord trauma is *not true*?

    A. Steroids must be administered within 8 hours of injury to provide a beneficial effect.
    B. The steroid protocol for reduction of spinal cord morbidity requires a period of administration that encompasses 24 hours.
    C. The steroid protocol for reduction of spinal cord morbidity requires a period of administration that encompasses 8 hours.
    D. High-dose corticosteroids have been shown to improve motor and sensory function after spinal cord injury.
    E. A short course of high-dose corticosteroids administered for spinal cord injury has not been shown to increase morbidity or mortality.

182. Abdominal Trauma

Select the best answer

1. Which of the following statements is *true*?

    A. Overwhelming postsplenectomy infection (OPSI) is more likely to occur among adults after splenectomy than among children.
    B. *Mycoplasma pneumoniae* infections are among those that commonly occur among patients who have undergone splenectomy.

C. Thrombocytosis following splenectomy should be managed with antiplatelet agents.

D. Administration of the Pneumovax vaccine is recommended for all patients who have undergone splenectomy.

E. Transient periods of hypotension among patients with known splenic trauma necessitate no operative intervention as long as intravenous fluid and blood administration can reestablish normal vital signs.

2. A 34-year-old woman is injured in a motor vehicle crash. Her hemodynamic condition is stable when she arrives at the hospital with normal vital signs, as is her neurologic condition. She is found to have a right clavicular fracture, fractures of the posterior aspects of right ribs 9 through 11, and a fracture of the right transverse process of the vertebra L2. Abdominal computed tomography (CT) shows no other abnormalities. The patient is admitted to the hospital for observation and recovery. Approximately 24 hours after the injury, a fever develops and rises to 103°F (39.5°C), associated with pulse of 140 beats/min, blood pressure 100/70 mm Hg, and respiratory rate 36 breaths/min. A chest radiograph reveals the presence of atelectasis at both bases. A flat plain radiograph of the abdomen reveals the presence of retroperitoneal air outlining the right kidney, raising the suspicion of duodenal rupture. What should be done at this point?

A. Laparotomy
B. Abdominal CT
C. Blood cultures
D. Nasogastric suction and bowel rest
E. Endoscopic retrograde cholangiopancreatography

3. Which of the following treatments is *not* generally recommended for the treatment of patients with rectal wounds?

A. Diverting colostomy
B. Performance of low rectal anastomosis with an EEA stapler
C. Distal rectal washout
D. Presacral drainage
E. Administration of systemic antibiotics

183. Burn Management

Select the best answer

1. The mean burn size associated with a 50% mortality among healthy young adults is:

A. 30%
B. 50%
C. 70%
D. 90%
E. 100%

2. The Parkland burn formula calls for resuscitation with:

A. Two milliliters of Ringer's lactate per kilogram of body weight per percentage of body surface area burned to be given in the first 8 hours after the burn.

B. Four milliliters of Ringer's lactate per kilogram of body weight per percentage of body surface area burned to be given in the first 8 hours after the burn.

C. Two milliliters of Ringer's lactate per kilogram of body weight per percentage of body surface area burned to be given in the first 24 hours after the burn.

D. Four milliliters of Ringer's lactate per kilogram of body weight per percentage of body surface area burned to be given in the first 24 hours after the burn.

E. Both **A** and **C** are correct.

3. Which of the following statements regarding nutritional support of burn injury is *not* true?

A. Immediately after sustaining a burn, patients need at least 50% to 60% of their calories in the form of carbohydrate.

B. Patients receiving calorie-to-nitrogen ratios of 100:1 have a better survival rate than patients receiving calorie-to-nitrogen ratios of 150:1.

C. Early wound closure immediately reverses the metabolic rate toward normal.

D. Large protein losses can occur through the burn wound.

E. Daily weight measurement often is inaccurate for burn patients.

4. Which of the following is an *incorrect* statement regarding pneumonia among burn patients?

A. It is emerging as a more frequent infectious cause of death.

B. It often can be prevented through the use of prophylactic antibiotics.

C. It usually is caused by penicillin-resistant staphylococci when it occurs in the first 3 days after the burn.

D. It usually is caused by gram-negative organisms when it occurs later in the postburn course.

E. Some studies have reported reduction in rates of pneumonia associated with use of sucralfate rather than H2-blockers for prophylaxis of stress ulcers.

184a. Sepsis and Other Shock States: Derangements of Oxygen Transport

Select the best answer

1. Systemic oxygen delivery is defined as:

A. The product of arterial P_{O_2} and mean arterial blood pressure

B. The product of the arterial P_{O_2} and cardiac output

C. The product of the arterial oxygen content and mean arterial blood pressure

D. The product of arterial oxygen content and cardiac output

E. The product of arteriovenous oxygen content difference and cardiac output

2. Pathologic supply dependency:

A. Exists only in animal models of sepsis

B. Describes a pattern in the oxygen consumption-delivery relation in which the plateau is higher and the critical oxygen delivery is right shifted

C. Can be found only among patients with the acute respiratory distress syndrome (ARDS)

D. Indicates the need for dopexamine infusion

E. Does not exist

184b. Septic Shock

Select the best answer

1. Which of the following conditions would not be considered essential in the definition of the systemic inflammatory response syndrome (SIRS)?

   A. Fever or hypothermia
   B. Tachycardia
   C. Tachypnea
   D. Alteration of the white blood cell count
   E. Hypotension

2. Which of the following statements is *true*?

   A. Lipopolysaccharide (LPS) appears to mediate septic shock, because anti-LPS antibody therapy administered to humans prevents it.
   B. Gram-negative bacteria appear to be the only microbial agents responsible for septic shock.
   C. Interleukin-6 is not an inflammatory cytokine.
   D. Tumor necrosis factor α (TNF-α) has no effect on nitric oxide synthesis.
   E. Humans rendered tolerant to LPS resist signs of illness when infected with viable gram-negative bacteria.

3. Which of the following substances is not thought to mediate the hypotension of septic shock?

   A. Naloxone
   B. Nitric oxide
   C. TNF-α
   D. Interleukin-1
   E. Prostaglandin E_2

184c. Multiple Organ Dysfunction Syndrome

True or False

1. Nonoperative diagnoses account for most instances of multiple organ dysfunction syndrome.
2. A larger number of dysfunctional organs is associated with increasing mortality.
3. Some studies indicate that nutritional interventions may affect mortality in multiple organ dysfunction syndrome.

185. Thoracic Trauma

Select the best answer

1. A 38-year-old man is thrown from his motorcycle at high speed onto a car in a parallel lane. At the scene of the collision, his initial vital signs show blood pressure 90/70 mm Hg, heart rate 112 beats/min, and respiratory rate 42 breaths/min.

He has a large, open pneumothorax involving the left chest. The paramedics apply an occlusive dressing over the wound, taping it tightly on only three of the four sides of the dressing. They also insert two 14-gauge intravenous (IV) catheters and infuse Ringer's lactate rapidly. During transport, after the infusion of 1500 mL IV solution, they find that the patient's blood pressure increases to 132/82 mm Hg, heart rate slows to 78 beats/min, and his breathing appears much easier at 16 breaths/min. The rate of IV infusion is decreased accordingly. On arrival in the emergency department, the patient is found to be acutely diaphoretic, cyanotic, and in respiratory distress with a blood pressure of 70/40 mm Hg, heart rate 140 beats/min, and respiratory rate 44 breaths/min. At the sternal notch, the trachea appears to be deviated to the right. What should be the initial response?

A. Emergency tracheostomy
B. Increase the rate of IV infusion once more, and type and cross match for blood
C. Administer IV epinephrine
D. Remove the dressing over the open pneumothorax
E. Perform emergency left thoracotomy

2. Which of the following radiologic signs is not strongly associated with mediastinal hematoma or traumatic tear of the thoracic aorta?

A. Fracture of the first rib
B. Mediastinal widening greater than 8 cm
C. Depression of the left main stem bronchus
D. Deviation of the trachea to the right
E. Presence of an apical cap

186. Compartment Syndromes

Select the best answer

1. Which of the following is most representative of the capillary perfusion pressure in the systemic circulation?

A. 5 mm Hg
B. 25 mm Hg
C. 45 mm Hg
D. 65 mm Hg
E. 85 mm Hg

2. A 21-year-old man is injured in a motorcycle accident in an isolated area of desolate country. At the scene of the accident, he is ventilating spontaneously and adequately, but he is hypotensive with a blood pressure of 86/56 mm Hg and a heart rate of 140 beats/min. He has an apparent closed pelvic fracture and closed fractures of the right tibia and fibula. Two large-bore intravenous catheters are placed by paramedics, and large volumes of Ringer's lactate are infused. Military antishock trousers (MAST) are applied, and both the abdominal and extremity segments are inflated. The nearest hospital is more than an hour away and the nearest trauma center even farther. The patient receives a total of 6500 mL of fluid during transport, arriving at the trauma center approximately 2½ hours after the paramedics arrived at the scene. On arrival, blood pressure is 92/62 mm Hg, but after administration of 4 units of packed red blood cells and application of a pelvic external fixator, blood pressure increases to 112/72 mm Hg and remains stable, even after removal of the MAST device. Computed tomographic scans of the head are unremarkable, and computed tomographic scans of the abdomen reveal only the pelvic fracture and a large surrounding pelvic hematoma. In addition to stabilizing the right tibia and fibula, which of the following should probably be performed?

A. A right leg fasciotomy
B. Measurement of intraabdominal pressure
C. Therapeutic embolization of the pelvic vessels
D. Bilateral leg fasciotomy
E. Measurement of bilateral lower extremity compartment pressures

3. A patient in stable condition with normal blood pressure who has sustained a tibial fracture has compartment pressures measured in the involved leg. The highest pressure recorded is 27 mm Hg. What should be done at this point?

A. Perform a fasciotomy in the involved leg
B. Administer 25 g mannitol intravenously
C. Continue to monitor the compartment pressures closely
D. Administer 2 ampules of sodium bicarbonate intravenously
E. Perform nerve conduction studies

Answers

Chapter 177

1. **D.**   Effectively identifying the pathophysiologic mechanisms responsible for producing the circulatory shock state in individual patients benefits effective clinical management. The general shock categories of hypovolemic, cardiogenic, and other (e.g., septic) appear relatively consistent among the shock classifications that have been proposed. Several potential causes can lead to the syndrome of hypovolemic shock. Acute pancreatitis produces massive sequestration of fluid in the peritoneal cavity and the retroperitoneum around the inflamed pancreas. This fluid is drawn from the circulating volume, often dropping circulatory performance to critical levels, producing a state of shock. Bilateral femur fractures can be associated with circulating volume losses primarily because of sequestration of blood and extracellular fluid from ruptured vessels around the fracture site. Intestinal obstruction sequesters fluid internally in the intestinal lumen and intraperitoneally; vomiting can exacerbate these fluid losses. Severe burns can cause loss of huge amounts of fluid through evaporative losses and cause some tissue sequestration, producing a hypovolemic state. Tension pneumothorax is not specifically linked to any deficit in circulating volume. Rather, the condition prevents effective venous return and limits the resulting cardiac output. This produces a cardiogenic type of shock even though the heart is not primarily dysfunctional. (*See textbook page* 1963.)

2. **B.**   The first stage of circulatory shock is considered a compensatory and reversible stage in which mechanisms are invoked that maintain adequate circulation without permanent tissue damage. As circulatory shock progresses to decompensation, permanent damage can develop and increase morbidity and mortality. Because of the favorable prognosis, resuscitation efforts should begin as early as possible while compensatory mechanisms are still effective. Though subtle, the signs of compensation can be detected clinically. Tachycardia provides evidence of increased myocardial activity to preserve cardiac output in the face of diminished circulatory volume. A narrowed pulse pressure can provide evidence of the vasoconstriction that helps to normalize the effective circulating volume and redistrib-

ute blood flow away from nonvital beds. The presence of cool, clammy skin also is evidence of this redistribution because flow to vital organs such as the brain and heart is preserved. (*See textbook pages* 1962, 1975.)

Chapter 178

1. **B.**   There has been a long and complex controversy in clinical medicine regarding the optimal fluid for circulatory resuscitation. To date, comparison studies have failed to show any substantial benefit in resuscitating patients from hemorrhagic shock or trauma with colloid solutions that would justify their higher cost. A meta-analysis of several clinical studies indicated that the mortality rate among trauma patients appears to be better when resuscitation is performed with crystalloid solutions, although there seemed to be a slight advantage to using colloid solutions for resuscitation of patients without traumatic injuries. Even though use of colloid solutions may enable more rapid resuscitation because of the smaller volumes needed, the outcomes are not obviously different, and thus the higher costs cannot be justified. Elevations in pulmonary microvascular pressure are the most important determinants governing the transvascular movement of fluid into the pulmonary interstitium, and thus pulmonary capillary wedge pressure monitoring can be crucial in ensuring a safe and effective resuscitation. Preliminary studies of the use of hypertonic saline solutions indicate that these solutions in relatively small volumes may be effective in resuscitation of patients who have hypovolemic shock. (*See textbook pages* 1981–1983.)

2. **E.**   The concept of prophylactic administration of blood components implies that the components are being given to prevent an undesired complication. To that end, physicians have traditionally administered platelets, fresh frozen plasma, or both during massive resuscitation efforts in an attempt to prevent serious coagulopathy from dilution. However, prospective studies have not shown that such regimens are effective at preventing the coagulopathies that develop in association with massive transfusion episodes. Coagulation status should be closely monitored, and replacement should be administered only if deficits actually develop rather than in anticipation of a potential problem. Trauma patients with severe thrombocytopenia (>20,000/mm3) may be at risk for hemorrhage due to known or undetected injuries, thus most clinicians still consider prophylactic platelet administration warranted under such circumstances. (*See textbook page* 1984.)

Chapter 179

1. **False.**   Trauma deaths are divided into immediate, early, and late deaths. Immediate deaths are unlikely to be affected by the availability of a trauma care system because these deaths occur before care arrives. Only prevention is likely to reduce these deaths. Persons at risk for early deaths are those most likely to benefit from provision of care and transport early in the postinjury period. (*See textbook page* 1987.)

2. **False.**   Blunt trauma distributes energy over a larger surface area of the body and is associated with acceleration or deceleration as a mechanism of action. (*See textbook page* 1987.)

3. **D.**   Immediate deaths constitute one half of all trauma deaths. They occur at the scene of the accident and are caused by severe cardiac, vascular, or brain injury. (*See textbook page* 1987.)

Chapter 180

1. **B.** Class I evidence supports the use of prophylactic anticonvulsants such as phenytoin or carbamazepine as a useful means of preventing early posttraumatic seizures. Class I evidence is the basis for a strong argument against systemic corticosteroid treatment. Maintenance of serum osmolality less than 320 mOsm has not been subjected to randomized prospective study. (*See textbook pages* 1993, 1994.)

2. **C.** The basilar skull is much more substantial than the other areas and rarely depresses into the cranial cavity after injury. The vulnerability of the basilar skull is that various cranial nerves traverse this area, and they may be injured. The most frequently injured cranial nerve is the olfactory nerve; the injury results in permanent loss of smell. (*See textbook page* 1994.)

Chapter 181

1. **B.** The determination whether a spinal injury is clinically stable is important in the treatment of patients with such injuries. Patients with stable injuries can be more readily mobilized, thus pulmonary and other complications that appear to develop during prolonged immobilization can be prevented. Patients with unstable injuries must have the spine adequately stabilized before safe mobilization can be undertaken. The three-column theory advanced by Denis helps in the understanding and application of the concept of clinical stability. The anterior column is considered to be made up of the anterior longitudinal ligament, the anterior annulus fibrosis, and the anterior part of the vertebral body. The middle column is formed by the posterior longitudinal ligament, the posterior annulus fibrosis, and the posterior half of the vertebral body. The posterior column is made up of the posterior bony arch, the posterior ligamentous complex (the supraspinous and interspinous ligaments), the capsules of the apophyseal joints, and the ligamentum flavum. Disruption of any two of the three columns produces clinical instability. Isolated middle column damage can be potentially unstable through herniation of material into the spinal canal. (*See textbook page* 2002.)

2. **E.** Cauda equina injury acts like peripheral nerve injury and carries a favorable prognosis. Conus medullaris injury is associated with a thoracolumbar junction injury and acts more like a spinal cord injury. Brown-Sequard is functional cord hemisection from penetrating injury. Anterior cord syndrome results from a flexion or anterior compression injury. (*See textbook page* 2003.)

3. **C.** The National Acute Spinal Cord Injury Study (NASCIS-2) demonstrated that a short (24-hour) course of high-dose methylprednisolone administered within 8 hours of spinal cord injury improved motor and sensory outcomes among patients who received the drug over the outcomes for those who received placebo. If the treatment was started more than 8 hours after injury, however, no benefit was seen. (*See textbook page* 2003.)

Chapter 182

1. **D.** Patients who undergo splenectomy are at risk for OPSI. Children who undergo splenectomy appear to be at greater risk for this complication than are adults. Encapsulated organisms, particularly *Streptococcus pneumoniae, Haemophilus influenzae,* and *Neisseria meningitidis* appear to be frequently involved in OPSI. *Mycoplasma pneumoniae* is not encapsulated. Because of this risk, the Pneumovax vaccine is generally recommended for all patients who have

undergone splenectomy. It provides immunity for many of the pneumococcal strains involved in OPSI. However, Pneumovax vaccine does not confer protection against all OPSI organisms, and long-term prophylactic antibiotics often are used, although the ultimate effectiveness of such an approach is not known. Patients who have undergone splenectomy frequently have postoperative thrombocytosis. Although this is a concern, it does not appear that risk for thrombosis is increased among these patients. Therefore, treatment with antiplatelet agents is not warranted unless other indications exist. One should always attempt to preserve the spleen whenever possible, and nonoperative treatment of a patient with a known splenic injury is certainly one way to achieve that goal. However, a patient with recurrent bouts of hypotension that necessitate repeated episodes of fluid and blood administration has a source of continued blood loss that should be controlled. If the spleen appears to be the source of bleeding, laparotomy should be performed, and hemostatic operative techniques often can be used to salvage the spleen. In many cases, it may be necessary to sacrifice the spleen to obtain hemorrhagic control. (*See textbook page* 2008.)

2. **A.**   The presence of retroperitoneal air outlining the right kidney in this patient who has sustained blunt abdominal trauma and appears to be in a state of sepsis indicates a ruptured duodenum. Although rare, it is a serious injury that can produce devastating infectious complications if untreated. The initial CT examination scan can easily miss such an injury in the early stages. CT is not necessary at this point, because a hollow viscus rupture is demonstrated by the presence of retroperitoneal air without any other obvious explanations. The most expedient measure in the care of this patient is to perform emergency laparotomy with repair and drainage of the injury. (*See textbook pages* 2009, 2010.)

3. **B.**   Rectal injuries represent a serious risk for infectious complications. Because of the huge bacterial concentrations resident in the rectal flora, pelvic infections are a likely consequence of rectal wounds unless the wounds are handled exceptionally well. Toward this end, several techniques are usually advocated as being beneficial in the treatment of patients with rectal wounds. These include (a) administration of large doses of broad-spectrum antibiotics, (b) placement of a proximal diverting colostomy, (c) thorough irrigation of the distal rectum, and (d) placement of perineal drains in the presacral space. Use of an EEA stapling device or any other technique for rectal anastomosis generally is not warranted, although most authorities recommend that the rectal wound be repaired if possible. (*See textbook page* 2011.)

Chapter 183

1. **C.**   The outcome from burn injury has improved greatly over the past century. Fifty years ago, the mean burn size associated with 50% mortality among healthy young adults was only about 30%, whereas today a burn size of approximately 70% is associated with 50% mortality. There are several contributing reasons for this improvement. They include a better understanding of the pathophysiologic mechanisms of burns, more effective management, improved methods of fluid administration and monitoring, improved antimicrobial agents, more effective nutritional maintenance, and an increased understanding of the need for early removal of necrotic burn tissue and skin grafting to minimize the degree and duration of physiologic stress. (*See textbook page* 2015.)

2. **D.**   Extracellular circulatory fluid losses through transudation, evaporation, and tissue edema are the natural consequences of burn injury. The amount of volume loss is directly related to the amount of skin surface area burned. If circulatory fluid losses are not replaced, hypovolemic underperfusion and its consequences

can occur. Several fluid management protocols have been advocated for burn resuscitation. The Parkland formula is one of the more commonly used regimens. It calls for 4 mL Ringer's lactate per kilogram of body weight per percentage of body surface area burned to be given in the first 24 hours after the burn; half of the total volume (2 mL of Ringer's lactate per kilogram of body weight per percentage of body surface area burned) is to be given in the first 8 hours after the burn. (*See textbook page* 2017.)

3. **C.**   Immediately after a burn a hypermetabolic state develops that can lead to a severely catabolic state. Effective nutritional support of these patients is often key to their survival. Monitoring of the nutritional requirements of burn patients is difficult, however. Daily weight measurements often are inaccurate because of the marked fluid shifts that can occur and the variable weight that can be provided by wound dressings. Nitrogen balance studies often are inaccurate because of the large protein losses that can occur through the burn wound. The burn wound appears to be an obligate glucose consumer. At least 50% to 60% of calories should be administered in the form of carbohydrate. Protein supplementation also is important. It has been observed over the years that patients receiving lower calorie-to-nitrogen ratios (100:1) experience an improved survival probability over those receiving more traditional ratios (150:1). Although early burn wound excision and closure appear to improve clinical outcome and may contribute to an ultimate reduction in hypermetabolism, reversal of the metabolic rate toward normal is not immediate after closure. (*See textbook pages* 2018, 2019.)

4. **B.**   Because of the declining incidence of burn wound sepsis, pneumonia is now emerging as a more frequent infectious cause of death among burn patients. Prophylactic use of antibiotics has failed to effectively prevent these pneumonias from occurring and often predispose the patient to infection by antibiotic-resistant bacteria. Better preventive measures include effectively clearing pulmonary secretions, avoidance of microaspiration around the endotracheal tube, and early extubation. Some authors believe that the use of sucralfate rather than H2-blockers for the prevention of stress ulcers reduces the incidence of pneumonia. When pneumonia occurs soon after a burn (within the first 3 days), it is commonly caused by penicillin-resistant staphylococci. When it occurs later in the postburn course, pneumonia is more likely to be caused by gram-negative enteric bacilli or *Pseudomonas* organisms. (*See textbook page* 2021.)

Chapter 184a

1. **D.**   Systemic oxygen delivery, also referred to as *oxygen transport,* is defined as the product of arterial oxygen content and cardiac output. Arterial oxygen content is the sum of hemoglobin-bound oxygen and dissolved oxygen in the blood. Hemoglobin-bound oxygen can be calculated with the product of the hemoglobin concentration, arterial oxygen saturation, and the hemoglobin-binding coefficient for oxygen (1.34). Dissolved oxygen is the product of arterial Po_2 and the solubility coefficient for oxygen in blood (0.003). The product of arteriovenous oxygen content difference and cardiac output defines oxygen consumption according to the Fick principle. (*See textbook page* 2024.)

2. **B.**   The relation between systemic oxygen delivery and oxygen consumption appears to be biphasic in controlled situations in which oxygen delivery can be progressively changed. An oxygen supply-dependent phase exists on the lower end of the spectrum, wherein the amount of oxygen consumed depends directly on the amount of oxygen delivery. On the higher end of the spectrum is an oxygen supply-independent phase in which the amount of oxygen delivered has no effect

on the amount of oxygen consumed. In clinical practice, it is more difficult to observe the biphasic relation between oxygen consumption and oxygen delivery because there is less independent control over the variables in question. It is likely that patients can change their oxygen consumption dependency state from moment to moment, distorting or skewing the observed pattern. In many cases, this can make it appear that critically ill patients are supply-dependent across the entire spectrum of oxygen delivery. Although such a relation appears commonly among patients with ARDS, it also occurs among patients who do not have ARDS. Many clinicians consider evidence of oxygen supply dependency as an indication for further circulatory support in the hope of achieving a supply-independent state. Inotropic agents such as dopamine, dobutamine, amrinone, milrinone, and dopexamine may be useful in this process. However, there is no clear consensus that this approach is completely beneficial or that the potential risks, such as arrhythmias, outweigh the potential benefits. (*See textbook pages* 2024, 2025.)

Chapter 184b

1. **E.**   SIRS is a new term used to designate a commonly appreciated clinical condition with infectious or noninfectious causes. It is defined by the presence of two or more of the following signs or symptoms: (a) abnormal body temperature, (b) tachycardia, (c) tachypnea, and (d) an alteration in white blood cell count. Hypotension is not a designated component of SIRS but would tend to indicate the presence of septic shock (when severe SIRS is caused by infection). (*See textbook page* 2031.)

2. **C.**   Gram-negative bacteria contain a substance known as LPS within their cell walls. This was once thought to be necessary for all cases of sepsis. It is now apparent that LPS is not the only toxic substance at work. In clinical trials, anti-LPS antibodies have been administered to humans with infections, sepsis, and septic shock. The findings were controversial at best and certainly there was no obvious curative effect. No results of studies of the preventive use of these agents have been published. The hemodynamic and metabolic manifestations of septic shock can occur when patients are infected with organisms other than gram-negative bacteria. Human volunteers who are rendered tolerant to LPS still manifest signs of illness when infected with viable gram-negative bacteria. It may be that many endogenous mediators such as TNF-α also participate in some of the phenomena observed among patients with septic shock. Among other things, TNF-α appears to induce nitric oxide synthase, especially in vascular smooth muscle, and promote at least some of the vasodilatation observed in sepsis. Interleukin-6 is not an inflammatory cytokine. Its presence does, however, correlate closely with the severity of the inflammatory response and patient outcome. (*See textbook pages* 2033, 2034, 2038.)

3. **A.**   One of the common features of early septic shock is hypotension associated with often elevated cardiac output and producing a dissociation between blood pressure and blood flow. Several agents have been implicated in this process of septic vasodilatation. TNF-α and interleukin-1 are two cytokines that have received a great deal of attention because they appear capable of producing many of the stigmata of septic shock. Among other effects, these cytokines appear to be able to induce nitric oxide synthase, the enzyme responsible for the production of nitric oxide, from smooth muscle cells. Nitric oxide is a potent vasodilator that increasingly appears to be highly involved in the septic shock response. Prostaglandin E_2 is a proinflammatory prostaglandin involved in the SIRS cascade. Naloxone is an opioid antagonist that was initially thought to be of potential benefit in the management of septic shock because of promising results from animal

studies, but it has failed to show benefit in clinical trails with human subjects. (*See textbook pages* 2032, 2033.)

Chapter 184c

1. **True.**   Seventy-six percent of patients in intensive care units with multiple organ dysfunction syndrome have nonsurgical illnesses. The most common are sepsis, pneumonia, congestive heart failure, cardiac arrest, and upper gastrointestinal bleeding. (*See textbook page* 2045.)
2. **True.**   The reported mortality rates are no organs affected 0.8% mortality, one organ 6.8%, two organs 26.2%, three organs 48.5%, four organs 68.8%, and organs 83.3%. (*See textbook page* 2047.)
3. **True.**   The institution of early enteral nutrition may be important in maintaining gastrointestinal mucosal barrier function and preventing the development of multiple organ dysfunction syndrome. It also has been demonstrated that therapy with a glutamine-supplemented enteral diet decreases bacterial translocation. (*See textbook page* 2046.)

Chapter 185

1. **D.**   Tension pneumothorax has just developed on the left side. Application of the semiocclusive dressing over the open pneumothorax is an effective way to aid lung expansion by producing a flap-valve mechanism. Ideally, air can escape the pleural space but not be sucked back into it. However, it is possible for such a dressing to trap air and produce tension pneumothorax if air leaks into the chest, as from injured lung tissue, and cannot escape as rapidly as it enters. The findings of acute hypotension and tracheal deviation away from the injured side support the diagnosis of left tension pneumothorax. Quick removal of the occlusive dressing from the left chest should relieve the tension and convert the left chest to simple pneumothorax, which should have considerably less severe hemodynamic consequences. (*See textbook pages* 2050, 2052.)
2. **A.**   The diagnosis of torn thoracic aorta in an injured patient can be life-saving if the aorta is repaired before it ruptures. Although infrequently encountered, for some patients who survive the initial accident, this condition provides a window of opportunity to make it to a hospital. The likelihood of presence of an aortic injury is based on the mechanism of injury (typically a deceleration force) and radio-graphic signs of mediastinal hematoma. The signs include mediastinal widening greater than 8 cm, indistinct aortic knob, opacification of the aortopulmonary window, depression of the left main stem bronchus, deviation of the trachea to the right, deviation of a nasogastric tube to the right indicating deviation of the esophagus, presence of an apical cap, and left pleural effusion. Although the presence of upper rib fractures indicates that a severe blow to the thorax has been sustained, studies of large series of patients indicate that there is no greater association with aortic injury among these patients than there is among patients who do not have upper rib fractures. (*See textbook page* 2054.)

Chapter 186

1. **B.**   Normal precapillary hydrostatic pressure is approximately 25 mm Hg and postcapillary 16 mm Hg. This information becomes important in conditions in

which tissue pressures can exceed perfusion pressure and limit nutrient blood flow. An example of such a situation is compartment syndrome, wherein intrafascial compartment pressures rise as a result of increased volume accumulation within a closed, nonexpansive space. Unless the compartment pressure is promptly released, tissue ischemia and eventually muscle necrosis occur. Other clinical situations in which systemic capillary pressure becomes important include management of intracranial hypertension, assessment of elevated abdominal pressure as a potential cause of oliguria, and the upper limit of endotracheal tube cuff pressure. (*See textbook page* 2059.)

2. **E.**   This patient is at great risk for compartment syndromes, not only in the injured right leg but also in the other leg as a result of the prolonged application of the MAST in the face of hypotension. Normal systemic hydrostatic pressure is about 25 mm Hg. When tissue pressure exceeds hydrostatic microvascular pressure (as occurs during MAST inflation), perfusion to the tissues may become impaired. In the case of this patient, the presence of hypovolemic shock, primarily caused by the large fluid losses imposed by the pelvic fracture, might have reduced systemic microvascular hydrostatic pressure even further. Thus, it is likely that perfusion pressures were exceeded for a long duration, rendering the leg muscles ischemic. With prolonged ischemia and venous and lymphatic compression, tissue edema can occur and aggravate the compartment syndrome. At the very least, expedient measurement of tissue pressures in all four compartments in both legs should be performed. This patient will likely need bilateral fasciotomy to preserve muscle and nerve viability. (*See textbook page* 2060.)

3. **C.**   A patient with a tibial fracture is at risk for compartment syndrome. This patient's compartment pressures are elevated, but not to severe levels. It appears that the threshold compartment pressure at which fasciotomy is warranted tends to vary from authority to authority. Most would not recommend fasciotomy in the care of a patient with normal blood pressure when compartment pressures are less than 30 mm Hg. Therefore, continued close monitoring of this patient would be important to ascertain whether compartment pressures increase so that prompt fasciotomy can be performed. Nerve conduction studies may provide information about the function of the nerves that run through the involved compartments and can demonstrate the presence of muscle viability. At these levels of compartment pressure, however, it is likely that the muscle is viable. Nerve conduction velocity measurements must be obtained by specially trained personnel and can produce false-positive results. Although such patients are at risk for myoglobinuria and acute renal failure, no evidence has been provided that this patient has increased levels of myoglobin release. A test for myoglobin in the urine should probably be performed before the administration of agents such as mannitol or sodium bicarbonate. (*See textbook pages* 2061, 2063.)

XIII. Neurologic Problems in the Intensive Care Unit

187. An Approach to Neurologic Problems in the Intensive Care Unit

Select the best answer

1. Which of the following does *not* represent a primary neurologic cause of depressed consciousness?

   A. Head trauma
   B. Diabetic ketoacidosis
   C. Intracranial hemorrhage
   D. Inapparent seizures

188. Evaluating the Patient with Altered Consciousness in the Intensive Care Unit

Select the best answer

1. The locked-in state:

   A. Describes a state of mild cerebral obtundation
   B. Is most commonly caused by a destructive process at the base of the pons
   C. Is characterized by having absolutely no muscle movement detectable
   D. Can be diagnosed only with electroencephalography
   E. Can be diagnosed only with computed tomography

189. Metabolic Encephalopathy

True or False

1. Rapid correction of hyperglycemic hyperosmolality with intravenous hydration and insulin results in cerebral water intoxication and signs of increased intracranial pressure.

2. Adrenocortical insufficiency, like many other metabolic encephalopathies, is associated with increased muscle tone and deep tendon reflexes.
3. For a patient with Wernicke's encephalopathy, prompt administration of 100 mg thiamine completely restores the impairment of ocular movements.

Select the best answer

4. Which of the following factors does *not* contribute to a poor outcome in Reye's syndrome?

   A. Age younger than 1 year
   B. Serum ammonia levels greater than five times normal at peak
   C. The presence of seizures
   D. Prothrombin time greater than 20 seconds
   E. Very rapid progression of liver failure in the first 48 hours

5. Which of the following statements regarding uremic encephalopathy is *true*?

   A. The results at electroencephalography (EEG) typically correlate with mental status changes.
   B. The level of blood urea nitrogen (BUN) is directly related to the cognitive state.
   C. Creatinine level is directly related to the cognitive state.
   D. EEG findings are not changed at higher levels of BUN.
   E. The pathophysiologic mechanism of uremic encephalopathy is not known.

190. Generalized Anoxia/Ischemia of the Nervous System

Select the best answer

1. In cases of out-of-hospital cardiac arrest:

   A. The prognosis for recovery is not related to cardiopulmonary resuscitation (CPR) time if the duration of untreated cardiac arrest is less than 6 minutes.
   B. More than half of patients make a good recovery when CPR is performed for more than 30 minutes if the duration of untreated cardiac arrest is less than 6 minutes.
   C. After out-of-hospital cardiac arrest, the overall probability of awakening is approximately 50%.
   D. Only 3% of patients recover if the untreated cardiac arrest time is longer than 6 minutes, even though actual CPR time is less than 5 minutes.
   E. Recovery is quite likely even if attempts fail to resuscitate patients before arrival in the emergency department.

2. In cases of nontraumatic coma:

   A. The absence of brainstem reflexes during the first 48 hours after an anoxic event has no effect on prognosis.
   B. The most valuable prognostic information is obtained from the physical examination.
   C. Only 30% of patients who do not regain at least two brainstem reflexes within 48 hours do not recover.
   D. The presence of decerebrate or decorticate posturing 24 hours after the event often portends a favorable outcome.
   E. Children have the same recovery rates as adults.

3. Seizures occur among what percentage of patients in anoxic coma?

    A. 5%
    B. 10%
    C. 25%
    D. 50%
    E. 90%

191. Status Epilepticus

True or False

1. Myoclonic status epilepticus among adults almost always is associated with mental retardation syndromes.
2. The most common cause of status epilepticus among adults is a change in antiepileptic drug serum levels.
3. Initial therapy for status epilepticus should be intravenous lorazepam with a loading dose of phenytoin.

Select the best answer

4. Approximately how much time is required on average for death to result from status epilepticus?

    A. 5 minutes
    B. 30 minutes
    C. 4 hours
    D. 13 hours
    E. 3 days

192. Cerebrovascular Disease

Select the best answer

1. Which of the following statements concerning heparin use in ischemic cerebrovascular disease is *not true*?

    A. Heparin therapy should be considered within 24 to 48 hours of the event for patients with cardioembolic stroke.
    B. It has been definitively demonstrated that heparin therapy impedes the progression of stroke in evolution.
    C. Patients with large cerebral infarcts generally should not receive heparin.
    D. Heparin should be administered as a continuous infusion.
    E. A randomized, double-blind trial of heparin versus placebo in the setting of acute partial stable stroke demonstrated no benefit.

2. Which of the following statements regarding primary intracranial hemorrhage is *not true*?

    A. In about 50% of cases it results from long-standing hypertension
    B. It is defined as bleeding within the brain parenchyma without an underlying cause such as a neoplasm, vasculitis, bleeding disorder, prior embolic infarction, aneurysm, vascular malformation, or trauma

C. Its incidence has increased over the last 30 years

D. It was probably misdiagnosed as bland infarcts in previous years

E. It carries a lower apparent fatality rate than seen in previous years

3. The most frequent site of occurrence of nontraumatic intracranial hemorrhage is:

A. The pons

B. The putamen

C. The cerebellum

D. The subcortical white matter

E. The thalamus

193. Neurooncologic Problems in the Intensive Care Unit

Match the term in the first column with the appropriate term in the second column.

1. Peritumoral edema

2. Vasogenic edema

3. Cytotoxic edema

4. Responsive to steroid therapy

A. Intracellular edema

B. Extracellular edema

5. The steroid most commonly used for the management of brain tumors is:

A. Methylprednisolone

B. Hydrocortisone

C. Dexamethasone

D. Aldosterone

E. Prednisone

194. The Guillain-Barré Syndrome

True or False

1. A surgical procedure can be an antecedent event that precedes the onset of Guillain-Barré syndrome (GBS).

2. Most patients have recurrent bouts of GBS after the initial episode.

3. More than half of patients with GBS need mechanical ventilation at some point in the clinical course.

4. Disturbances of the autonomic nervous system are common and potentially lethal.

5. A cerebrospinal fluid (CSF) analysis typically shows an elevated protein level, minimal cellularity, normal glucose level, and normal opening pressure.

6. Plasmapheresis has been shown to offer no benefit to patients with GBS.

Select the best answer

7. GBS:

A. Was first described by Dr. Strohl Guillain-Barré 1902

B. Has an annual incidence of 1 case per 1,000,000 population

C. Is a congenital disorder of neurons
D. Often occurs 2 to 4 weeks after a flulike illness
E. Is a weakness that classically descends from the arms to the legs

195. Myasthenia Gravis in the Intensive Care Unit

True or False

1. Respiratory muscles are the most frequently involved.
2. Edrophonium hydrochloride (Tensilon) is a fast, short-acting parenteral cholinesterase inhibitor that transiently accentuates muscle weakness among persons with myasthenia gravis.
3. Antiacetylcholine receptor antibody titer correlates well with the severity of the disease.
4. Arterial blood gas values are the best indicators of impending respiratory failure among persons with myasthenia gravis.
5. Neuromuscular blocking agents should never be administered to patients in the intensive care unit with myasthenia gravis.
6. Corticosteroids are beneficial to most patients with myasthenia gravis in whose care use of these agents is attempted.
7. Thymectomy should be considered early in the course of myasthenia gravis.

Select the best answer

8. Myasthenia gravis:

   A. Is an autosomal dominant disorder
   B. Affects men four times more frequently than women
   C. Is an exceedingly rare disorder, occurring once among every 4,000,000 persons
   D. Is produced when circulating antibodies react with parts of acetylcholine receptors in postsynaptic membranes, block receptor activation, and accelerate receptor degradation
   E. Is usually a disease of children

9. Plasmapheresis for myasthenia gravis:

   A. Offers little benefit
   B. Often is followed by increased sensitivity to cholinesterase inhibitors
   C. Helps by removing abnormal neurotoxins that cannot be metabolized by patients with myasthenia gravis
   D. Requires several weeks of therapy to show a favorable response for most patients

196. Miscellaneous Neurologic Problems in the Intensive Care Unit

True or False

1. A patient who appears dead after apparent suicidal hanging cannot be resuscitated.
2. Hanging is the third most common means of committing suicide.

3. Hyperthermia can develop after hanging as a result of hypoxic damage to the hypothalamus.
4. Complete or partial recovery is rare among most patients who survive after hanging.
5. Direct current is more dangerous than alternating current.
6. Spinal cord injury is the most common neurologic sequela of electric injury.
7. Myoglobinuria and acute renal failure can result from muscle damage due to electric injury.
8. Seizures are common after electric injury.

Select the best answer

9. Carbon monoxide:

   A. Can be lethal at a concentration of 0.001%
   B. Has a distinctive odor
   C. Can be emitted from charcoal-burning grills
   D. Is not elevated in the bloodstream of cigarette smokers
   E. Is not normally formed *in vivo*

10. Which of the following statements regarding carbon monoxide poisoning is *false*?

    A. Headaches can occur with concentrations of less than 10%.
    B. The classic cherry-red color on the lips usually requires carboxyhemoglobin levels of 30% to 40% to be evident.
    C. One hundred percent oxygen should be administered immediately to any patient believed to have carbon monoxide poisoning.
    D. Steroids have been shown to be effective at controlling the intracranial hypertension resulting from carbon monoxide poisoning.
    E. Roughly 75% of persons with carbon monoxide poisoning recover within a year of the insult.

11. Which of the following statements regarding decompression sickness is *false*?

    A. The onset of symptoms occurs within 12 hours of the decompression event for 97% of patients.
    B. Four fifths of patients with decompression sickness have neurologic symptoms.
    C. The patient should be placed in the head-up position lying on the right side to prevent systemic gas embolization.
    D. Air embolism is a serious form of decompression injury, producing symptoms within 5 minutes of decompression.
    E. Recompression is the primary definitive treatment.

197. Subarachnoid Hemorrhage

True or False

1. Saccular aneurysms occur mainly in the posterior circulation.
2. Most subarachnoid hemorrhages are preceded by a sentinel hemorrhage that may be mistaken for a migraine or muscle tension headache.

Select the best answer

3. Which of the following studies is the most appropriate first investigation to perform when subarachnoid hemorrhage is suspected?

    A. Lumbar puncture
    B. Four-vessel cerebral angiography
    C. Noncontrast computed tomography (CT) of the head
    D. Contrast-enhanced CT of the head
    E. Magnetic resonance imaging and angiography

Answers

Chapter 187

1. **B.** Causes of depressed consciousness often are separated into primary neurologic causes and secondary causes from other medical illnesses. Included in the latter category are many metabolic causes such as ketoacidosis, drug intoxication, and anoxia. (*See textbook page* 2069.)

Chapter 188

1. **B.** The locked-in state is a state of paralysis without loss of consciousness. It is commonly caused by destruction of the base of the pons. Less frequent causes include acute polyneuritis (Guillain-Barré syndrome), acute poliomyelitis, exposure to toxins that block transmission at the neuromuscular junction, and myasthenia gravis. The patient is completely paralyzed except for vertical eye movements and blinking, which operate by means of muscles innervated by midbrain structures. Consciousness is preserved through the ascending reticular activating system, which is located in the tegmentum of the pons and is therefore dorsal to the damaged area. The diagnosis is commonly made through clinical neurologic examination. (*See textbook page* 2073.)

Chapter 189

1. **True.** The hyperosmolality that accompanies hyperglycemia causes a shift of water from the intracerebral tissue space to the intravascular space. This produces brain tissue shrinkage that makes the brain susceptible to water intoxication. Signs of increased intracranial pressure develop if rehydration is accomplished too rapidly. (*See textbook page* 2083.)
2. **False.** Unlike other metabolic encephalopathies, adrenocortical insufficiency produces decreased muscle tone and deep tendon reflexes that do not clear until cortisone replacement is given with therapy for any associated electrolyte imbalances. (*See textbook page* 2084.)
3. **True.** Wernicke's encephalopathy develops acutely among persons with alcoholism or malnutrition. It produces striking impairment of ocular movements. Ocular function can be completely restored with prompt intravenous and oral administration of 100 mg thiamine. Cerebral symptoms resolve more slowly with thiamine therapy. (*See textbook page* 2085.)
4. **C.** Reye's syndrome is a morbid form of acute hepatic encephalopathy among children, usually between the ages of 1 and 10 years, that follows a viral infection combined with aspirin therapy. Therapy for Reye's syndrome is directed at decreasing intracranial hypertension through aggressive reduction of cerebral edema and at controlling seizures and providing adequate nutritional and metabolic support during the period of liver failure. The prognosis for Reye's syndrome

has improved considerably in recent years, with a mortality and morbidity of 10% to 20% at present compared with 40% to 50% in previous decades. Factors that appear to contribute to a poor outcome are patient age younger than 1 year, serum ammonia level that peaks higher than five times the normal level, prothrombin time longer than 20 seconds, rapid progression of liver failure within the first 48 hours, and the presence of renal failure. (*See textbook page* 2081.)

5. **E.** Uremic encephalopathy is one of the many metabolic encephalopathies that can occur among patients in intensive care units. It is often a complication of systemic diseases that independently affect the central nervous system, such as collagen vascular disease, malignant hypertension, drug overdoses, diabetes mellitus, or bacterial sepsis. The clinical presentation is quite variable, with no direct correlation between the cognitive state and level of BUN or any other biochemical marker. The EEG is slower at higher levels of BUN, but it also does not correlate with mental status. The pathophysiologic mechanism of uremic encephalopathy remains unknown. (*See textbook page* 2082.)

Chapter 190

1. **C.** For all patients resuscitated from out-of-hospital cardiac arrest, the probability of awakening is 50%. It is vital that circulation to the brain be restored as promptly as possible. Prognosis is related to the duration of CPR efforts if the duration that the arrest goes untreated is less than 6 minutes. Thus, when CPR lasts less than 30 minutes before circulation is restored, more than half of patients make a good neurologic recovery. If CPR lasts longer than 30 minutes, only 3% of patients make a good neurologic recovery. If the duration of the untreated arrest is longer than 6 minutes, as many as 50% of patients can still recover if the CPR time is less than 5 minutes. Longer periods of CPR are associated with poorer outcomes. If resuscitation efforts fail before the patient's arrival in the emergency department, the prognosis is bleak. (*See textbook pages* 2086, 2087.)

2. **B.** The best prognostic information about nontraumatic coma is acquired through the physical findings. The presence of brainstem reflexes (pupillary light, corneal, and vestibuloocular) within the first 48 hours after an anoxic event, provides a more favorable prognosis than if they are absent. Essentially no patients recover who do not regain at least two of these brainstem reflexes within 48 hours. The persistence of decerebrate or decorticate posturing 24 hours after the event, militates against a favorable outcome. In general, children appear to have better prospects for return of neurologic function than do adults. (*See textbook page* 2087.)

3. **C.** Approximately 25% of patients in anoxic coma have seizures. These seizures can usually be managed as are other seizures with loading, and then maintenance doses of phenytoin or fosphenytoin. In rare cases it may be necessary to use phenobarbital because of cardiac conduction abnormalities. In most cases, however, phenobarbital should be avoided because of its sedative effects and long half-life. (*See textbook page* 2088.)

Chapter 191

1. **False.** Myoclonic status epilepticus is a rare form of convulsion. Among children, it usually occurs in association with chronic epilepsy and mental retardation. Among adults, myoclonic states almost always are caused by toxic, metabolic, viral, or degenerative causes of acute or subacute encephalopathy. (*See textbook page* 2090.)

2. **False.** The most common cause of status epilepticus among adults, causing more than 25% of the cases in one series, is stroke, accounting for over 25% of cases in one study. Another important cause, especially among persons known to have epilepsy, appears to be a change in serum levels of antiepileptic drugs. The incidence of status epilepticus has increased over the past century despite the introduction of antiepileptic drugs, implying a link between the use of these drugs and status epilepticus. (*See textbook page* 2091.)

3. **True.** The initial management of status epilepticus is best approached with intravenous lorazepam for immediate, short-term arrest of any ongoing seizure activity. A loading dose of phenytoin should be administered simultaneously with the lorazepam to establish maintenance therapy. If these drugs do not control the seizures, phenobarbital should be added, and if necessary, barbiturate coma should be induced. (*See textbook page* 2092.)

4. **D.** The duration of status epilepticus profoundly affects patient outcome. The mean duration of status epilepticus for patients who died of status epilepticus was 13 hours in one clinical study. Patients who had no neurologic sequelae of status epilepticus had an average duration of status of 90 minutes, whereas those with neurologic sequelae had an average status duration of 10 hours. (*See textbook page* 2091.)

Chapter 192

1. **B.** Although anticoagulants have been used for many years as therapy for ischemic cerebrovascular disease, definitive proof of their efficacy is lacking. Short-term anticoagulation is considered for patients with cardioembolic strokes; it is generally given within 24 to 48 hours of the event to prevent recurrence. Heparin therapy often is given to patients with stroke in evolution to prevent progression, although there is no definitive proof that it works. Heparin therapy also often is given to patients with multiple transient ischemic attacks to prevent stroke, although there is no proof of efficacy. A randomized, controlled, double-blind clinical trial in the setting of acute partial stable strokes demonstrated no benefit of heparin over placebo. When given, heparin should be administered as a constant infusion with the general aim of maintaining partial thromboplastin time at 1.5 to 2 times control. (*See textbook page* 2099.)

2. **C.** Primary or spontaneous intracranial hemorrhage, rupture of saccular aneurysms, arteriovenous malformations account for most cases of nontraumatic intracranial hemorrhage. Primary intracranial hemorrhage is defined as bleeding within the brain parenchyma without an underlying cause such as a neoplasm, vasculitis, bleeding disorder, prior embolic infarction, aneurysm, vascular malformation, or trauma. It does appear, however, that about half of the cases of primary intracranial hemorrhage are caused by long-standing and uncontrolled hypertension, suggesting it is a secondary process. The incidence of spontaneous intracranial hemorrhage has dropped over the past 30 years, in large part because of the aggressive modern approach to systemic hypertension. This reduction in incidence has occurred, even though computed tomographic scans now more readily depict small hemorrhages that were once misdiagnosed as bland infarcts. Because of the inclusion of these small spontaneous hemorrhages, the apparent fatality rate for nontraumatic intracranial hemorrhage has declined. (*See textbook page* 2100.)

3. **B.** The most frequent site of occurrence of nontraumatic intracranial hemorrhage is the putamen, where it occurs in 30% to 50% of cases. The bleeding is from a lenticulostriate vessel, and the clinical syndrome typically produced is one of sudden flaccid hemiplegia, hemisensory disturbances, homonymous hemianopsia, and paralysis of conjugate gaze to the side opposite the lesion. The subcortical

white matter is involved in 15% of cases, in which the condition often is called *lobar hemorrhage.* These hemorrhages produce syndromes dependent on the location of the bleeding and generally have the lowest mortality and best prognosis. Thalamic intracranial hemorrhages account for 10% of cases and produce unilateral sensorimotor deficits in which sensory findings predominate. Pontine intracranial hemorrhages carry the highest mortality and account for 10% of intracranial hemorrhages. Cerebellar hemorrhages account for 10% of cases and have a mortality as high as 60%. (*See textbook page* 2101.)

Chapter 193

1. **B**
2. **B**
3. **A**
4. **B.**   In addition to cellular growth, brain neoplasms tend to increase extracellular edema. Consequently, this form of edema also is called *peritumoral edema,* and because of its association with altered capillary permeability it is known as *vasogenic edema.* Vasogenic edema typically is highly responsive to steroid therapy. Intracellular edema, however, usually is caused by cellular membrane pump failure and thus is called *cytotoxic edema.* (*See textbook page* 2104.)
5. **C.**   Dexamethasone is the most commonly used steroid in the management of brain tumors. It is a potent glucocorticoid and yet has minimal mineralocorticoid effects. It also, however, has a relatively long onset of action and is therefore not as useful for immediate reduction of elevated intracranial pressure as are other measures, such as hyperventilation or mannitol administration. (*See textbook page* 2106.)

Chapter 194

1. **True.**   Several clinical conditions appear to precede the onset of GBS. These include flulike illnesses, viral infections, including human immunodeficiency virus, immunization, surgical intervention, and renal transplantation. (*See textbook page* 2115.)
2. **False.**   The nadir of the clinical course occurs among most patients within 1 month. Only 2% to 5% have recurrent GBS. (*See textbook page* 2115.)
3. **False.**   Between 10% and 25% of patients need ventilator assistance within 18 days after the onset of the condition. (*See textbook page* 2115.)
4. **True.**   About 50% of patients can have disturbances of the autonomic nervous system that are potentially lethal, taking the form of cardiac arrhythmias, hypotension, and hypertension. (*See textbook page* 2115.)
5. **True.**   The CSF typically shows an albuminocytologic dissociation (elevated protein level with minimal pleocytosis). The CSF glucose and opening pressure typically are normal. (*See textbook page* 2116.)
6. **False.**   Plasmapheresis appears to improve the course of GBS. Patients who receive plasmapheresis walk sooner on average than those who do not. (*See textbook page* 2119.)
7. **D.**   GBS was first described by Guillain, Barré, and Strohl in 1916. It is the most common cause of rapidly progressive weakness, with an annual incidence of roughly 1 case per 100,000 population. It appears to have an immunologically mediated mechanism and classically occurs 2 to 4 weeks after a flulike illness. The

typical presentation is progressive ascending weakness that moves from the legs to the arms, then the respiratory and bulbar muscles. (*See textbook page* 2115.)

Chapter 195

1. **False.** The ocular muscles are the most frequently involved muscle group in myasthenia gravis, which commonly produces ptosis. Respiratory muscle involvement is not rare; respiratory insufficiency occurs with frequency. (*See textbook page* 2122.)
2. **False.** The Tensilon test is evoked by edrophonium hydrochloride (Tensilon), a short, fast-acting parenteral cholinesterase inhibitor that transiently strengthens the affected muscles of a patient with myasthenia gravis. (*See textbook page* 2123.)
3. **False.** Because myasthenia gravis is an autoimmune disease, the presence of antiacetylcholine receptor antibodies is a strong indication of the presence of the disease, although they often are absent among patients with purely ocular myasthenia. Antibody titer does not correlate with severity of the disease or response to treatment. (*See textbook page* 2123.)
4. **False.** The best measurements for monitoring patients with myasthenia gravis for potential respiratory failure are forced vital capacity, maximum inspiratory pressure, and maximum expiratory pressure. (*See textbook pages* 2123, 2124.)
5. **True.** Neuromuscular blocking agents should never be administered to patients in the intensive care unit with myasthenia gravis because these agents usually have prolonged and excessive effects. (*See textbook page* 2124.)
6. **True.** Because of the immunologic nature of myasthenia gravis, immunotherapy has become the mainstay of therapy for myasthenia. Use of corticosteroids is associated with a response rate of 80%. (*See textbook page* 2125.)
7. **True.** Because of the excellent response to thymectomy, this procedure should be considered early in the course of myasthenia gravis, except in the care of patients who are too unstable or too frail to undergo an operation. (*See textbook page* 2126.)
8. **D.** Myasthenia gravis is an autoimmune disease caused by production of circulating antibodies that attack parts of acetylcholine receptors in the postsynaptic membranes of muscles. This blocks the acetylcholine receptors from full activation and may accelerate degradation of receptors. It is a relatively common disorder, affecting approximately 1 in 20,000 persons. The female-to-male ratio is 3 : 2. The incidence peaks among women in the third decade of life and among men in the fifth and sixth decades of life. (*See textbook page* 2122.)
9. **B.** Because of the immunologic nature of myasthenia gravis, plasmapheresis has been attempted with favorable results. Most patients respond within 48 hours of the initiation of plasmapheresis, although therapy must be continued on an intermittent basis. Many patients eventually have increased sensitivity to cholinesterase inhibitors after plasmapheresis, mandating reduction in the maintenance dosage of these drugs. (*See textbook page* 2125.)

Chapter 196

1. **False.** A patient who appears dead after hanging can be resuscitated and likely needs endotracheal intubation, mechanical ventilation, restoration of a normal cardiac rhythm and circulation, and control of intracranial hypertension. (*See textbook page* 2128.)

2. **True.**   Hanging is the third most common means of committing suicide and is more common among men (3:1). (*See textbook page* 2127.)

3. **True.**   Hyperthermia can occur after hanging as a result of hypoxic damage to the hypothalamus. (*See textbook page* 2128.)

4. **False.**   Despite the initially poor appearance, most patients who survive the initial event recover partially or completely. (*See textbook page* 2128.)

5. **False.**   Because of tetanic contractions that prevent voluntary release from the current source, alternating current is more dangerous than direct current. It also is more likely to produce cardiac arrhythmia and respiratory arrest. (*See textbook page* 2128.)

6. **True.**   Neurologic sequelae occur among more than 25% of patients with electric injuries. Spinal cord injury is most commonly involved because of the common occurrence of extremity-to-extremity current flow, which goes through at least some part of the cord. (*See textbook page* 2128.)

7. **True.**   Myoglobinuria and acute renal failure can be caused by the extensive muscle damage that can occur. (*See textbook page* 2129.)

8. **False.**   Seizures are uncommon after electric injury. (*See textbook page* 2129.)

9. **C.**   Carbon monoxide is a colorless, tasteless, odorless gas that is normally present in the atmosphere in concentrations less than 0.001%. Concentrations of 0.1% can be lethal. Carbon monoxide can be emitted from charcoal-burning grills and from automobile exhaust. It also is found in fires, methylene chloride, volcanic gas, and cigarette smoke. Because of the latter, carbon monoxide levels in the bloodstream (normally present in concentrations of 1% to 3% from the degradation of hemoglobin) can be elevated in cigarette smokers to levels of 6% to 7%. (*See textbook page* 2130.)

10. **D.**   Headaches are a frequent symptom after carbon monoxide poisoning and can occur with concentrations of less than 10%. Although well-known, the classic cherry-red color on the lips is rarely seen, because it usually requires carboxyhemoglobin levels of 30% to 40%. For any patient believed to have experienced carbon monoxide poisoning, 100% oxygen should be administered immediately. Such therapy can shorten the half-life of carbon monoxide in the bloodstream from 320 minutes to 80 to 90 minutes. Steroids have not been proved effective for the management of carbon monoxide poisoning and may reduce the oxygen toxicity seizure threshold if hyperbaric oxygen treatments are used. About 75% of persons with carbon monoxide poisoning have recovered within 1 year of the insult. (*See textbook page* 2130.)

11. **C.**   For most patients, symptoms after decompression occur within 6 hours. Symptoms occur within 12 hours among 97% of patients. Nearly 80% of patients with decompression sickness have neurologic symptoms, the most common being paresthesia. The patient should be placed in a slight Trendelenburg position on the left side to prevent left ventricular coalescence of gas bubbles and systemic embolization. Air embolism is a more serious form of decompression injury, probably resulting from lung injury and producing symptoms within 5 minutes of decompression because of occlusion of large vessels. Recompression is the only real definitive treatment. (*See textbook page* 2131.)

Chapter 197

1. **False.**   Eighty-five percent of saccular aneurysms are located in the anterior circulation; 15% are along the vessels of the posterior circulation. Common sites of aneurysms are the junction of the anterior cerebral and anterior communicating arteries, the origin of the posterior communicating artery, the mid-

dle cerebral artery trifurcation, and the top of the basilar artery. (*See textbook page* 2136.)

2. Sentinel hemorrhage occurs in only approximately 20% of cases. In 20% to 40% of those cases, it is misdiagnosed as a more benign cause of headache such as migraine or muscle tension headache, sinusitis, viral syndrome, viral meningitis, or malingering. (*See textbook page* 2136.)

3. C.   If subarachnoid hemorrhage is suspected, the initial study should be non-contrast CT of the head. A lumbar puncture is indicated if the CT examination provides no diagnostic information. The other studies may be used at some point in the evaluation, but not as the first step. (*See textbook pages* 2136, 2137.)

XIV. Transplantation

198. Transplant Immunology and the Use of Immunosuppressive Agents in Solid Organ Transplantation

True or False

1. Cyclosporine acts by inhibiting interleukin-2 synthesis through inhibition of messenger RNA transcription.
2. Cyclosporine levels are best obtained as a peak dose after oral administration to best guard against nephrotoxicity.

Select the best answer

3. Which of the following statements regarding cyclosporine is *true*?

   A. Cyclosporine is primarily excreted in the urine.
   B. Oral cyclosporine has a mean bioavailability of 80%.
   C. Adequate cyclosporine absorption depends on the presence of bile salts.
   D. Cyclosporine dosing usually has to be increased with time after transplantation.

4. Which of the following is a *correct* statement regarding drug interactions with cyclosporine?

   A. Drugs that induce the P-450 IIIA enzyme (phenytoin, rifampin) can cause increased cyclosporine levels.
   B. Drugs that are metabolized by the same enzymes as cyclosporine, such as erythromycin, show competitive enhancement and lead to decreased cyclosporine levels.
   C. P-450 IIIA enzymes have been isolated from the intestine and may influence oral cyclosporine absorption.
   D. Cyclosporine metabolism cannot be influenced advantageously.

5. Which of the following is a *correct* statement regarding the side effects of treatment with cyclosporine?

   A. The main side effect of cyclosporine administration is hepatotoxicity.
   B. Cyclosporine dosing must be carefully adjusted to avoid nephrotoxicity among patients with renal failure.
   C. Cyclosporine nephrotoxicity only develops acutely.
   D. Calcium channel blocking agents may be the drugs of choice for the management of hypertension among recipients of transplants.

6. Which of the following statements correctly describes the role of corticosteroids in posttransplant management?

  A. Corticosteroids inhibit interleukin-2 synthesis.
  B. Corticosteroids inhibit chemotaxis of inflammatory cells.
  C. Optimal dosing of corticosteroids has been established over the 30 years of their use in management of transplant rejection.
  D. Steroids can reverse only 30% to 40% of rejection episodes among kidney and heart transplant patients.

7. Which of the following is a *correct* statement regarding the use of muromonab-CD3 (Orthoclone OKT3)?

  A. Muromonab-CD3 is effective in the management of acute cellular rejection episodes.
  B. Muromonab-CD3 is effective in blunting chronic humoral rejection.
  C. Muromonab-CD3 is not effective in the management of rejection episodes refractory to conventional treatment.
  D. Muromonab-CD3 is administered by means of slow intravenous drip for the purpose of minimizing capillary leak syndrome.

199. Critical Care Problems in Kidney Transplant Recipients

Select the best answer

1. Which of the following is a *true* statement regarding complications following kidney transplantation?

  A. Prevention of acute tubular necrosis (ATN) after transplantation begins immediately in the intensive care unit.
  B. Patients with low postoperative output of urine should undergo vigorous volume resuscitation regardless of renal response.
  C. Dialysis impairs graft function and is not indicated in the care of recipients of renal transplants.
  D. Recipients of kidneys from living related donors are prone to fewer postoperative complications because of a lesser requirement for immunosuppression.

2. Which of the following statements correctly describes acute tubular necrosis (ATN) among recipients of renal transplants?

  A. The prevalence of ATN averages 15% among recipients of cadaveric kidneys.
  B. Prognostic factors for ATN are ischemic and immunologic.
  C. ATN has no influence on graft rejection.
  D. ATN and acute rejection are managed similarly.

200. Specific Critical Care Problems in Heart, Heart-Lung, and Lung Transplant Recipients

True or False

1. The most common indication for heart-lung transplantation is pulmonary vascular disease.

2. After transplantation into recipients with pulmonary hypertension, a transplanted lung remains hypoperfused.

Select the best answer

3. Which of the following is a *correct* statement?

   A. Acute failure of a transplanted heart occurs more commonly than acute failure of a transplanted lung.

   B. Lung graft failure can be manifested by hypoxemia, pulmonary edema, and even perihilar infiltrates on a chest radiograph.

   C. Prophylaxis against the development of deep venous thrombosis is not required.

   D. An inferior vena caval filter should not be used in recipients of lung transplants because of the possibility of filter migration and disruption of the pulmonary arterial anastomosis.

4. Which of the following statements regarding airway complications is *correct*?

   A. Airway complications are common after heart-lung transplantation.

   B. Early airway complications after transplantation generally are attributed to delayed healing caused by steroids.

   C. Intraoperative bronchoscopy is not indicated because of risk for disruption of the newly made anastomosis.

   D. Dehiscence of the airway anastomosis occurs 1 week after transplantation.

201. Care of the Pancreas Transplant Recipient

True or False

1. The initial postoperative care of a recipient of a pancreatic transplant involves maintenance of blood glucose levels less than 250 mg/dL.

2. Steroids are useful in the management of rejection among recipients of pancreatic transplants.

Select the best answer

3. Which of the following statements regarding simultaneous cadaveric pancreas-kidney allograft rejection is *correct*?

   A. Episodes of rejection often are accompanied by hypoglycemia.

   B. The first laboratory derangement seen in rejection of a pancreas-kidney allograft is a rise in serum sodium level.

   C. Most rejection episodes among recipients of simultaneous kidney-pancreas transplants are heralded by a rise in serum creatinine level.

   D. Urinary amylase level is not useful in the monitoring of pancreatic allograft function.

4. Which of the following is a *correct* statement regarding complications after pancreatic transplantation?

   A. Early pancreatitis after transplantation usually is the result of gallstone obstruction.

   B. University of Wisconsin (UW) solution has contributed to a lower incidence of graft-related complications in pancreatic transplantation.

C. Pancreatic allograft thrombosis occurs in as many as 9% of cases.

D. Because bleeding is a more common occurrence than thrombosis, the use of antiplatelet and anticoagulant drugs is contraindicated in pancreatic transplantation.

202. *Management of the Organ Donor*

True or False

1. Each year in the United States, 50,000 brain-dead persons are potential organ donors, but the AIDS epidemic and the 55 mile an hour speed limit have decreased the number of actual donations.

2. The overall consent rate for organ donation is rising.

3. Transmission of malignant disease is rare and has occurred in fewer than 100 of 150,000 transplantation procedures.

Select the best answer

4. The order of priority for next of kin in obtaining consent for organ donation is:

   A. (1) Spouse, (2) adult son or daughter, (3) either parent, (4) adult brother or sister, and (5) legal guardian.

   B. (1) Spouse, (2) adult brother or sister, (3) adult son or daughter, (4) either parent, and (5) legal guardian.

   C. (1) Spouse, (2) legal guardian, (3) adult brother or sister, (4) adult son or daughter, and (5) either parent.

   D. (1) Legal guardian, (2) spouse, (3) either parent, (4) adult brother or sister, and (5) adult son or daughter.

5. Which of the following is a *correct* statement regarding the pathophysiologic mechanism of brain death?

   A. Resting vagal tone is preserved after brain death.

   B. Hypotension after brain death is caused by loss of vasomotor tone and peripheral venous pooling.

   C. Cardiac dysfunction is uncommon after brain death.

   D. The Cushing reflex occurs with brain herniation and consists of hypertension and tachyarrhythmia.

6. Regarding the care of a potential organ donor:

   A. Hypertension is the most common hemodynamic abnormality among brain-dead organ donors.

   B. The usual cause of hypotension among brain-dead organ donors is loss of endogenous catecholamine response to stress.

   C. β-Blockade with short-acting agents is useful in managing the tachyarrhythmias associated with brain death.

   D. Electrolyte abnormalities are uncommon among organ donors.

203. *Diagnosis and Treatment of Rejection, Infection, and Malignancy among Recipients*

True or False

1. Ten percent of renal transplant recipients experience at least one episode of acute rejection in the first 6 months after transplantation.
2. The early clinical signs of acute rejection are subtle.

Select the best answer

3. Regarding immunosuppressive agents, which of the following statements is *false*?

   A. Corticosteroids bind to a steroid receptor and migrate as a complex to the nucleus, where the action is to upregulate specific messenger RNA production.
   B. Corticosteroids block the production of inflammatory cytokines.
   C. Muromonab-CD3 (Orthoclone OKT3) binds to the CD3 molecule, which leads to downregulation of T-cell activity.
   D. Azathioprine interferes with nucleic acid synthesis.

4. Which of the following is *true* about chronic rejection?

   A. Chronic rejection is a slow process that is inevitable, well characterized, and well understood.
   B. Chronic rejection is characterized by acute graft dysfunction followed by slow return of function that rarely achieves baseline levels.
   C. The histologic characteristics of chronic rejection are primarily vascular.
   D. Chronic rejection is the consequence of tissue-destructive mechanisms that are distinct from acute rejection.

5. Which of the following is a true statement regarding cytomegalovirus (CMV) infection?

   A. CMV is easy to identify directly in urine and blood.
   B. Immunocytochemical identification of CMV is sensitive and specific, but unfortunately it requires several days to see results.
   C. Biopsy can be a useful diagnostic tool in the diagnosis of CMV infection.
   D. Therapy for CMV infection is the same regardless of the clinical state of the patient.

204. *Critical Care of the Liver Transplant Recipient*

True or False

1. Fulminant hepatic failure is a contraindication to liver transplantation.
2. More than two-thirds of liver transplant patients have at least one episode of infection after transplantation.

Select the best answer

3. Which of the following manifestations of chronic liver disease does not imply a decompensated state?

    A. Ascites
    B. Hepatopulmonary syndrome
    C. Spider angiomas
    D. Recurrent variceal bleeding
    E. Hepatic encephalopathy

Answers

Chapter 198

1. **True.**   Cyclosporine acts by interrupting the signal transduction of cytokine synthesis in antigen-primed T lymphocytes. Cyclosporine brings about immunosuppression through binding to calcineurin, which is responsible for proper assembly of transcription factor NF-AT. This precludes proper binding of NF-AT to the interleukin-2 gene in the cell nucleus, and this inhibits transcription of messenger RNA for interleukin-2 and other cytokines. (*See textbook page* 2145.)

3. **False.**   Monitoring of cyclosporine level is most commonly performed with a steady-state predose level. The time to peak cyclosporine level after oral administration is variable, and peak level is therefore unreliable and is not usually measured. In addition to allowing for maintenance of cyclosporine levels within therapeutic ranges, measurement and monitoring of cyclosporine levels help ascertain patient compliance and allow differentiation between allograft dysfunction, allograft rejection, and drug toxicity. (*See textbook page* 2147.)

3. **C.**   Oral cyclosporine has a mean bioavailability of 30%, but adequate absorption depends on the presence of bile salts. Less than 1% of unchanged cyclosporine is excreted in the urine. Factors that impair cyclosporine absorption include cholestasis, short-bowel, diarrhea, ileus, gastroparesis, and biliary diversion. These generally occur early in the postoperative period, so the dosage of cyclosporine must often be reduced with time as the availability of cyclosporine increases. (*See textbook pages* 2145–2147.)

4. **C.**   Drugs such as phenytoin and rifampin that induce P-450 IIIA enzymes can cause marked decreases in cyclosporine levels, and use of these agents can lead to allograft rejection. Drugs that are similarly metabolized, such as erythromycin, can cause elevated cyclosporine levels. P-450 IIIA enzymes have been found in the human intestinal mucosa, and either induction or inhibition of these enzymes can impair or enhance cyclosporine absorption. Inhibitors of cyclosporine metabolism, such as ketoconazole and diltiazem have been shown to decrease cyclosporine dose requirements by 80% and 50%, respectively. There is a suggestion of renal protection with diltiazem. (*See textbook page* 2147.)

5. **D.**   Although the proper adjustment of cyclosporine dosing is critical to avoid the complication of nephrotoxicity, dosage adjustment is not needed by a patient with preexisting renal failure, because 1% of cyclosporine is excreted in the urine. Cyclosporine nephrotoxicity may develop at any time in the posttransplantation period. The acute form is mediated by altered intrarenal hemodynamics. Longterm cyclosporine administration has been associated with histologic evidence of interstitial fibrosis and tubulointerstitial injury. Preliminary evidence suggests that calcium channel blockers may help to ameliorate cyclosporine nephrotoxicity. (*See textbook pages* 2147, 2148.)

6. **B.**   Corticosteroids suppress both the alloantigen-specific and nonspecific immune responses through intracytoplasmic binding to a receptor. The steroid-

receptor complex then binds to nuclear DNA and modifies messenger RNA transcription of enzymes and cytokines. Interleukin-1 is the most important cytokine inhibited by corticosteroids. Corticosteroids inhibit chemotaxis of inflammatory cells and production of proinflammatory molecules. In spite of 30 years of steroid use in the management of graft rejection, optimal dosages associated with maximum efficiency and minimum toxicity are not well established. Intravenous methylprednisolone reverses 75% to 85% of rejection episodes among recipients of kidney and heart transplants. (*See textbook pages* 2148, 2149.)

7. **A.** Muromonab-CD3 is effective in the management of acute cellular rejection. It is more effective than steroids as first-line antirejection therapy in the treatment of patients who have received kidney and liver transplants. Muromonab-CD3 also has been used effectively to reverse rejection episodes that are refractory to conventional therapy. Muromonab-CD3 typically is administered as an intravenous bolus of less than 1 minute. Low-dose therapy has been associated with less severe side effects but must be coupled with CD3+ cell monitoring to ensure adequate levels of immunosuppression. (*See textbook page* 2151.)

Chapter 199

1. **D.** Prevention of ATN after transplantation begins intraoperatively with liberal hydration, including crystalloid and colloid products to avoid hypotension from intravascular volume depletion at the time of unclamping. Cardiac status always must be borne in mind during fluid replacement for recipients of renal transplants. If there is no cardiac dysfunction, high-output diuresis is managed with milliliter for milliliter replacement. With cardiac dysfunction, replacement should be less than milliliter for milliliter. Patients with low-urine output should not be overhydrated, because this can result in volume overload, congestive heart failure, and pulmonary edema. Hyperkalemia and volume overload are indications for dialysis in the care of recipients of renal transplants. (*See textbook page* 2158.)

2. **B.** ATN is the most common cause of impaired renal function immediately after transplantation. ATN is rare among recipients of kidneys from living related donors. The incidence among recipients of cadaveric transplants is 35%. Prognostic factors for the development of ATN are ischemic (cold and warm ischemic time, hypertension, hypotension, and vasopressor use) and immunologic (high percentage of antibodies, retransplantation, and poor matching). ATN has an early effect on graft function and has a detrimental effect on graft survival and postoperative morbidity. Patients with posttransplantation ATN have a higher incidence of acute rejection than do other recipients. (*See textbook page* 2158.)

Chapter 200

1. **True.** Heart-lung transplantation is performed almost exclusively for patients with pulmonary vascular disease with either primary or secondary pulmonary hypertension. Heart-lung transplantation occasionally may be performed for septic lung disease with cardiomyopathy, as in the care of a patient with cystic fibrosis and cardiomyopathy. (*See textbook page* 2167.)

2. **False.** Single lung transplantation initially was performed for patients with pulmonary fibrosis. It is now also undertaken for patients with chronic obstructive pulmonary disease and has recently been performed in conjunction with repair of congenital heart defects. Reperfusion edema can occur among patients who undergo single lung transplantation for pulmonary hypertension. This is

the result of elevated blood flow through the transplanted lung. Perfusion scan show that as much as 80% of the total blood flow goes to the transplanted lung. (*See textbook page* 2169.)

   3. **B.**   Acute failure of a transplanted lung is more common than acute failure of a transplanted heart. Many of the reasons are related to preoperative considerations, such as suboptimal graft condition, unrecognized injury to the donor lung, and reperfusion edema in the transplanted lung. Lung graft failure can be manifested by infiltrates on a chest radiograph, hypoxemia, and edema with reperfusion. Prophylaxis for pulmonary embolism is routine in the care of lung transplant recipients, because pulmonary embolism is a devastating complication. Insertion of inferior vena caval filters is advocated in the care of patients with a history of deep venous thrombosis. (*See textbook page* 2169.)

   4. **B.**   Airway complications are more common after single lung or bilateral lung transplantation because the vascular supply to the anastomosis is more tenuous than in heart-lung recipients. Early complications are related to use of steroids and delayed healing. It is important to perform intraoperative bronchoscopy to establish a baseline appearance of the bronchial anastomosis. Dehiscence usually occurs 3 to 6 weeks after transplantation. Early signs of dehiscence include pallor at the site, gray or black mucosa at the suture line, suture material apparent within the airway, and herniation of externally wrapped tissue into the lumen of the airway. (*See textbook page* 2170.)

Chapter 201

   1. **False.**   Laboratory monitoring for a recipient of a pancreatic transplant involves glucose determinations every 1 to 2 hours during the first postoperative day and then every 2 hours. In the early postoperative period, an infusion of regular insulin is used to maintain plasma glucose levels less than 150 mg/dL because it has been demonstrated that chronic hyperglycemia is detrimental to β cells. (*See textbook page* 2179.)

   2. **True.**   Methylprednisolone initially is given intravenously in doses of 250 to 500 mg/day. If this is not effective within 48 hours, antilymphocyte antibody therapy is given. Because the total amount of antilymphocyte antibody therapy in the first 4 months after transplantation is limited to 21 doses, a second episode of rejection during that period would be treated with steroids alone. (*See textbook page* 2180.)

   3. **C.**   The acute rejection of a pancreatic or simultaneous kidney-pancreas transplant is heralded by a decrease in urine amylase level and hyperglycemia. However, for recipients of simultaneous kidney-pancreas transplants, the first indication of rejection often is a rise in serum creatinine level. (*See textbook pages* 2175, 2180.)

   4. **C.**   The pancreas is prone to a unique series of complications because of its exocrine function and relatively low blood flow. Thrombosis is a particularly devastating complication occur caused by preservation edema from pancreatitis. To minimize graft thrombosis, low-dose heparin and antiplatelet drugs are used in the immediately postoperative period. The risk of bleeding among these patients is not trivial, but it is significantly lower than the risk for thrombosis of the graft (1% versus 6%). (*See textbook page* 2180.)

Chapter 202

   1. **False.**   The number of brain-dead persons who are potential organ donors is 10,000 to 13,700. Of these potential donors, 5,416 actually became organ donors

in 1996. The single most commonly cited reason for lack of organ retrieval is inability to obtain consent. Family refusal or inability to locate and contact family members remains the leading cause of nonuse of potential organ donors. (*See textbook page* 2186.)

2. **False.** The overall consent rate for organ donation is dropping. This is an especially acute consideration for intensive care unit physicians, who may be an important liaison between a grieving family and the primary care team. A recent public opinion survey suggested that 69% of persons would be interested in donating their own organs and that 93% would honor the wishes of a family member if these wishes were clearly stated. The problem is that only 52% of these persons had communicated their wishes to family members. A critical statistic shows that 37% of these same persons did not comprehend that a brain-dead person should be considered dead, and 42% did not know that organ donation costs the family of the deceased nothing. (*See textbook page* 2186.)

3. **True.** Transplantation of malignant disease in donor organs is extremely rare; it has occurred in fewer than 100 of 150,000 transplantation procedures. Donor selection is particularly important in this regard; use of organs from potential donors with most types of cancer is contraindicated. The exceptions are low-grade malignant lesions of the skin, carcinoma in situ of the uterine cervix, and primary low-grade nonglioblastoma of the brain. It is especially important to ensure that a donor with what is assumed to be a primary malignant tumor of the central nervous system does not have a metastatic brain lesion. Use of organs from a person with a primary malignant tumor of the brain who has undergone radiation therapy, chemotherapy, shunting, or craniotomy also is contraindicated because of increased risk for systemic dissemination of tumor cells. (*See textbook page* 2193.)

4. **A.** Rates of consent for organ donation are markedly higher if brain death is discussed and the family is allowed time to assimilate the loss of the loved one. The proper order for consent is specified in the Uniform Anatomical Gift Act of 1968 for a donor older than 18 years: (a) spouse, (b) adult son or daughter, (c) either parent, (d) adult brother or sister, and (e) legal guardian. (*See textbook page* 2194.)

5. **B.** The pathophysiologic mechanism of brain death has been derived from observation and through animal models. Hemodynamic instability with brain herniation is the result of autonomic dysfunction caused by loss of central neuro-humeral regulatory control of vital functions. Increased intracranial pressure leads to worsening brain ischemia and severe systemic hypertension resulting from an excess of catecholamines. A period of transient bradycardia associated with the hypertensive response occurs early in the process of brain herniation and is called the *Cushing reflex*. Cardiac dysfunction is common during and after brain death, and impairment of coronary blood flow can occur that results in cardiac microinfarction. Within 15 minutes after brain herniation and brain death, catecholamine levels decrease to less than baseline. (*See textbook page* 2194.)

6. **C.** The care of a potential organ donor is an important part of intensive care. Hypotension and tachyarrhythmias are common among the brain-dead patients. The usual cause of hypotension among these patients is relative hypovolemia caused by vasomotor collapse and common therapies for increased intracranial pressure, which require minimizing hydration and the use of osmotic diuretics. The state of hydration is critical in the care of these patients. Drugs used to treat dysrhythmias should be short acting, such as esmolol and nitroprusside. Another commonly used agent is dopamine, which should be used in low doses. Electrolyte abnormalities are common, and hypophosphatemia, hypokalemia, hypocalcemia, and hypomagnesemia should be anticipated and managed. High-dose inotropic support is to be avoided because of vasoconstrictive effects and the potential for end-organ damage. (*See textbook pages* 2194, 2196.)

Chapter 203

1. **False.**   Acute rejection occurs among 18% to 60% of kidney recipients, depending on allograft and recipient risk factors and the immunosuppressive regimen. Among patients who experience an episode of acute rejection, it is known that the 1-year graft survival rate is decreased. (*See textbook page* 2203.)

2. **True.**   The diagnosis of acute rejection is based on clinical, biochemical, and histologic features in biopsy specimens. Since the introduction of cyclosporine in the 1980s, the clinical signs of acute rejection, such as graft tenderness and graft swelling have become less obvious. The biochemical markers of a rise in serum creatinine and blood urea nitrogen levels with a fall in urine output are helpful indices of acute rejection, but the differential diagnosis should always include other causes of graft dysfunction, such as hypovolemia, acute tubular necrosis (delayed graft function), ureteral obstruction or urinary leak, and cyclosporine nephrotoxicity. (*See textbook page* 2203.)

3. **C.**   The most common immunosuppressive agents act at various sites within the immune system to prevent and manage acute rejection. Adrenal corticosteroids such as oral prednisone and intravenous methylprednisolone bind to a steroid receptor, which migrates intracellularly to the nucleus, where the complex acts to downregulate specific production of messenger RNA. Production of interleukin-2 is severely impaired by corticosteroids. Azathioprine is an antimetabolite that interferes with rapidly dividing cells such as lymphocytes through interfering with nucleic acid synthesis. Muromonab-CD3 is a murine monoclonal antibody that binds to the CD3 molecule and interferes with the actions of T cells in the immune cascade. It is effective in management of ongoing rejection because it can inhibit the activity of established effector T cells. (*See textbook page* 2204.)

4. **C.**   The cellular mechanisms responsible for chronic rejection are less well understood than those responsible for acute rejection. Chronic rejection usually occurs months to years after transplantation. It is a process characterized by progressive functional deterioration thought to stem from repeated episodes of acute rejection or from small subclinical foci of acute rejection within a graft. Both immunologic and nonimmunologic mechanisms are thought to be involved. The histologic finding is vascular changes with fibrointimal thickening and interstitial fibrosis. (*See textbook page* 2203.)

5. **C.**   Early diagnosis of CMV infection is critical because early treatment may limit or decrease the severity of infection. CMV is coated with a β2-microglobulin in the blood and urine, so it is not simple to identify its presence directly. Immunocytochemical detection can be accomplished in less than 24 hours with a sensitivity and specificity in active CMV infection of 90% or greater. CMV infection also may be identified by means of histologic analysis of biopsy specimens from the lung, esophagus, liver, or stomach. Identification of intranuclear vital inclusions and giant cells is characteristic of CMV infection. Management of CMV infection ranges from observation of a patient who has no symptoms during minimal immunosuppression, to administration of ganciclovir with or without reduction in immunosuppression, and finally to the addition of CMV hyperimmune globulin to ganciclovir therapy in the most severe cases. (*See textbook pages* 2210, 2211.)

Chapter 204

1. **False.**   Fulminant hepatic failure is a major indication for transplantation. With medical therapy it carries a mortality approaching 75%. With transplantation the survival rate approaches 80%. (*See textbook page* 2220.)

2. **True.**   More than two thirds of patients who undergo liver transplantation experience at least one episode of infection after transplant. This is the highest rate among patients who undergo solid organ transplantation. The following factors account for this: the length and magnitude of the operation; the high potential for biliary and enteric colonization; and the poor overall condition of many recipients. The mortality for these infections has dropped from 25% to 50% reported earlier to less than 10% recently. Nonetheless infections remain the most common cause of early death after transplantation. (*See textbook page* 2230.)

3. **C.**   Chronic liver disease by itself is not an indication for transplantation. In a well-compensated state, patients may live 10 years or longer without intervention. When chronic liver disease decompensates, prognosis diminishes considerably. Examples of such decompensation include hepatic encephalopathy, refractory ascites, hepatorenal syndrome, hepatopulmonary syndrome, recurrent or refractory variceal bleeding, recurrent infections such as cholangitis or spontaneous bacterial peritonitis, intractable pruritus, and severe malnutrition. (*See textbook page* 2220.)

XV. Metabolism and Nutrition

205a. The Basic Principles of Nutrition Support in the Intensive Care Unit

True or False

1. After resuscitation, the only contraindication to the initiation of enteral feeding is a nonfunctioning intestine.

Select the best answer

2. Which of the following is an appropriate component of the nutritional support of most critically ill patients?

   A. Protein delivery of 2.0 to 2.6 g/kg per day
   B. Glucose constituting 60% to 80% of the total calories administered per day
   C. Lipids providing 30% to 40% of the total calories administered per day
   D. Approximately 25 kcal/kg usual body weight per day
   E. All of the above

205b. Enteral and Parenteral Nutrition

True or False

1. Enteral nutrition can reduce risk for postoperative complications.
2. Nutritional support should be provided beyond the ligament of Treitz.

206. Disease-Specific Nutrition

True or False

1. Parenteral formulations designed for use by hypermetabolic patients include high-dose arginine and glutamine.
2. Regarding dietary manipulation in renal failure, clinical trials comparing essential amino acids alone to a mixture of nonessential and essential amino acids have shown a need of more than 40 g essential amino acids per day.

207. The Inflammatory Response, Immune Dysfunction, and Immunonutrition

True or False

1. Nosocomial infections are typical in the systemic inflammatory response syndrome and multiple organ dysfunction syndrome, which usually begin 7 days after injury and involve skin organisms.
2. The mechanism hypothesized in the development of nosocomial infections with gastrointestinal flora involve failure of gastrointestinal barrier functions.
3. There is no benefit to early enteral feeding regarding timing or route that can improve patient outcome.

Answers
Chapter 205a

1. **True.** Enteral feeding has been shown to reduce infection, preserve gastrointestinal integrity, and maintain barrier and immune function. It is the preferred route of nutrient administration. Current recommendations support initiation of enteral feeding as soon as possible after resuscitation. (*See textbook page* 2240.)
2. **D.** Approximately 25 kcal/kg usual body weight per day is a typical and appropriate caloric intake for a critically ill patient. Protein delivery should be approximately 1.2 to 1.5 g/kg per day. Glucose constituting 30% to 70% of the total calories and lipids providing 15% to 30% of the total calories administered per day also are appropriate. (*See textbook page* 2241.)

Chapter 205b

1. **True.** For patients undergoing operations on the colon or rectum, administration of 1 L nutritional solution directly into the small intestine over the first 4 postoperative days reduces the incidence of postoperative complications and infectious complications in comparison with a similar volume of saline solution. (*See textbook page* 2243.)
2. **False.** This statement is clearly an oversimplification. Gastric feeding stimulates all aspects of gastrointestinal secretion, enzyme production, and digestion. On the other hand, many patients have some component of gastroparesis that impairs gastric feeding. For those patients distal access is necessary. (*See textbook page* 2245.)

Chapter 206

1. **True.** Specialty amino acid solutions marketed for use in the care of patients with severe metabolic stress include essential, semiessential, and nonessential amino acids with higher concentrations of branched-chain amino acids. Other modifications under investigation include high-dose arginine and glutamine. Arginine is provided in standard amino acid products in amounts lower than doses demonstrating immunomodulating properties. Glutamine has limited solubility and stability in solution and so is not available in standard amino acid solutions.

It is available as a supplement for an essential amino acid solution marketed for use in renal failure. (*See textbook page* 2263.)

2. **False.**   Nitrogen metabolism in renal failure is an area of great interest in which both quantity and quality of protein must be considered. Patients who need hemodialysis or peritoneal dialysis have increased catabolism and loss of protein into the dialysate; therefore protein restriction is not appropriate. Clinical trials comparing essential amino acids alone to a mixture of nonessential and essential amino acids have had conflicting results. Excessive amounts (>40 g essential amino acids) may cause hyperammonemia. Nonessential acids, such as arginine, ornithine, and citrulline, are necessary for ammonia detoxification, through the urea cycle, without which there may be increased serum ammonia levels. (*See textbook page* 2271.)

Chapter 207

1. **False.**   Nosocomial infections are typical of systemic inflammatory response syndrome and multiple organ dysfunction syndrome. The infection usually begins 7 to 10 days after injury. The main sites are the sinuses, lower respiratory tract, invasive lines, prosthetic devices, and the urinary tract. The organisms involved tend to be those harbored in the gastrointestinal tract. Within a few days of injury, the enteral flora have colonized the skin, upper gastrointestinal tract, and respiratory tract in as many as 80% of patients. (*See textbook page* 2276.)

2. **True.**   Two mechanisms are hypothesized through which colonization of sites with gastrointestinal flora can occur, both originating from a failure of gastro-intestinal barrier function. In the first, organisms move up the gastrointestinal tract from the colon, to the small intestine, to the stomach, and to the respiratory tract by means of direct migration. In the second, organisms translocate through the wall of the gastrointestinal tract into regional lymph nodes and then into the systemic circulation. (*See textbook page* 2277.)

3. **False.**   There appears to be a window of opportunity in the treatment of criti-cally ill patients in which enteral feeding can improve patient outcome. This win-dow appears to be between the injurious event and establishment of the systemic inflammatory response. The reduction in infection rate appears to be for both line sepsis and infections other than line sepsis. (*See textbook page* 2280–2283.)

XVI. Rheumatologic and Immunologic Problems in the Intensive Care Unit

208. Rheumatologic Disorders in the Intensive Care Unit

True or False

1. Diuresis with furosemide may precipitate an attack of gout.
2. A synovial fluid leukocyte count less than 10,000/mm³ excludes a diagnosis of septic arthritis.

209. Anaphylaxis

Select the best answer

1. Characteristics of anaphylaxis include which of the following?

   A. It is a life-threatening form of delayed hypersensitivity.
   B. A mast cell mediator release requires immunoglobulin E (IgE) binding to cell surface Fab receptor.
   C. Preformed mediators are released on cell activation.
   D. Mediator release is suppressed by cyclic guanosine monophosphate (GMP) and enhanced by cyclic adenosine monophosphate (AMP).

2. A 12-year-old girl arrives in the emergency department approximately 15 minutes after being stung by a yellow jacket. She is anxious and flushed and exhibits rhinorrhea and a rapid pulse. She reported chest tightness and shortness of breath immediately after the sting, but her breathing seemed to improve on the way to the hospital. A true statement about her condition is:

   A. The danger of a severe reaction has passed because her breathing has improved.
   B. The most common cause of death of anaphylaxis is hemodynamic collapse.
   C. This patient should receive epinephrine.
   D. Rapid onset of symptoms is a favorable prognostic sign.

3. Penicillin allergy is:

    A. The most common cause of anaphylaxis in the United States
    B. Associated with cross reactivity to cephalosporins among 20% to 30% of patients
    C. Rarely associated with cross reactivity to carbapenems
    D. Unlikely with a negative skin test response to cephalosporins

210. Dermatologic Problems in the Intensive Care Unit

True or False

The following statements relate to the toxic shock syndrome:

1. Vomiting and diarrhea are common.
2. Skin erythema usually is localized.
3. Diffuse muscle pain is present.

Select the best answer

4. Brown recluse spider bites:

    A. Occur primarily in the spring and summer months
    B. May produce a large area of ischemic necrosis surrounding the bite
    C. May produce life-threatening systemic disease
    D. May be associated with urticaria
    E. All of the above

211. Collagen Vascular Diseases in the Intensive Care Unit

Select the best answer

1. Scleroderma renal crisis is characterized by:

    A. Microangiopathic hemolytic anemia
    B. Urinary red blood cell casts
    C. Low plasma renin level
    D. Nonoliguric renal failure

2. A common manifestation of antiphospholipid syndrome is:

    A. Increased bleeding tendency
    B. Presence of active vasculitis
    C. Thrombocytosis
    D. Spontaneous abortion

212. Vasculitis in the Intensive Care Unit

True or False

1. Most patients with polyarteritis nodosa have been found to have antibodies to hepatitis C virus.
2. At the time of presentation, the most common site of involvement of Wegener's granulomatosis is the upper respiratory tract.

Select the best answer

3. Which of the following statements regarding the response to therapy for Wegener's granulomatosis is correct?

    A. Oral azathioprine can generate complete remission among 93% of patients.
    B. Oral cyclophosphamide can generate complete remission among 93% of patients.
    C. Oral methotrexate can generate complete remission among 93% of patients.
    D. A combination of high-dose pulse steroid (1 g methylprednisolone a day for 3 days) and azathioprine can generate complete remission among 93% of patients.
    E. A combination of oral azathioprine and oral methotrexate can generate complete remission among 93% of patients.

Answers
Chapter 208

1. **True.** Drug-induced hyperuricemia is one of the most frequently identifiable causes of gout. Although thiazide diuretics were the first diuretic to be implicated, furosemide, acetazolamide, ethacrynic acid, and diazoxide all have been reported to cause hyperuricemia. This may be the result of a decrease in effective arteriolar blood volume or inhibition of the secretion of uric acid. (*See textbook page* 2290.)
2. **False.** Leukocyte counts generally exceed 50,000/mm³, although counts as low as 5,000/mm³ occasionally are found. Other findings are a low synovial fluid glucose level (serum glucose exceeding synovial fluid glucose by 40 to 50 mg/dL or more) and poor mucin clot formation. All of these findings also may occur with rheumatoid arthritis, making the diagnosis of septic arthritis difficult in the care of patients with rheumatoid arthritis. (*See textbook page* 2294.)

Chapter 209

1. **C.** Anaphylaxis is a form of immediate hypersensitivity. Initial antigen contact stimulates generation of IgE antibodies with Fab segments that recognize the antigen. These preformed antibodies bind by means of Fc receptors to mast cells and basophils. The antibodies may remain unbound for weeks. Subsequent antigen exposure can cause release of mediators from mast cells and basophils by binding to the Fab portion of two IgE molecules. This bridging activates secretion of pre-

formed primary mediators such as histamine, heparin, neutrophil chemotactic factor, and proteolytic enzymes. The release of mediators is modulated by cyclic AMP and enhanced by cyclic GMP. (*See textbook pages* 2298, 2299.)

2. **C.**   The anaphylactic reaction is severe in this patient. Epinephrine is the drug of choice, and she should receive 0.3 to 0.5 mL of 1:1,000 solution (0.3 to 0.5 mg) subcutaneously. The injections should be repeated every 5 to 10 minutes if symptoms do not improve. Rapid onset of symptoms correlates with severity of reaction. The leading cause of death of anaphylaxis is respiratory failure caused by laryngeal edema and bronchospasm. Noncardiogenic edema also may occur. (*See textbook pages* 2301–2303.)

3. **A.**   Penicillin is the most common cause of anaphylaxis in the United States. Approximately 10% of the population has a positive skin test reaction to penicillin. Cross reactivity to cephalosporins occurs among 5.4% to 16.5% of the population who are allergic to penicillin. Skin testing for cephalosporin hypersensitivity is unreliable. Monobactams such as aztreonam do not cross react with penicillins, but carbapenems such as imipenem show a high degree of *in vivo* cross reactivity. (*See textbook pages* 2304, 2305.)

Chapter 210

1. **True.**   Toxic shock syndrome is characterized by the acute onset of high fever, diffuse skin erythema, profound hypotension, and vomiting or diarrhea. (*See textbook page* 2320.)

2. **False.**   A diffuse sunburn-like rash is most common, although this may evolve into discrete macules that are localized or generalized. (*See textbook page* 2320.)

3. **True.**   Muscle pain and neurologic symptoms are common. (*See textbook page* 2320.)

4. **D.**   Severe systemic problems, including hemolysis and disseminated intravascular coagulopathy, may occur after a brown recluse spider bite. The bite initially may go unnoticed, but it may evolve into a necrotic, ischemic full-thickness lesion over 24 to 48 hours. Enzymes in the spider venom are responsible. Most bites occur between April and October. (*See textbook page* 2322.)

Chapter 211

1. **A.**   Scleroderma renal crisis is characterized by accelerated hypertension and renal insufficiency. Oliguria is typical. Increased renin release is triggered presumably by decreased renal cortical blood flow. Vascular constriction and intimal necrosis and fibrosis lead to microangiopathic hemolytic anemia. Modest proteinuria is common, but urinary red blood cell casts typical of glomerulonephritis are not found. The hypertension and renal insufficiency often respond to angiotensin-converting enzyme inhibitors, sometimes with the addition of calcium channel blockers. (*See textbook page* 2354.)

2. **D.**   Antiphospholipid antibodies are present in some patients with systemic lupus erythematosus, in those with some other connective tissue disease syndromes, and in some with no identifiable underlying disease. Antiphospholipids have prothrombotic effects believed to be caused by promotion of platelet aggregation and thrombus formation or effects on plasminogen-activating factor or activation of protein C. The pathologic lesion is thrombosis and embolization, not vasculitis. Thrombocytopenia is common. Spontaneous abortion occurs more frequently among women with antiphospholipid antibodies than among

other woman because of vascular insufficiency and thrombosis in placental vessels. (*See textbook page* 2352.)

Chapter 212

1. **False.** Approximately 20% of patients with polyarteritis nodosa have antibodies to hepatitis C virus. In contrast, there is a much stronger association between hepatitis C virus infection and mixed cryoglobulinemia. (*See textbook page* 2368.)

2. **True.** When they come to medical attention, 85% to 90% of patients have symptoms referable to the upper respiratory tract, including sinusitis, nasal obstruction, rhinitis, otitis, hearing loss, ear pain, gingival inflammation, epistaxis, sore throat, laryngitis, and nasal septal deformity. Renal manifestations are present among 80% of patients. Lung involvement is found among only one-third of patients when they come to medical attention, although lower respiratory tract disease almost always occurs at some time during the illness. (*See textbook page* 2371.)

3. **B.** Oral cyclophosphamide can generate complete remission among 93% of patients. The usual dose is 1 to 2 mg/kg per day, although for patients with rapidly progressive renal disease, a dose of 2 to 4 mg/kg per day sometimes is used. Azathioprine has not been as helpful in inducing remissions but may be helpful in maintaining cyclophosphamide-induced remission among patients unable to continue taking cyclophosphamide. Corticosteroids have not improved the prognosis of Wegener's granulomatosis, although they may be helpful for the control of constitutional symptoms caused by arthritis, pericarditis, and vasculitic skin rash. Methotrexate is used for less severe disease, and use of this agent results in remission for 69% of patients. (*See textbook page* 2372.)

XVII. Psychiatric Issues in Intensive Care

213. Diagnosis and Treatment of Agitation and Delirium in the ICU Patient

True or False

1. The electroencephalogram (EEG) of a delirious patient is usually abnormal.
2. The delirium associated with narcotic withdrawal can be so severe as to be lethal.
3. Haloperidol is not recommended for the management of delirium because it lacks U.S. Food and Drug Administration (FDA) approval for such an indication.
4. Extrapyramidal symptoms are common after intravenous administration of haloperidol.

Select the best answer

5. Delirium is:

   A. Identical to dementia
   B. Irreversible
   C. An organic mental disorder
   D. Differentiated from dementia because dementia also has an altered level of consciousness

6. Which of the following drugs is least likely to produce delirium in a patient in an intensive care unit?

   A. Meperidine
   B. Naloxone
   C. Lidocaine
   D. Cimetidine
   E. Penicillin

214. Recognition and Treatment of Anxiety in the Intensive Care Unit Patient

True or False

1. Anxiety is defined as the sense of dread and foreboding that may occur in response to an external threatening event.

2. An organic cause of anxiety is suggested by its occurrence in conjunction with discrete physical events or in the absence of a psychologically charged situation.
3. Panic disorders have been found among 40% to 60% of patients with chest pain and normal coronary angiograms.
4. Ventilator weaning often can provoke anxiety in a patient in an intensive care unit (ICU).

Select the best answer

5. Anxiety in the ICU:

   A. Is the most common reason for psychiatric consultation soon after admission to the coronary care unit
   B. Is experienced by 10% of patients recovering from coronary artery bypass graft operations
   C. Has no effect on hemodynamic status
   D. Does not contribute at all to mortality after myocardial infarction
   E. Is not associated with plasma catecholamine levels

6. Which of the following benzodiazepines is least likely to produce substantial interdose rebound?

   A. Oxazepam
   B. Midazolam
   C. Clonazepam
   D. Lorazepam

215. Recognition and Treatment of Depression in the Intensive Care Unit

True or False

1. Tricyclic antidepressant medications have type I or quinidine-like antiarrhythmic properties.
2. Polycyclic antidepressant medications are not recommended in the acute post-myocardial infarction phase.
3. Orthostatic hypotension from tricyclic antidepressants is infrequently observed among medically healthy patients.

Select the best answer

4. Which of the following conditions is *not* a common cause of depression among patients in intensive care units (ICUs)?

   A. A reaction to an acute medical illness
   B. A manifestation of a primary affective disorder
   C. A mood disorder associated with organic disease
   D. A result of the overlap of somatic symptoms of depression and the symptoms of medical illness
   E. A side effect of catecholamine infusion

5. Which of the following conditions has been shown to be associated with depression?

    A. Increased cardiac beat-to-beat variability
    B. Relative insulin resistance
    C. Immune system changes
    D. Decreased ventilatory response to carbon dioxide
    E. All of the above

6. Which of the following statements regarding the diagnosis of depression is *false*?

    A. The evaluating physician should specifically screen for each of the eight symptoms of depression.
    B. An increase in appetite makes the diagnosis of depression unlikely.
    C. A potentially depressed patient should be evaluated for the presence of suicidal thoughts.
    D. The evaluating physician should ask if the patient has a specific plan for a suicide attempt.
    E. The evaluating physician should assess the feasibility of the patient's suicide plan.

7. Which of the following conditions can be accompanied by depression? (1) Hypothyroidism. (2) Cushing's disease. (3) Post-stroke state. (4) Human immunodeficiency virus infection. (5) Parathyroid disturbance.

    A. 1, 2, and 3
    B. 1 and 3 only
    C. 2 and 4 only
    D. 4
    E. All

216. Suicide

True or False

1. The most important risk factor for suicide is the presence of psychiatric illness.
2. Increasing age is correlated with decreased suicidal risk.
3. Asking a patient about the possibility of suicide can have the adverse effect of planting the idea in the patient's mind.
4. Most suicidal intoxicated patients still are suicidal when the effects of the intoxicants have worn off.

Select the best answer

5. The least likelihood for suicidal potential is present in which of the following groups?

    A. Those who have never married
    B. Patients with panic attacks
    C. Married persons with children
    D. Unemployed persons
    E. Patients with substance abuse problems

6. Which of the following principles is least important in treating a suicidal patient?

    A. Management of the underlying problem
    B. Allowing the passage of time

C. Maintenance of patient safety through the use of physical or chemical restraints
D. Respect for the patient's wishes to refuse treatment
E. Allowing an intoxicated patient to become sober before completing the evaluation

217. Problematic Behaviors of Patients, Family, and Staff in the Intensive Care Unit

Select the best answer

1. Which of the following items does *not* contribute to feelings of helplessness and anxiety on the part of intensive care unit (ICU) patients?

    A. Limited communication from the ICU staff regarding the patient's condition
    B. Use of physical or chemical restraints
    C. Being placed in a dependent situation
    D. Open communication regarding the patient's situation and treatment involving both the patient and the family
    E. The absence of denial mechanisms

2. A patient with which of the following personality types is likely to pit ICU staff members against each other?

    A. Oral-dependent (or borderline)
    B. Histrionic
    C. Obsessive
    D. Noncompliant
    E. None of the above

218. Recognition and Management of Staff Stress in the Intensive Care Unit

True or False

1. There appears to have been more research on burnout among intensive care unit (ICU) nurses than among physicians.
2. Studies have shown that ICU nurses have higher burnout rates than nurses who do not work in ICUs.
3. A lack of opportunity to share experiences and feelings with other staff members is a leading source of stress for ICU personnel.

Select the best answer

4. Which of the following features of the house officer syndrome is not ubiquitous among house officers at one time or another?

    A. Chronic anger
    B. Pervasive cynicism
    C. Suicidal ideation
    D. Episodic cognitive impairment
    E. Family discord

219. Neuropsychiatric Aspects of Cancer and AIDS in the Intensive Care Unit

True or False

1. Patients who have previously received chemotherapy that provokes vomiting may become conditioned to avoid treatment.
2. Complex partial seizures are easier to diagnose than are generalized seizures.
3. Generalized seizures are common among cancer patients.
4. Akathisia can occur as a side effect of neuroleptic medications.
5. The most common psychiatric diagnoses among patients with human immunodeficiency virus (HIV) infection are adjustment disorders, major depression, and organic mental disorders.
6. Magnetic resonance imaging is more sensitive than computed tomography in the evaluation of patients with HIV encephalopathy because of its superior capability to depict evidence of white matter disease.
7. Seizures among patients with HIV infection can be attributed to a mass lesion in nearly all cases.
8. The suicide rate among patients with acquired immunodeficiency syndrome (AIDS) is equivalent to that of the general population.

Select the best answer

9. Which of the following statements regarding the primary infection syndrome in HIV infection is true?

   A. Seroconversion usually occurs several weeks before the appearance of a primary infection syndrome.
   B. Primary infection syndrome is insidious in onset.
   C. The illness usually takes several months to resolve.
   D. The symptoms are similar to those of mononucleosis.
   E. Headaches are rare and are mild whenever they occur.

Answers

Chapter 213

1. **True.** The EEG of a delirious patient is typically abnormal, suggesting a state of cerebral insufficiency and failure of the normal cerebral metabolic processes. The EEG characteristically shows diffuse, generalized slowing the severity of which usually parallels the intensity of the delirium. It is this typical EEG abnormality that is most responsible for characterization of delirium as an organic defect. (*See textbook page* 2386.)
2. **True.** Failure to identify the correct substance from which a patient is withdrawing can lead to worsening delirium, seizures, or death of untreated withdrawal. (*See textbook page* 2387.)
3. **False.** Nonspecific delirium is best managed with a neuroleptic agent such as haloperidol. Although the intravenous use of haloperidol lacks FDA approval, haloperidol has been shown to be effective therapy for delirium and has a high degree of safety among patients in ICUs. (*See textbook page* 2388.)
4. **False.** Extrapyramidal symptoms, which commonly occur after oral and intramuscular haloperidol use, appear to be uncommon when the drug is administered intravenously. (*See textbook page* 2388.)

5. **C.**   Delirium occurs often among patients in ICUs. It is a reversible organic mental disorder characterized by the acute onset of confusion and an altered level of consciousness. This altered level of consciousness is what differentiates delirium from dementia, in which confusion exists with a normal level of consciousness. (*See textbook page* 2383.)

6. **B.**   Several drugs have been shown to be capable of producing delirium syndrome. Most of these appear to evoke the condition through anticholinergic effects. Narcotics such as meperidine and morphine are common and often unrecognized causes of delirium among patients in ICUs. Naloxone often is an effective antidote for management of delirium under these circumstances. Other classes of drugs that can produce delirium are antiarrhythmics (e.g., lidocaine, procainamide, and quinidine), antibiotics (e.g., penicillin and rifampin), antihistamines (e.g., diphenhydramine, promethazine, cimetidine, and ranitidine), and β-blockers (e.g., propranolol). (*See textbook page* 2385.)

Chapter 214

1. **False.**   Fear is defined as the sense of dread and foreboding that may occur in response to an external threatening event. Anxiety differs from fear, in that the same sense of foreboding instead derives from an unknown internal stimulus, and either is inappropriate or excessive to the reality of the external stimulus or is concerned with a future one. (*See textbook pages* 2393, 2394.)

2. **True.**   An organic cause of anxiety is suggested by its occurrence in the absence of a psychologically charged situation or in conjunction with discrete physical events such as a run of ventricular tachycardia while receiving vasopressors. (*See textbook page* 2394.)

3. **True.**   Panic disorders can be so severe as to be confused with acute myocardial infarction. The condition has been found among 40% to 60% of patients with chest pain and normal coronary angiograms. (*See textbook page* 2395.)

4. **True.**   The presence of mechanical ventilation often can provide psychologic support to a patient, and weaning can therefore provoke marked anxiety, often severe enough to interfere with the weaning process itself. (*See textbook page* 2398.)

5. **A.**   Anxiety is the most common reason for psychiatric consultation within the first 2 days after admission to a coronary care unit. There are many reasons for this. Anxiety is common among patients in ICUs. Sixty percent of patients recovering from coronary artery bypass operations and 65% to 85% of patients who have had acute myocardial infarction are estimated to experience anxiety. Anxiety can have profound effects on a patient in an ICU and can cause increased cardiac output from sympathetic nervous system activity. Elevated levels of catecholamines, free fatty acids, and cortisol often accompany the anxiety associated with acute myocardial infarction. There is evidence that psychiatric consultation and management of anxiety are associated with decreased urinary levels of catecholamines and free fatty acids, decreased incidence of ventricular arrhythmias, and possibly a reduction in mortality. (*See textbook page* 2393.)

6. **C.**   Interdose rebound is less likely with drugs that have a relatively long half-life in relation to dosing frequency. Drugs with an especially short half-life, such as midazolam, therefore are quite likely to produce interdose rebound. Oxazepam has a half-life of 5 to 15 hours, and lorazepam has a half-life of 10 to 20 hours, making them relatively short-acting agents. Of this list, clonazepam has the longest half-life, ranging from 15 to as long as 50 hours, making it least likely to produce an interdose rebound phenomenon. (*See textbook page* 2398.)

Chapter 215

1. **True.** Tricyclic antidepressant medications have many potent cardiovascular effects. They exhibit type I (quinidine-like) antiarrhythmic properties and can decrease the rate of premature ventricular contractions. Among patients with bundle branch block, there is greater risk for second-degree or third-degree block when tricyclic antidepressants are used. (*See textbook page* 2406.)

2. **True.** Because of the many adverse cardiovascular effects that tricyclic antidepressants can produce, these agent are not recommended for use during the acute phase following myocardial infarction. (*See textbook page* 2407.)

3. **False.** Orthostatic hypotension is the most serious and frequently encountered cardiovascular side effect of tricyclic antidepressants among medically healthy patients. It occurs among as many as 20% of patients receiving tricyclic antidepressants. (*See textbook page* 2406.)

4. **E.** Depression occurs among patients in ICUs and can frequently complicate critical care. There is evidence that depressed patients have poorer survival statistics than do patients who are not depressed. Depression can occur in an ICU as a reaction to an acute medical illness. Patients with this type of depression include driven persons who are suddenly confronted with their own mortality, as after acute myocardial infarction, or young, vigorous persons stunned by permanent traumatic spinal cord paralysis. Depression also can be a manifestation of a primary affective disorder in a patient with a critical illnesses. Depression can emerge as a manifestation of organic disease, as may occur with some brain tumors, and can produce somatic symptoms that may mimic those of a medical illness. (*See textbook pages* 2401, 2404.)

5. **E.** Depression is associated with many physiologic changes that can have important consequences for critically ill patients. Severe cardiac effects can occur among depressed patients. Recent data suggest that unmanaged depression is associated with increased cardiac mortality. A possible mechanism for the increase in cardiac deaths is suggested by the finding that depressed patients often have increased cardiac beat-to-beat variability. Many endocrine alterations have been identified among depressed patients. These include increased plasma cortisol level, increases in plasma and central nervous system metabolites of norepinephrine, and a relative resistance to insulin. Changes in the immune system, specifically decreased T-cell and B-cell mitogen responses, have been observed, as has a decreased ventilatory response to carbon dioxide levels. (*See textbook page* 2401.)

6. **B.** Either an increase or a decrease in appetite may be associated with depression. The diagnosis of depression is based on several clinical findings. To qualify as clinically depressed, a patient must have had a sustained period of a depressed mood for at least 2 weeks in association with at least four (of a total of eight) neurovegetative symptoms. A patient should be asked specifically about each of the eight possible symptoms, and the symptoms should be evaluated. A mnemonic device is SIG E CAPS for (a) *s*leep alteration, (b) decreased *i*nterest, (c) *g*uilt, (d) decreased *e*nergy, (e) decreased *c*oncentration, (f) altered *a*ppetite, (g) *p*sychomotor retardation or agitation, and (h) *s*uicidal ideation. The presence of suicidal ideation, especially if the physician can determine that an actual suicide plan exists, mandates psychiatric consultation. (*See textbook page* 2402.)

7. **E.** Various medications and medical conditions can cause depression and other organic affective disorders. Endocrine disorders (e.g., hypothyroidism, Cushing's disease, and parathyroid diseases) often are accompanied by depression. After cerebrovascular accidents, as many as 60% of patients with left hemispheric lesions and 15% of those with right hemispheric disorders can experience depres-

sion. Depression may be the first manifestation of infection with human immuno-deficiency virus. (*See textbook page* 2404.)

Chapter 216

1. **True.**   Suicide and suicide risk can vary significantly from patient to patient. The most important risk factor for suicide is the presence of a psychiatric illness. Patients with depression, psychosis, substance abuse, character disorders, and panic disorders are at risk to attempt suicide. (*See textbook page* 2416.)

2. **False.**   The elderly and patients with chronic medical conditions are in high-risk groups for suicide. (*See textbook page* 2416.)

3. **False.**   Contrary to popular belief, questioning a patient about whether he or she has ever had suicidal thoughts does not produce or promote such ideas. Because of the great risk to life that suicide represents, such questions should not be avoided. (*See textbook page* 2415.)

4. **False.**   Intoxicated patients who exhibit suicidal behavior during a period of intoxication often no longer are suicidal once they are sober. (*See textbook page* 2418.)

5. **C.**   The potential for suicide attempts should be carefully evaluated when certain behaviors suggest that a person may be having suicidal thoughts. Statistics show that different persons have variable likelihood of attempting suicide. Persons with depressive symptoms are at greatest risk. Other groups at risk are those who are substance abusers, those with psychotic illnesses, and those with character disorders and panic disorders. Persons who have never married, those who have been widowed, the unemployed, and those without children are at greater risk to attempt suicide than are married persons with children. (*See textbook pages* 2416, 2417.)

6. **D.**   Maintenance of patient safety is the key element that must guide the approach to a suicidal patient. Management of the underlying problem and allowing the passage of time usually reduce suicidal potential. Patients who are intoxicated cannot be fairly evaluated for suicidal risk and should be allowed to become sober before the evaluation is completed. If a patient is judged to be at high risk for harming himself or herself, physical or chemical restraints are appropriate if restraint reduces risk. That a patient may not want any treatment or attention to his or her problems, should not influence the decision about how to protect the safety of a self-destructive persons. (*See textbook pages* 2417, 2418.)

Chapter 217

1. **D.**   Being in an intensive care setting places a patient in a dependent situation by its very nature. Adjunctive use of chemical and physical restraints may be necessary to protect the patient from harming himself or herself but may accentuate the sense of helplessness and anxiety. Inadequately dealing with the patient's or family's concerns and anxieties by not fully informing them of the patient's status and likely course can contribute to feelings of helplessness. However, denial may provide some protection against anxiety, and there is evidence that deniers have more favorable outcomes than nondeniers. Thus there may be no benefit in emphasizing bad news, although in general the more informed and involved are the patient and family, the less anxiety and helplessness are produced. (*See textbook page* 2420.)

2. A. Different personality types bring different coping styles to the experience of intensive care. Patients with oral-dependent or borderline personalities are impulsive, afraid of being alone, and expect total care. These patients are able to present different sides of themselves to different staff members to maintain each relationship at the appropriate emotional distance. This can cause the staff to have opposing views regarding the patient's status and care needs. The divisiveness these patients cause can be one of the strongest clues to the presence of a borderline personality type. Histrionic patients tend to manifest their insecurity by dramatizing everything and encouraging staff members to reveal more of themselves. Obsessive patients tend to become paralyzed by anxiety through their excessive analysis of every detail. Noncompliant behaviors on the part of patients tend to evoke collusion, sadism, or denial among staff members. (*See textbook page* 2420.)

Chapter 218

1. True. Burnout among ICU staff members can be a serious problem affecting hospital resources, morale, and patient care. Burnout appears to develop as the culmination of a sustained and intense response to negative stress. Both physicians and nurses can experience burnout, although the effect can be different because of the different natures of the jobs involved. Because nurses can be exposed to the stressful environment of an ICU on a continuous basis, whereas physicians in training tend to rotate through an ICU for more limited exposure, there has been a greater amount of study and interest regarding burnout among nurses than among physicians. (*See textbook page* 2430.)

2. False. Studies comparing ICU workers with those who do not work in an ICU have been unable to identify significant differences in stress levels between the two environments, although the types of conditions producing the stresses may differ. For example, ICU nurses may be more often stressed by changing shifts or schedules, whereas non-ICU nurses are more likely to be stressed when confronting an emergency situation. (*See textbook page* 2430.)

3. True. Among the many conditions that can produce stress among health care workers are a lack of opportunity to share experiences and emotions with other staff members, the death of a patient, insufficient dedication of time for a patient's emotional support, inadequate training to help with a patient's emotional needs, and unfamiliarity with the use of specialized equipment. (*See textbook page* 2430.)

4. C. The stressful environment and intense pressures that exist during residency training can produce marked effects on the participants. In 1981, Small described the house officer syndrome, which consists of seven features: episodic cognitive impairment, chronic anger, pervasive cynicism, family discord, depression, suicidal ideation, and substance abuse. It is likely that the first four are present in all house officers at one time or another. Depression, suicidal ideation, and substance abuse are serious conditions that should be identified and effectively managed to avoid serious harm to the resident and to patients. (*See textbook page* 2429.)

Chapter 219

1. True. The treatment that cancer patients receive can produce a variety of neuropsychiatric behaviors. Patients who have previously received chemotherapy that produces nausea and vomiting as a side effect can later become nauseated at the prospect of a recurrent treatment, becoming conditioned on occasion to avoid therapy altogether. (*See textbook pages* 2433, 2434.)

2. **False.** Complex partial seizures, manifested by psychic phenomena, autonomic changes, or unusual sensory experiences, are more common than are generalized seizures, although they are more difficult to diagnose. (*See textbook page* 2434.)

3. **True.** Patients with cancer commonly have generalized seizures because of the physiologic effects of tumor, infection, or drug treatments. (*See textbook page* 2434.)

4. **True.** Akathisia, a sense of restlessness, can be produced by neuroleptic medications such as phenothiazines, butyrophenones, and metoclopramide used for the management of nausea, anxiety, or agitation among cancer patients. (*See textbook page* 2434.)

5. **True.** The nature of HIV infection and its treatment often promotes the development of myriad neuropsychiatric symptoms. The most common neuropsychiatric disorders among patients with HIV infection are adjustment disorders, major depression, and organic mental disorders. (*See textbook page* 2436.)

6. **True.** HIV encephalopathy is a syndrome involving affective, behavioral, cognitive, and motor abnormalities. Magnetic resonance images can depict evidence of white matter disease better than can computed tomography, and thus may be preferable in the evaluation of patients with HIV encephalopathy. (*See textbook page* 2437.)

7. **False.** Seizures that develop among patients with HIV infection do so in approximately one-third of instances as a result of a mass lesion, in another third as a result of HIV encephalopathy, and in another third as the result of unknown causes. (*See textbook pages* 2437, 2438.)

8. **False.** The suicide rate among patients with AIDS was shown in one study to be as much as 66 times higher than that for the general population and 36 times that among persons of the same sex and age. The exact incidence is not known. (*See textbook page* 2438.)

9. **D.** Primary infection syndrome in HIV infection is an acute mononucleosis-like illness. It occurs within a few weeks of exposure to HIV. Seroconversion usually occurs several weeks after the resolution of the acute syndrome. The illness usually is self-limited after its acute onset and usually resolves within 3 weeks. Headaches may be severe enough to be consistent with the diagnosis of meningitis. (*See textbook page* 2436.)

XVIII. Moral, Ethical, Legal, and Public Policy Issues in the Intensive Care Unit

220. An Economic, Ethical, and Legal Analysis of Problems in Critical Care Medicine

True or False

1. A recent position statement by the American College of Surgeons supports suspending all do not resuscitate (DNR) orders when a patient is in the operating room.

Select the best answer

2. Which of the following was not a finding of the Study to Understand Prognosis and Preferences for Outcomes and Risks of Treatment (SUPPORT)?

   A. The presence and intervention of specially trained nurse practitioners working to improve physicians' understanding of patients' levels of care preferences improved the physicians compliance with patients' wishes.

   B. Only 47% of physicians accurately reported their patients' DNR wishes.

   C. Twenty-two percent of patients reported being in moderate to severe pain at least half the time.

   D. Nearly half of patients who wanted cardiopulmonary resuscitation withheld did not have a written DNR order.

221. Public Policy-Making for Intensive Care Units

Select the best answer

1. According to Kingdon, which of the following is not one of the three main conditions that must be present for an issue to receive a spot on the health policy agenda?

   A. Appropriate unfolding of political events

   B. Recognition of the problem

C. Consensus on the ethical justification of a policy
D. Policy proposal generation

222. Health Care Reform and Cost Containment

True or False

1. Microallocation is a set of duties within the domain of the medical director of an intensive care unit.
2. The Clinton health reform proposal of 1993 established the following as goals of national health care policy: access to care for all, access to the best care for all, patients' freedom of choice, and cost containment.

223. Current Directions in Severity Modeling: Limitations Leading to a New Definition of a High-Performance Intensive Care Unit

True or False

1. In many intensive care unit (ICU) scoring systems, an individual patient with a predicted 40% mortality has a 60% likelihood of survival.
2. A high-performance ICU is defined as an ICU with the lowest mortality rates.

224. Beyond Technology: Caring for the Critically Ill Patient

Select the best answer

1. Which of the following are goals of case management?

   A. Achievement of expected or standardized patient outcomes
   B. Early discharge of patients or discharge within appropriate lengths of stay
   C. Improved professional development and personal satisfaction on the job
   D. Encouragement of contributions by all care providers to the achievement of improved patient outcomes
   E. All of the above

225. Rural Critical Care

True or False

1. The most important aspect of transferring a patient from a community hospital to a tertiary care center is doing it quickly.

226. Managing Risk, Performance, and Information

True or False

1. Accreditation of a hospital by the Joint Commission for Accreditation of Health-care Organizations (JCAHO) indicates that the hospital meets the national standard for provision of quality care.

Select the best answer

2. Which of the following is *not* one of the crucial elements in proving negligence?

   A. The provider owed a duty to the patient.
   B. The provider failed to meet his or her duty to the patient.
   C. The outcome that was achieved was adverse.
   D. The patient sustained damages as a result of the provider's failure to meet his or her duty to the patient.
   E. The direct cause of the damages was the failure of the provider to meet their accepted duty.

227. Organization and Management of Critical Care Units

True or False

1. The Joint Commission for Accreditation of Healthcare Organizations (JCAHO) mandates that critical care units have a designated physician director.
2. In a semiclosed unit organization structure, the physician director or associate consults on the care of all patients and manages issues related to hemodynamics, respiratory failure, multiple organ system failure, and fluid balance.

Answers

Chapter 220

1. **False.** A recent American College of Surgeons statement concluded, "Policies that lead either to automatic enforcement of all DNR orders and requests or to disregarding or automatic cancellation of such orders and requests during an operation and recovery period may not sufficiently address a patient's right to self determination." (*See textbook page* 2447.)
2. **A.** The Study to Understand Prognosis and Preferences for Outcomes and Risks of Treatment (SUPPORT) involved 9,000 patients with life-threatening illnesses. In a 2-year initial observation period, the investigators found what they thought were glaring inadequacies in the care of these patients. Among these were that only 47% of physicians accurately reported their patients' DNR wishes, 22% of patients reported being in moderate to severe pain at least half the time, and nearly half of patients who wanted CPR withheld did not have a written DNR order. For patients who ultimately did have a DNR order before death, most orders were written in the few days before death. When an attempt was made to intervene and correct these deficits, the presence and intervention of specially trained nurse

practitioners working to improve physicians' understanding of patients' levels of care preferences had no effect on physician compliance with patients' wishes. (*See textbook page 2443.*)

Chapter 221

1. **C.**   Appropriate unfolding of political events, recognition of the problem, and policy proposal generation must converge for an issue to take a place on the national policy stage. Consensus on the ethical justification of a policy often is difficult to generate and even when present may not help determine the fate of an issue. (*See textbook page 2451.*)

Chapter 222

1. **True.**   *Macroallocation* refers to health care policy issues such as deciding what percentage of available funds goes to critical care as opposed to primary care. *Microallocation* refers to cost management issues in a specific intensive care unit. *Mesoallocation* falls to the specialty of critical care medicine in determining how the profession allocates resources assigned to it. (*See textbook page 2460.*)
2. **True.**   Many involved in the health care policy debate believe these goals to be inherently unattainable because achievement of one goal tends to impede achievement of others. (*See textbook page 2457.*)

Chapter 223

1. **False.**   Most ICU prediction models do not entail prediction of the odds of survival for individual patients. A 40% predicted mortality indicates that among 100 similar patients, 40 are expected to die and 60 to survive. (*See textbook page 2472.*)
2. **False.**   One of the main categories of poor performance includes ICUs that try too hard to save every patient. This ICU has a lower than expected mortality but high severity-adjusted resource use, a high percentage of patients who die with cardiopulmonary resuscitation, long stays for patients who die, low family satisfaction, and rare use of DNR orders. (*See textbook page 2476.*)

Chapter 224

1. **E.**   Case management is a clinical system for the strategic management of cost and quality outcomes. In addition to the goals listed, goals of case management include appropriate or reduced utilization of resources, collaborative practice and coordination, and continuity of care. (*See textbook page 2482.*)

Chapter 225

1. **False.**   There is a process designed to enhance the appropriateness of patient transport through selection of the best receiving center, bed availability, cost,

patient preference, mode of transport, and stability of patient's condition for transport, among other factors. Transport always should be delayed until the patient's condition for transport has been stabilized to the best ability of the referring center. (*See textbook page* 2482.)

Chapter 226

1. **False.**   Accreditation by the JCAHO is meant to attest that a hospital "can provide quality health care." That a hospital can provide quality care does not assure that it does. (*See textbook page* 2489.)
2. **C.**   The four elements necessary to prove negligence are (a) the provider owed a duty to the patient (in the case of a physician, a doctor-patient relationship was established); (b) the provider failed to meet that duty; (c) the patient sustained damages as a result of the provider's failure to meet his or her duty to the patient; and (d) the direct cause of the damages was the failure of the provider to meet his or her accepted duty. That an adverse outcome occurred by and of itself does not contribute to the determination of negligence. (*See textbook page* 2497.)

Chapter 227

1. **True.**   The JCAHO mandates that all special care units be directed by "a physician member of the active medical staff who has received special training, acquired experience, and demonstrated competence in a specialty related to the care provided in the unit." (*See textbook page* 2507.)
2. **False.**   In a semiclosed unit, the physician director or associate must review and approve all admissions, taking into consideration appropriateness of care and staffing levels. All final decisions regarding admission, discharge and triage rest with the director. The physician director may consult on the care of all patients, do so only when requested, or consult only in the case of an emergency situation. In an open unit, the director or associates consult only when requested to do so. All qualified attending physicians may admit and care for patients in the intensive care unit. In a closed unit, the director or associate is responsible for all admissions and discharges. When a patient is admitted to the intensive care unit that patient's care is turned over to the unit team. (*See textbook page* 2506.)

Appendix

Calculations Commonly Used in Critical Care

Table of Contents

Abbreviations Used in the Appendix

A	Alveolar	atm	Atmosphere
D	Dead	BSA	Body surface area
E	Expiration	cap	Capillary
I	Inspiration	cr	Creatinine
P	Pressure	dyn	Dynamic
Q̇	Net liquid flow	is	Interstitium
R	Respiratory quotient	st	Static
T	Tidal	ICP	Intracranial pressure
V	Volume	a	Arterial
Δ	Change	d	Distribution
η	Viscosity	l	Length
π	Oncotic pressure	r	Radius
σ	Permeability	t	Time
		v̄	Mixed venous

Fahrenheit and Celsius Temperature Conversions

°C	°F
45	113.0
44	111.2
43	109.4
42	107.6
41	105.8
40	104.0
39	102.2
38	100.4
37	98.6
36	96.8
35	95.0
34	93.2
33	91.4
32	89.6
31	87.8
30	86.0
29	84.2
28	82.4
27	80.6
26	78.8
25	77.0
24	75.2
23	73.4
22	71.6
21	69.8
20	68.0

Dosage and Action of Common IV Vasoactive Drugs

	Dosage	α	β₁	β₂
Dopamine	1–2 µg/kg/min	+	+	0
	2–10 µg/kg/min	+ +	+ + +	0
	10–30 µg/kg/min	+ + +	+ +	0
Dobutamine	2–30 µg/kg/min	+	+ + +	+ +
Norepinephrine	2–80 µg/min	+ + +	+ +	+
Epinephrine	1–200 µg/min	+ +	+ + +	+ + +
Isoproterenol	2–10 µg/min	0	+ + +	+ + +
Metaraminol	>20 µg/min	+ +	+	+
Phenylephrine	>30 µg/min	+ + +	0	0
Amrinone	2–15 µg/kg/min	0	0	0
Phentolamine	1–2 mg/min	—	0	0
Labetolol	>2 mg/min	—	—	—
Esmolol	50–400	—	—	—

Hemodynamic Calculations

MEAN BLOOD PRESSURE (mm Hg)

$$= \overline{BP}$$

$$= \frac{Systolic\ BP + (2\ \times\ Diastolic\ BP)}{3}$$

$$= Diastolic\ BP + \tfrac{1}{3}\ (Systolic\ BP - Diastolic\ BP)$$

Normal values: 85–95 mm Hg

THE FICK EQUATION FOR CARDIAC INDEX (L/min/m²)

$$= CI$$

$$= \frac{CO}{BSA}$$

$$= \frac{Oxygen\ consumption}{Arterial\ O_2\ content - Venous\ O_2\ content}$$

$$= \frac{10 \times \dot{V}o_2\ (ml/min/m^2)}{Hgb\ (g/dl) \times 1.39 \atop \times\ (Arterial\ \%\ saturation - Venous\ \%\ saturation)}$$

Normal values: 2.5–4.2 L/min/m²

STROKE INDEX (ml/beat/m²)

$$= \frac{CI\ (L/min/m^2) \times 1000}{Heart\ rate\ (beats/min)}$$

Normal values: 33–47 ml/beat/m²

SYSTEMIC VASCULAR RESISTANCE (dyne-sec-cm⁻⁵)

$$= SVR$$

$$= \frac{80 \times (arterial\ \overline{BP} - right\ atrial\ \overline{BP})}{CO\ (L/min)}$$

Normal values: 770–1500 dyne-sec-cm⁻⁵

PULMONARY VASCULAR RESISTANCE (dyne-sec-cm⁻⁵)

$$= PVR$$

$$= \frac{80 \times (Pulmonary\ artery\ \overline{BP} - Pulmonary\ capillary\ wedge\ pressure)}{CO\ (L/min)}$$

Normal values: 20–120 dyne-sec-cm⁻⁵

TOTAL PULMONARY RESISTANCE (dyne-sec-cm⁻⁵)

$$= TPR$$

$$= \frac{80 \times Pulmonary\ artery\ \overline{BP}}{CO\ (L/min)}$$

CAPILLARY FLUID FILTRATION

$$= \dot{Q}_f$$

$$= k(P_{cap} - P_{is}) - k\sigma(\pi_{cap} - \pi_{is})$$

Nutritional Calculations

BODY MASS INDEX

$$= BMI$$

$$= \frac{Weight\ (kg)}{(Height\ (cm))^2}$$

CALORIC CONTENT OF FOODS

Foodtype	Kcal/g	
Carbohydrate	3.4	Range 3.4–4.1
Protein	4.0	Range 3.3–4.7
Fat	9.1	Range 9.1–9.5

RESPIRATORY QUOTIENT

$$= \frac{CO_2\ production\ (ml/min)}{O_2\ consumption\ (ml/min)}$$

$$= \frac{\dot{V}_{CO_2}}{\dot{V}_{O_2}}$$

RELATIONSHIP OF FUEL BURNED TO RESPIRATORY QUOTIENT

Fuel	R
Ketones	<0.6
Fat	0.7
Carbohydrate	1.0
Lipogenesis	>1.0

NITROGEN BALANCE

$$= Nitrogen\ consumed - Nitrogen\ excreted$$

$$= \frac{Protein\ calories\ (kcal/day)}{25}$$

$$- Urine\ nitrogen\ (g/day) - 5\ (g/day)$$

HARRIS-BENEDICT EQUATION OF RESTING ENERGY EXPENDITURE (kcal/day)

$$Males = 66 + (13.7 \times Weight\ [kg]) + (5 \times Height\ [cm]) - (6.8 \times Age)$$

$$Females = 655 + (9.6 \times Weight\ [kg]) + (1.8 \times Height\ [cm]) - (4.7 \times Age)$$

WEIR EQUATION (MODIFIED) OF ENERGY EXPENDITURE (kcal/day)

$$= (3.94 \times \dot{V}o_2\ [ml/min]) + (1.11 \times \dot{V}_{CO_2}\ [ml/min])$$

Typical Intravenous Drug Dosages for Rapid Intubation

Muscle relaxants
    Rocurium   0.6–1.2 mg/kg
    Succinylcholine   1 mg/kg
    Vecuronium   0.1–0.28 mg/kg
Sedatives
    Thiopental   3–4 mg/kg
    Ketamine   1–2 mg/kg
    Etomidate   0.3–0.4 mg/kg

Pulmonary Calculations

TIDAL VOLUME

$$= V_T$$

$$= Dead\ space + Alveolar\ space$$

$$= V_D + V_A$$

ALVEOLAR GAS EQUATION

$$P_{AO_2} = P_{IO_2} - \frac{P_{aCO_2}}{R}$$

$$= F_{IO_2}(P_{atm} - P_{H_2O}) - \frac{P_{aCO_2}}{R}$$

$$= 150 - \frac{P_{aCO_2}}{R}\ (room\ air,\ sea\ level)$$

ALVEOLAR ARTERIOLAR GRADIENT

$$= A - a\ gradient$$

$$= P_{AO_2} - P_{aO_2}$$

Normal values (upright): 2.5 + (0.21 × age)

ALVEOLAR VENTILATION (L/min)

$$= \dot{V}_E$$

$$= k\ \frac{\dot{V}_{CO_2}}{P_{aCO_2}}$$

$$= \frac{0.863 \times \dot{V}_{CO_2}\ (ml/min)}{P_{aCO_2}(1 - V_D/V_T)}$$

Normal values: 4–6 L/min

BOHR EQUATION OF DEAD SPACE

$$V_D/V_T = \frac{P_{aCO_2} - P_{ECO_2}}{P_{aCO_2}}$$

Normal values: 0.2–0.3

PHYSIOLOGIC DEAD SPACE

$$V_D/V_T = \frac{P_{aCO_2} - P_{ECO_2}}{P_{aCO_2}}$$

Normal values: 0.2–0.3

OXYGEN DISSOLVED IN BLOOD (ml/dl)

$$= D_{O_2}$$

$$= 0.003\ (ml\ O_2/dl) \times P_{aO_2}\ (mm\ Hg)$$

OXYGEN CAPACITY OF HEMOGLOBIN (ml O_2/dl)

$$= 1.39\ (ml\ O_2) \times Hgb\ (g/dl)$$

Normal values: 17–24 ml/dl

OXYGEN CONTENT OF THE BLOOD (ml/dl)

$$= C_{O_2}$$

$$= D_{O_2} + (1.39 \times Hgb\ [g/dl] \times [\%\ Hgb\ saturated\ with\ O_2])$$

$$= D_{O_2} + (1.39 \times Hgb\ [g/dl] \times S_{O_2})$$

Normal values: 17.5–23.5 ml/dl

PERCENTAGE OF SATURATION OF HEMOGLOBIN WITH OXYGEN

$$= S_{O_2}$$

$$= 100 \times \frac{C_{O_2} - D_{O_2}}{1.39 \times Hgb\ (g/dl)}$$

Normal values: >95%

PHYSIOLOGIC SHUNT

$$= \dot{Q}_S/\dot{Q}_T$$

$$= \frac{C_{capO_2} - C_{O_2}}{C_{capO_2} - C_{\bar{v}O_2}}$$

$$= \frac{1.39 \times Hgb\ (g/dl) + 0.003 \times P_{aO_2} - C_{aO_2}}{1.39 \times Hgb\ (g/dl) + 0.003 \times P_{aO_2} - C\bar{v}O_2}$$

Normal values: <5%

COMPLIANCE

$$= \Delta V/\Delta P\ (ml/cm\ H_2O)$$

On Mechanical Ventilation

$$Static\ compliance = C_{st} = \frac{V_T}{P_{plateau} - P_{end\ exp}}$$

$$Dynamic\ effective\ compliance = C_{dyn} = \frac{V_T}{P_{peak} - P_{end\ exp}}$$

During Spontaneous Breathing

$$Compliance\ of\ the\ lung = C_L = \frac{V_T}{P_{alveolus} - P_{pleura}}$$

$$Compliance\ of\ the\ chest\ wall = CW_{cw} = \frac{V_T}{P_{pleura} - P_{atm}}$$

$$Compliance\ of\ the\ respiratory\ system = C_{rs} = \frac{V_T}{P_{alveolus} - P_{atm}}$$

Normal values: $C_{st} > 60$ ml/cm H_2O; $C_{dyn} > 60$ ml/cm H_2O
$C_L > 200$ ml/cm H_2O; $C_{rs} > 100$ ml/cm H_2O

RESISTANCE—OHM'S LAW

$$= \Delta P/flow = \Delta P/\dot{Q}$$

Normal values: airway resistance of the lung at functional residual capacity (FRC) = 2 cm H_2O/L/sec

WORK OF BREATHING

$$W_{Thorax} = \int_{t_1}^{t_2} (P_{aw} - P_{atm}) \dot{V} dt$$

$$W_{Lung} = \int_{t_1}^{t_2} (P_{aw} - P_{es}) \dot{V} dt$$

$$W_{Chest\ wall} = \int_{t_1}^{t_2} (P_{es} - P_{atm}) \dot{V} dt$$

Normal values: W_{thorax} = 0.5 kg-M/min

LAPLACE'S LAW OF SURFACE TENSION OF A SPHERE

$$P = 2T/r$$

POISEUILLE'S LAW OF LAMINAR FLOW

$$\dot{V} = \frac{P\pi r^4}{8\eta l}$$

Composition and Properties of Common Intravenous Solutions

Solution	Na^+	Cl^-	K^+	Ca^+	Lactate	Kcal/L	mOsm/L
D5W	0	0	0	0	0	170	252
D10W	0	0	0	0	0	240	505
D50W	0	0	0	0	0	1700	2530
½ NS	77	77	0	0	0	0	154
NS	154	154	0	0	0	0	308
3% NaCl	513	513	0	0	0	0	1026
Ringer's lactate	130	109	4	3	28	0	308
20% mannitol	0	0	0	0	0	0	1098

Electrolyte and Renal Calculations

ANION GAP

$$= [Na^+] - [Cl^-] - [HCO_3^-]$$

Normal values: 9–13 mEq/L

EXPECTED ANION GAP IN HYPOALBUMINEMIA

$$= 3 \times (albumin\ [g/dl])$$

CALCULATED SERUM OSMOLALITY

$$= 2[Na^+] + \frac{[Glucose]}{18} + \frac{[BUN]}{2.8}$$

Normal values: 275–290 mOsm/kg

OSMOLAR GAP

$$= Serum\ osmolality\ measured - Serum\ osmolality\ calculated$$

Normal values: 0–5 mOsm/kg

Na^+ AND GLUCOSE
$[Na^+]$ decreases 1.6 mEq/L for each 100 mg/dl increase in [glucose]

Ca^+ AND ALBUMIN
$[Ca^+]$ decreases 0.8 mg/dl for each 1.0 gm/dl decrease in albumin

GLOMERULAR FILTRATION RATE = GFR

$$Measured = creatinine\ clearance = \frac{U_{Creat}V}{P_{Creat}}$$

$$= \frac{[Creatinine]_{urine}\ (g/dl) \times \dfrac{Urine\ volume\ (ml/day)}{1440\ (min/day)}}{[Creatinine]_{plasma}\ (mg/dl)}$$

$$Estimated\ for\ males = \frac{(140 - Age) \times (Lean\ body\ weight\ [kg])}{P_{Creat} \times 72}$$

$$Estimated\ for\ females = 0.85 \times Male\ estimate$$

Normal values: 74–160 ml/min

WATER DEFICIT IN HYPERNATREMIA (L)

$$= 0.6 \times (Body\ weight\ [kg]) \times \left(\frac{[Na^+]}{140} - 1\right)$$

WATER EXCESS IN HYPONATREMIA (L)

$$= 0.6 \times (Body\ weight\ [kg]) \times \left(1 - \frac{[Na^+]}{140}\right)$$

FRACTIONAL EXCRETION OF SODIUM

$$= F_E Na$$

$$= \frac{Excreted\ Na^+}{Filtered\ Na^+} \times 100$$

$$= \frac{U_{Na^+} \times V}{GFR} \times [Na^+] \times 100$$

$$= \frac{U_{Na^+}/[Na^+]}{U_{Creat}/[Creat]}$$

Uses incomprehensible sounds	2
Nil	1

CEREBRAL PERFUSION PRESSURE (mm Hg)

$$= \overline{BP} - ICP$$

Acid-Base Formulas

HENDERSON-HASSELBALCH EQUATION

$$pH = pK + \log \frac{[HCO_3^-]}{0.03 \times Paco_2}$$

HENDERSON'S EQUATION FOR CONCENTRATION OF H+

$$[H^+] \text{ (nM/L)} = 24 \times \frac{Paco_2}{[HCO_3^-]}$$

METABOLIC ACIDOSIS
Bicarbonate deficit (mEq/L) = 0.5 × (*body weight* [kg]) × (24 − [HCO_3^-])
Expected Pco_2 = 1.5 × [HCO_3^-] + 8 ± 2

METABOLIC ALKALOSIS
Bicarbonate excess = 0.4 × (*Body weight* [kg]) × ([HCO_3^-] − 24)

RESPIRATORY ACIDOSIS

$$Acute: \frac{\Delta H^+}{\Delta Paco_2} = 0.8$$

$$Chronic: \frac{\Delta H^+}{\Delta Paco_2} = 0.3$$

Body Surface Area Formula and Nomogram

BODY SURFACE AREA (BSA)

$$= (height \text{ [cm]})^{0.718} \times (weight \text{ [kg]})^{0.427} \times 74.49$$

Neurologic Calculations

GLASGOW COMA SCALE (3–15)

= *Eyes* (1–4) + *Motor* (1–6) + *Verbal* (1–5)

Normal value: 15

Table A-1. Specific Components of the Glasgow Coma Scale

Eye opening	
Spontaneous	4
To speech	3
To pain	2
Nil	1
Motor response	
Obeys commands	6
Localizes	5
Withdraws	4
Exhibits abnormal flexion	3
Exhibits abnormal extension	2
Nil	1
Verbal response	
Oriented	5
Confused, conversant	4
Uses inappropriate words	3

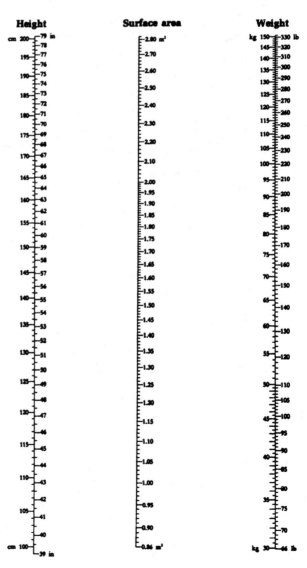

Fig. A-1. Nomogram for calculation of body surface area (BSA) in square meters by height and weight.

Calculation of APACHE II Score

PHYSIOLOGIC VARIABLE	HIGH ABNORMAL RANGE					LOW ABNORMAL RANGE			
	+4	+3	+2	+1	0	+1	+2	+3	+4
TEMPERATURE — rectal (°C)	≥41°	39°-40.9°		38.5°-38.9°	36°-38.4°	34°-35.9°	32°-33.9°	30°-31.9°	≤29.9°
MEAN ARTERIAL PRESSURE — mm Hg	≥160	130-159	110-129		70-109		50-69		≤49
HEART RATE (ventricular response)	≥180	140-179	110-139		70-109		55-69	40-54	≤39
RESPIRATORY RATE — (non-ventilated or ventilated)	≥50	35-49		25-34	12-24	10-11	6-9		≤5
OXYGENATION: A-aDO₂ or PaO₂ (mm Hg) a. FIO₂ ≥ 0.5 record A-aDO₂	≥ 500	350-499	200-349		<200				
b. FIO₂ <0.5 record only PaO₂					PO₂ >70	PO₂ 61-70		PO₂ 55-60	PO₂ <55
ARTERIAL pH	≥7.7	7.6-7.69		7.5-7.59	7.33-7.49		7.25-7.32	7.15-7.24	<7.15
SERUM SODIUM (mMol/L)	≥180	160-179	155-159	150-154	130-149		120-129	111-119	≤110
SERUM POTASSIUM (mMol/L)	≥7	6-6.9		5.5-5.9	3.5-5.4	3-3.4	2.5-2.9		<2.5
SERUM CREATININE (mg/100 ml) (Double point score for acute renal failure)	≥3.5	2-3.4	1.5-1.9		0.6-1.4		< 0.6		
HEMATOCRIT (%)	≥60		50-59.9	46-49.9	30-45.9		20-29.9		<20
WHITE BLOOD COUNT (total/mm3) (in 1,000s)	≥40		20-39.9	15-19.9	3-14.9		1-2.9		<1
GLASGOW COMA SCORE (GCS): Score = 15 minus actual GCS									
[A] Total ACUTE PHYSIOLOGY SCORE (APS): Sum of the 12 individual variable points									
Serum HCO₃ (venous-mMol/L) [Not preferred, use if no ABGs]	≥ 52	41-51.9		32-40.9	22-31.9		18-21.9	15-17.9	< 15

[B] AGE POINTS:
Assign points to age as follows:

AGE(yrs)	Points
≤44	0
45-54	2
55-64	3
65-74	5
≥75	6

[C] CHRONIC HEALTH POINTS
If the patient has a history of severe organ system insufficiency or is immuno-compromised assign points as follows:
a. for nonoperative or emergency postoperative patients — 5 points
or
b. for elective postoperative patients — 2 points

DEFINITIONS
Organ Insufficiency or immuno-compromised state must have been evident prior to this hospital admission and conform to the following criteria:

LIVER: Biopsy proven cirrhosis and documented portal hypertension; episodes of past upper GI bleeding attributed to portal hypertension; or prior episodes of hepatic failure/encephalopathy/coma.

CARDIOVASCULAR: New York Heart Association Class IV.
RESPIRATORY: Chronic restrictive, obstructive, or vascular disease resulting in severe exercise restriction, i.e., unable to climb stairs or perform household duties; or documented chronic hypoxia, hypercapnia, secondary polycythemia, severe pulmonary hypertension (>40mmHg), or respirator dependency.
RENAL: Receiving chronic dialysis.
IMMUNO-COMPROMISED: The patient has received therapy that suppresses resistance to infection, e.g., immuno-suppression, chemotherapy, radiation, long term or recent high dose steroids, or has a disease that is sufficiently advanced to suppress resistance to infection, e.g., leukemia, lymphoma, AIDS.

APACHE II SCORE
Sum of [A] + [B] + [C]

[A] APS points _____

[B] Age points _____

[C] Chronic Health points _____

Total APACHE II _____

From ref. 1, with permission.

See Fig. A–1 for the nomogram for calculating BSA.

Pharmacologic Calculations

DRUG CLEARANCE

$$= V_d \times K_{el}$$

DRUG HALF-LIFE

$$= t^{1/2}$$

$$= \frac{0.693}{K_{el}}$$

DRUG ELIMINATION CONSTANT

$$= K_{el}$$

$$= \frac{\ln\left(\frac{[Peak]}{[Trough]}\right)}{t_{peak} - t_{trough}}$$

DRUG LOADING DOSE
$$= V_d \times [Target\ peak]$$

DRUG DOSING INTERVAL

$$= \frac{-1}{K_{el}} \times \ln\left(\frac{[Desired\ trough]}{[Desired\ peak]}\right) + Infusion\ time\ (hr)$$

See Fig. A–2 for the calculation of APACHE scores.

Normal Values of Expiratory Peak Flow [2]

There is a wide variability in peak expiratory flows due to individual differences. Values also vary slightly depending on the peak flow meter used.